MIRACLES

MIRACLES

God, Science, and Psychology
in the Paranormal

VOLUME 1
Religious and Spiritual Events

Edited by J. Harold Ellens

Psychology, Religion, and Spirituality

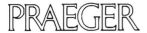

Westport, Connecticut
London

Library of Congress Cataloging-in-Publication Data

Miracles : God, science, and psychology in the paranormal / edited by
J. Harold Ellens.
      p. cm. — (Psychology, religion, and spirituality, ISSN 1546–8070)
   Includes bibliographical references and index.
   ISBN 978–0–275–99722–9 (set : alk. paper) — ISBN 978–0–275–99724–3
(v. 1 : alk. paper) — ISBN 978–0–275–99726–7 (v. 2 : alk. paper) —
ISBN 978–0–275–99728–1 (v. 3 : alk. paper)
   1. Miracles. 2. Medicine—Religious aspects. 3. Religion and science.
4. Parapsychology—Religious aspects. I. Ellens, J. Harold, 1932–
   BT97.M49 2008
   202'.117—dc22   2008011269

British Library Cataloguing in Publication Data is available.

Library of Congress Catalog Card Number: 2008011269
ISBN: 978–0–275–99722–9 (set)
      978–0–275–99724–3 (vol. 1)
      978–0–275–99726–7 (vol. 2)
      978–0–275–99728–1 (vol. 3)
ISSN: 1546–8070

First published in 2008

Greenwood Press, 88 Post Road West, Westport, CT 06881
An imprint of Greenwood Publishing Group, Inc.
www.greenwood.com

Printed in the United States of America

This work on miracles is dedicated
To Rebecca and Brenda
Because they work miracles of healing
Every day.

I wish to express intense gratitude and high esteem for the meticulous and devoted labor of Beuna C. Carlson who read all the proofs with a sharp eye and sturdy hand for ferreting out errors. Surely the devil is in the details and she has mastered the devil.

CONTENTS

SERIES FOREWORD

The interface between psychology, religion, and spirituality has been of great interest to scholars for a century. In the last three decades a broad popular appetite has developed for books that make practical sense out of the sophisticated research on these three subjects. Freud expressed an essentially deconstructive perspective on this matter and indicated that he saw the relationship between human psychology and religion to be a destructive interaction. Jung, on the other hand, was quite sure that these three aspects of the human spirit: psychology, religion, and spirituality, were constructively and inextricably linked.

Anton Boisen and Seward Hiltner derived much insight from both Freud and Jung, as well as from Adler and Reik, while pressing the matter forward with ingenious skill and illumination. Boisen and Hiltner fashioned a framework within which the quest for a sound and sensible definition of the interface between psychology, religion, and spirituality might best be described or expressed.[1] We are in their debt.

This series of general interest books, so wisely urged by Praeger Publishers, and particularly by its editors, Deborah Carvalko and Suzanne I. Staszak-Silva, intends to define the terms and explore the interface of psychology, religion, and spirituality at the operational level of daily human experience. Each volume of the series identifies, analyzes, describes, and evaluates the full range of issues, of both popular and professional interest, that deal with the psychological factors at play (1) in the way religion takes shape and is expressed, (2) in the way spirituality functions within human persons and shapes both religious formation and expression, and (3) in the ways that spirituality is shaped and expressed by religion. The interest is psychospiritual. In terms of the rubrics of the disciplines and the science of psychology and spirituality this series of volumes investigates the *operational dynamics* of religion and spirituality.

The verbs *shape* and *express* in the above paragraph refer to the forces that prompt and form religion in persons and communities, as well as to the manifestations of religious behavior (1) in personal forms of spirituality, (2) in acts of spiritually motivated care for society, and (3) in ritual behaviors such as liturgies of worship. In these various aspects of human function the psychological and/or spiritual drivers are identified, isolated, and described in terms of the way in which they unconsciously and consciously operate in religion, thought, and behavior.

The books in this series are written for the general reader, the local library, and the undergraduate university student. They are also of significant interest to the informed professional, particularly in fields corollary to his or her primary interest. The volumes in this series have great value for clinical settings and treatment models, as well.

This series editor has spent an entire professional lifetime focused specifically on research into the interface of psychology in religion and spirituality. This present set, *Miracles: God, Science, and Psychology in the Paranormal,* is an urgently needed and timely work, the motivation for which is surely endorsed enthusiastically by the entire religious world today, as the international community searches for strategies that will afford us better and deeper religious self-understanding as individuals and communities. This project addresses the deep psychosocial, psychospiritual, and biological sources of human nature that shape and drive our psychology and spirituality. Careful strategies of empirical, heuristic, and phenomenological research have been employed to give this work a solid scientific foundation and formation. Never before has such wise analysis been brought to bear upon the dynamic linkage between human physiology, psychology, and spirituality in an effort to understand the human mystification with apparent miraculous events in our experience and traditions.

For 50 years such organizations as the Christian Association for Psychological Studies and such graduate departments of psychology as those at Boston University, Fuller, Rosemead, Harvard, George Fox, Princeton, and the like, have been publishing important building blocks of research on issues dealing with religious behavior and psychospirituality. In this present project the insights generated by such patient and careful research are synthesized and integrated into a holistic psychospiritual worldview, which takes seriously the special aspect of religious tradition called miracle. This volume employs an objective and experience-based approach to discerning what happens in miracle stories, what that means, and in what ways that is an advantage or danger to our spiritual life and growth, as we pursue the irrepressible human quest for meaning.

Some of the influences of religion upon persons and society, now and throughout history, have been negative. However, most of the impact of the great religions upon human life and culture has been profoundly redemptive and generative of great good. It is urgent, therefore, that we discover and understand better what the psychological and spiritual forces are that empower people of faith and genuine spirituality to open their lives to the transcendent connection and give themselves to all the creative and constructive enterprises that, throughout the centuries, have made of human life the humane, ordered, prosperous, and aesthetic experience it can be at its best. Surely the forces for good in both psychology and spirituality far exceed the powers and proclivities toward the evil.

This series of Praeger Publishers volumes is dedicated to the greater understanding of *Psychology, Religion, and Spirituality,* and thus to the profound understanding and empowerment of those psychospiritual drivers that can help us (1) transcend the malignancy of our earthly pilgrimage, (2) open our spirits to the divine spirit, (3) enhance the humaneness and majesty of the human spirit, and (4) empower our potential for magnificence in human life.

J. Harold Ellens
Series Editor

NOTE

1. L. Aden and J. H. Ellens (1990), *Turning Points in Pastoral Care: The Legacy of Anton Boisen and Seward Hiltner,* Grand Rapids: Baker.

INTRODUCTION

J. Harold Ellens

Miracle stories live forever. They appear in all religious traditions and though the traditions change greatly over the centuries, the miracle stories stay the same. Krister Stendahl, professor of biblical studies at Harvard Divinity School and bishop of the Lutheran Church of Sweden, wrote the foreword to Anton Fridrichsen's *The Problem of Miracle in Primitive Christianity.* In it he approved of Fridrichsen's "theological conviction that genuine faith and vital religion is and will remain mythical, miraculous, and resistant to theological reductionism—orthodox, conservative, liberal, or radical."[1] Regardless of the perspective one takes on the faith tradition that holds one's attention, the miracle stories remain the same kind of enigma from generation to generation.

The questions asked today by devoted believers and agnostic critics, by theological scientists and empirical scientists, by mythologists and rationalists, are the same questions as the ancient Greeks, Romans, and Christians were asking about the miracles reported and celebrated in their world 2,000 years ago. Numerous explanations of miracle stories have filled uncountable volumes over the centuries. None, so far, quite satisfies the hunger of the human mind and spirit for a final answer to the question, "Are miracles real, or a chimera of our imaginations? What really happened and what does it mean?"

Is it possible to devise thoroughly rational and naturalistic interpretations of this mystifying phenomenon? Possibly, but then when that is said and done we have the sense that while the rationale holds up well enough, the intriguing center of the issue has not been exploded. Likewise, we may provide a literal, psychological, or mythological explanation of the miracle stories and discover in the end that we have not quite understood the depth of the narrative that gives us the ultimate clue. We cannot escape the haunting suspicion that in the miracle stories the transcendent world has somehow touched our mundane existence. That is true whether it is a biblical narrative or a newspaper report of some spontaneous remission of disease in the twenty-first century. Paul J. Achtemeier observed that, as regards our understanding or accounting for the biblical miracles, particularly those performed by Jesus and recorded in the synoptic Gospels, in the end we must face the fact that Jesus really did heal that demon-possessed boy in Mark 9, for example, and if our explanation does not reflect that forthrightly we have distorted the forthright Gospel report.[2]

It is a good thing, therefore, that we have been able to assemble a company of the brightest and best scholars from around the world today to examine this profoundly important issue. The contributors to these volumes on *Miracles: God, Science, and Psychology in the Paranormal* are esteemed scholars whose life's calling and professional specialty it is to know the New Testament thoroughly and scientifically. They have agreed to address, in this volume, the issue of biblical miracles from every conceivable perspective we could imagine. Here follows in 16 chapters the rather rich fruit of our devoted labor.

NOTES

1. Anton Fridrichsen (1972), *The Problem of Miracle in Primitive Christianity*, Minneapolis: Augsburg, 8. This work was originally published in 1925 as *Le Problème du Miracle dans le Christianisme Primitif*, by the Faculty of Protestant Theology at the University of Strasbourg.

2. Paul J. Achtemeier (1975), Miracles and the Historical Jesus: Mark 9:14–29, *Catholic Biblical Quarterly*, 37 (4), 424–51.

CHAPTER 1

BIBLICAL MIRACLES AND PSYCHOLOGICAL PROCESS: JESUS AS PSYCHOTHERAPIST

J. Harold Ellens

In his recent volume, *Jesus the Village Psychiatrist: Disabling Anxiety in a World of Insecurity*, Donald Capps finally addressed definitively what psychologists and theologians have been dancing around for 20 centuries.[1] He has looked squarely in the face the issue of the psychological nature and method of Jesus' healing ministries. Those ministries are more than adequately documented by the witnesses in the numerous New Testament miracle stories. It is clear from those narratives that people who were close to Jesus, or knew those who were, were wholly persuaded that Jesus cured sicknesses and impairments.

Furthermore, when you have a couple of generations of people standing around who were well aware of the person and work of Jesus of Nazareth, there is only so much hyperbole you can use in describing such a personage, and get away with it. Since the stories of Jesus' miracles were so popular and so widespread within 50 years of his death, there must be something very important about them. If not, there would have been significant numbers of voices raised to counter the claims of the biblical stories. It is possible to make a heroic figure out of an ordinary man or woman simply by telling stories about them that embellish their reputation. However, even then one can only get away with telling stories that ring true to some characteristic of the person's nature or behavior. If the stories are wildly exaggerated, beyond that which is believable about that character, they will be countered, contradicted, falsified, and forgotten.

If I told you that Jules Verne's stories about trips to the moon or to the bottom of the sea were not fiction but truth, I might be able to get away with it if I could convince you that he is alive today, but I certainly could not get away with that regarding a man who you know lived in the eighteenth or nineteenth century. You would immediately falsify my claim because you could prove that the technology did not exist then. Likewise, if I told you that the Wright brothers flew an airship for a few hundred feet at Kitty Hawk at about the turn of the nineteenth to the twentieth century, you would probably believe it. However, if I expanded that story to persuade you that they also created a space ship and visited the moon or Mars, you would laugh at me because the metals, tools, chemicals, and technology for such operations could not have been available to the Wright brothers under any circumstances. What were available were bicycles, primitive internal combustion engines, rather unrefined iron bars, canvas, and such stuff out of which to rig a rickety airframe for rather rustic experimentation. Their real story is only marginally believable. Anything wilder than that would not be believable at all! It was the same with Jesus' miracle stories.

The nature, behavior, and equipment of the heroic character in a story must be such that he or she can authentically carry the freight that the reports heap upon him or her. So the question about Jesus as miracle worker is not really so much the question of whether he performed healings, but rather the question of what kind of character he must have been that this particular set of narratives, this meaning freight, could be placed upon him and become immediately believable regarding him. Apparently people who knew him or knew about him readily responded with something like, "Yes! That is the sort of thing he did or surely would and could have done." The stories seem to have been affirmed from the outset without reservation, not because people were particularly gullible but because people knew something about Jesus that made the stories believable.

SPIRITUAL DYNAMICS AND SOCIAL DYNAMICS

A great deal of footwork has been employed by biblical scholars, other scientists, and popularizers over the centuries, dancing around the issue of biblical miracle reports; and a lot of ink has been spilled to explain away the fact or the meaning of Jesus' miracles. Those perspectives generally leave one feeling less than satisfied, because they give the impression that they do not take the biblical narratives with adequate seriousness. Whether the miracles are explained in a sacred or secular manner, as divine or human acts, or denied altogether, one has the suspicion that something more should be said. One feels that the attempts to divinize, psychologize, or negativize the miracle stories in the Bible are simply leaving something out. The haunting sense persists that what is being missed in the explanation really has to do with the core of the matter.

That is the issue addressed in Capps's fine book. It is worth our while and wholly appropriate that we should begin here, then, with a summary and assessment of Capps's thesis and argument. Capps's important volume begins with a discussion of the way in which the miracles of Jesus have been psychologized or rationalized away by scholars since the eighteenth-century Enlightenment. He discusses, for example, Albert Schweitzer's argumentation about whether Jesus was delusional. In the fifth chapter of this work, Capps moves from a discussion of conversion hysteria as an explanation of some spontaneous healings to the issue itself of Jesus as the village psychiatrist.

Capps suggests that Jesus should be taken seriously as a member of our helping professions, particularly those focused primarily upon psychotherapy. Jesus would not have recognized the term *psychotherapy*, but might well have been conscious of that category, described in standard dictionaries as healing that deals with the treatment and prevention of mental illness such as psychoses and neuroses. Mental illness in Jesus' day was caused by many things, just as it is today. Capps thinks that the normal emotional stress and strain for Jewish villagers in Palestine in Jesus' time was greatly increased by Roman occupation of their land. That would have jeopardized their village livelihood since the wealthy Roman cities that sprang up, with their voracious appetites, would have dominated the landscape, economy, and politics. He suggests that these sociocultural factors would have worsened personal stress, family tensions among the villagers of established families, and intergenerational conflicts. Jesus was a rural psychiatrist, in the sense that he ministered in and to the junctures of conflict between rural and urban cultures, between families and social groups, and between parents and children.

Capps notes that having been a carpenter, Jesus was more accustomed to building up than tearing down. So his interest in the well-being of those around him would have enticed him into the helping professions. It is not surprising that he, like so many of us, saw that as a calling in ministry that was both material and spiritual, related to matters mundane and religious. The anxiety and dysfunction of the people around him would have attracted his attention.

Anxiety is the driver behind most mental illness, frequently leading to irrational thoughts and behavior. Free-floating anxiety, which is not focused upon a real source of danger, may lead to the behavior of denial, exaggeration of the perceived threat, or projection of a danger where there is none. Capps believes that anxiety was the underlying cause of the disorders that Jesus treated successfully. Some forms of neurotic or psychotic acting out of anxiety can lead to hysteria and its psychophysical manifestations, as Freud contended. In his explication of this perspective, Capps focuses first upon two biblical narratives, both having to do with paralyzed persons (Mk 2:1–12; Jn 5:1–9).

Everyone knows well the story of the paralytic who was let down through the roof in Capernaum so that Jesus would be compelled to notice him. We know this is a case of hysterical paralysis because of the way the cure worked. Jesus undoubtedly knew this man and his family history since Jesus vacationed regularly in Capernaum on the shores of the Sea of Galilee. In fact, he eventually had a home in that city. He surely would have noticed the fellow or heard his story frequently, understood his family or life story, and realized the sources of the poor fellow's dysfunction. When the four friends presented the man to Jesus, he addressed him immediately in a familiar manner by saying, "Your sins are forgiven. Get up and walk." Carl Jung thought that half the healing power of a therapist lay in the aura and authority of healer that the patient projected upon the therapist. Jesus spoke with authority to inform the paralytic man that his fear, guilt, and shame had been removed by God from the equation of his life, so he could let go of his symptomatology and function normally. The point is that it worked. Jesus was an effective village psychotherapist.

The end of this story is a joke, of course, played on those who challenged Jesus' right to forgive sins since that is God's domain. It was obviously impossible to discredit the effectiveness for the healed man of Jesus' intervention, because the man began to walk home. So Jesus asked whether the complainers thought it easier to heal the fellow by saying his sins were forgiven, which was obviously effective, or by telling him to get up and walk, which he was already doing? It is interesting that in the second narrative about the man at the pool in Jerusalem, Jesus simply instructed him to get up and walk. The authority in his voice led the man to believe he could, and so he did, throwing off his psychological dysfunction. Nothing here about removal of fear, guilt, and shame! Obviously, Jesus knew that the causes were different in each case, and that suggests that he knew the case history well enough to understand the causes in each case.

THE PSYCHODYNAMICS

Capps observes correctly that such cases of anxiety-induced hysterical paralysis develop from a person's perception of a severely threatening danger, translated into conscious anxiety, internalized as free-floating unconscious anxiety that is disconnected from the danger source, and then somatized in psychophysiological dysfunction. At that point the original danger may have disappeared or been discovered as nonexistent in the first place; and the original anxiety may have dissipated. However, the unconscious anxiety persists, together with the psychosomatic dysfunction it induced, because the person has developed unrelated payoffs for persisting in the dysfunction. Such secondary gains, as we call them, can be the attention the handicap incites, the fear that acting against the symptoms might induce the original danger to recur, malingering, or other psychosocial payoffs. The person remains disabled because there are unconscious peripheral incentives. In such cases, the person usually wishes at the conscious level to be well; but at the unconscious level has numerous reasons to remain dysfunctional.

The effectiveness of a therapist's intervention in such cases has to do with the action of a trusted authority, upon whom the patient has projected the aura of healer, who gives the patient permission to act on his conscious desire to transcend his or her dysfunction. Jesus outflanked the suffering person's anxiety, inviting him to be free of psychospiritual imprisonment to both internalized and externalized fear, guilt, and shame. That act on the part of Jesus, as healer, permitted the patient a different perspective and hence a new master story, so to speak. Of course, we must remember that Jesus was not alone in that. The gospel records that there were others casting out demons in his society, at least one of whom was doing it by citing the authority of Jesus himself and Jesus commended him for doing so (Lk 9:49–50 and Mk 9:38–41).

It is interesting that when Jesus healed the man at the pool, he first asked him whether he wished to be healed. Undoubtedly, this suggests that Jesus was aware of the man's ambivalence about his imprisonment to his symptomatology with all its unconscious secondary gains, on the one hand; and his conscious claim that he wished to be healed but could never quite manage the optimal timing for it, on the other. One would think that after lying there for 38 years, as he claimed, he would have figured out how to seize the moment, if he were really thoroughly persuaded that he wanted to be healed. Obviously, in both this man's case and that of the paralytic let through the roof by his friends, Jesus' invitation to act on whatever motive each man had for being well tipped the psychospiritual scales in favor of freedom and health.

Capps would like to know what was wrong with these fellows and why. Cases of conversion hysteria resulting in paralysis are quite numerous. Familiar ones, for example, tend to appear regularly in the literature. An adolescent boy in a repressively moralistic family discovers the delights of masturbation and is repeatedly caught at it by his abusively scolding parent; and is so filled with fear, guilt, and shame that he converts these terrors of the soul into a paralysis of the arm and hand he uses to masturbate. I have a patient who not only developed such paralysis, but moved across the line into a psychotic episode in which he cut off the offending limb with his band saw. The men in Jesus' two stories may not have had sex-related hysteria, but may have faced physical threats they considered beyond their ability to defend against, and so saved their lives by retreating into dysfunction. So many dynamics can cause this kind of dysfunction that we cannot adequately speculate about or analyze what the operational sources of their suffering were. We only know what psychopathological category it is into which they neatly fit: classic hysterical paralysis.

In his chapter on "Jesus the Village Psychiatrist," Capps expends a great deal of analysis upon setting the social and psychophysiological setting for the suffering of the two Jewish men in these very Jewish stories. This turns out to be pure speculation, however, and not very useful. We cannot adequately reconstruct the psychosocial setting in ancient Galilee or Jerusalem. Capps relates the two healings of the paralytics to the stories of the healing at Jericho of the blind man Bartimaeus in Mark 10:46–50, and the healing at Bethsaida of another blind man in Mark 8:22–26. These too, he suggests, are cases of conversion hysteria. His judgment is based upon the fact that the stories indicate that the men both want to see, that both are spontaneously healed when Jesus invites or commands it, and that Jesus instructs one of them to go home and avoid the village.

Capps's assumption is that something in the village was so difficult for the man that it caused his dysfunction, and he could relapse. Did he have eyes for a forbidden woman of the village? Social censure in small villages is unmerciful. Moreover, was there not an injunction afloat in those days that said that every one who looks at a woman lustfully thereby commits adultery with her? Moreover, what about Jesus' observation that if your eye causes you to sin you should pluck it out and dispose of it, since it is better to dispose of one eye than lose yourself in hell (Mt 5:27–29)? That may not have been original with Jesus. It probably was a commonly known proverb of that day in that culture. Capps tops off his discussion with the additional observation that the length of average life in Jesus' day was so short as to obviate most causes of blindness that we see today, such as macular degeneration, hence psychosomatic causes are more likely. Capps's rationale regarding these two blind men is speculative, but of considerable interest.

Hysterical blindness is common, though usually temporary. I experienced it in one eye at about age 12 and it lasted for one night, though the trauma only lasted for a few hours. Capps reports that Ralph Waldo Emerson (1803–92) was blind for nine months at age 22. The dysfunction was not unrelated to his chronic tuberculosis, but the onset of the blindness seems to have been induced by his attempt, in developing his Unitarian theological rationale, to prove that if a demonic god does not exist the good God is the source of evil. In mid-sentence, so to speak, while penning that thought, he was struck blind. He left his studies and left Cambridge to work as a farm laborer. There he met another laborer who persuaded him of the empirical evidence for the efficaciousness of prayer. He undertook to pray for his eyesight, which began to return in December and was fully restored by February so he could go back to his studies and his Cambridge podium. He never revisited the psychospiritual impasse on the occasion of which he went blind. Instead of his perspective of religious doubt he shifted to a constructive quest of theological reflection. In commenting on this, Capps reports that Emerson acknowledged that his psychospiritual stress and associated anxiety had a significant role to play in his affliction.

Emerson's writings are filled with metaphors about eyes, vision, seeing, illumination, sight, and insight. His journals testify to the fact that Emerson began to recognize in college that he had an intense attraction response to glancing at some other persons, both male and female, for whom he felt an immediate sense of erotic longing and intimate connection. This caused him much anxiety, he acknowledges, probably in response to the glances of males more than those of females, though we do not know with certainty. He first reports noticing it with regard to a male friend in his class at Harvard. Emerson was about 19 and was experiencing the awakenings of love in a way that was rather standard at his age for that time, and had to work through some gender confusion at first, as everyone does in puberty. This confusion dissipated for Emerson in young adulthood. Capps relates this to intense levels of anxiety in Emerson, likely related to his conversion hysteria blindness. The reason that it caused problems with his eyes, Capps implies, is that they were the offending organs inducing the anxiety and triggering the psychosomatic symptomatology that was used to manage his psychospiritual problem in a psychopathological manner.

CASTING OUT DEMONS

Contrary to many biblical scholars, Capps holds that Jesus' miracles of casting out demons were healing miracles, similar to those of the healing of the paralytics and blind men. It is interesting that the persons whom Jesus cured of demon possession seem to have been predominantly males, though of course Luke 8:2 refers to women who were cured of evil spirits. Mary Magdalene was cured of seven demons, and both Mathew (15:21–28) and Mark (7:24–28) refer to a girl cured of demon possession. The cured males were mostly young males and adolescents, and Capps focuses primarily on these young men, who were brought to Jesus by their fathers. Capps does not address the case of the girl possessed of a demon and brought to Jesus by her mother (Mt 15:21–28, Mk 7:24–28). Only the two Gadarene demoniacs, found near the Sea of Galilee, seem to have been independent of close family. Probably because of the severity of their disorders, they seem to have been living in a cemetery. That would mean that they lived on the edge of the Jewish community, marginalized in their own region. This is confirmed by that fact that there was a herd of pigs close at hand, animals that Jews assiduously avoided.

Most scholars believe the biblical stories of demon possession are evidences of classic epilepsy. Capps argues for conversion hysteria or a combination of the two, a condition we might call automatism in which a person is induced to behavior over which he seems to have no control and which he cannot himself explain. He suggests the Freudian interpretation that a combination of sexual anxiety and role confusion anxiety can induce such hysteria. Jewish males in Jesus' day, says Capps, would have been suffering from a sense of being unempowered by the ignominy inflicted upon them and their nation by Roman dominance.

This would have undercut their sense of phallic prowess and would have forced sublimation or repression of their sexual energies, causing a struggle with problems of sexual diversion such as incest, adultery, and perversion; as well as a hysterical conversion of their normal assertiveness. The anxiety associated with this for a young man can induce the psychological parody of a conversion disorder that looks like demon possession or epilepsy; severely self-destructive and self-punishing behavior, such as casting him into the water and fire or throwing him violently upon the ground. Josephus says that Galilean boys were inured to war from infancy by harsh discipline and brutal training. Lack of maternal warmth and the presence of strong patriarchal discipline, in a context of male powerlessness and sexual repression and confusion, could prompt a child or adolescent to elect unconsciously for such a conversion reaction hysteria.

The implication of this state of affairs seems to be that males, particularly in Galilee, who were demasculinized by various forces including Roman disempowerment and harsh parental demeanment, would have had little opportunity for fighting back against this oppression as they gained the strength of late adolescence and young manhood. Jesus himself seems to have come to his unconventional break with that society very late. Only in his thirties did he finally find his voice and his true empowerment, and that was in a role and expression of a contrarian who rejected his family, community, vocation, and religious traditions.

To consider such unconventional choices as Jesus made in declaring himself to be the Messiah, or the decision of the Essenes to withdraw from the general society, or even more seriously the choice that the Zealots made to kill Romans, one by one, wherever they could catch one out, would have both raised and expressed enormous anxiety in individual males and in the society in general. Most of the time for most Jewish males those choices would have had to be rejected and repressed, sublimated into other channels of expression. For some, the impasse proved so serious, intense, and unresolvable, Capps claims, that it turned into the psychological conversion reaction of hysterical and self–destructive automatism; a severe psychospiritual pathology.

Instead of the aggressive expression being directed toward the "enemy" it would be directed against the self, just as in hysterical blindness or paralysis. Capps suggests that we have reason to believe that this was a fairly common state of affairs with young men in Jesus' day and later. He cites a document from the third century after Christ, which relates a mother's petition regarding the condition of her son, remarkably similar to the demon possessions cured by Jesus.

THE LARGER WORLD OF MIRACLES

Miracle stories decorate ancient literature of all cultures more elaborately than we generally realize. They are always assumed to be unexpected and abnormal events caused by divine action in this material world, either directly by a god or by someone who acts for God. This tradition goes back to the very earliest legends or reports of human experience, and they bedeck the memories of primitive cultures and of the most sophisticated societies. Howard Clark Kee says that these events raise the questions about what happened and what it means; specifically, what divine message is intended to be conveyed by the event.[2] Kee confirms Capps' approach to the biblical miracles in insisting that it is inappropriate to describe a miracle as a violation of natural law. Surprising events in ancient societies were described as miracles because their worldview, technology, and science had no paradigm within which to manage this unusual data. Even the Stoics, who posited the notion of natural law, left room for direct divine action, and they thought they observed such interventions associated with major turning points in history such as those associated with Julius and Augustus Caesar.

According to Brown, it was only since the rise of modern science and its model of the pervasive lawfulness of the material universe that "miracles came to be defined increasingly in terms of violations of the laws of nature. This led Spinoza to seek natural explanations for the biblical miracles . . . and Hume to claim that the whole idea of miracles was self-refuting."[3] Since Spinoza the struggle to understand the nature and meaning of miracles or of the miracle stories in the Bible has fueled an ongoing debate as to whether a given miraculous event was extraordinary in the fortuitous nature and timing of the way the event unfolded, or in the overt violation of natural law. The former case might be a night-long "strong east wind" that parted the water in the Exodus (Ex 14:21). The latter case would be that of raising a dead person to life. In both cases, the event might be understood, indeed, was seen in the biblical world, as a divine intervention.

Kee cites biblical miracles that have the function of divine confirmation of some course of human action; divine illumination of someone's sense of guidance and destiny; judgment upon some misbehavior; deliverance from dire circumstances; revealing divine purposes; and inauguration in this world of the divine rule of grace that works and love that heals. Jesus' healings were miracles of deliverance that inaugurated the breaking in of the reign of God in human affairs. Kee concludes his article by declaring that the biblical miracles are presented as divine instruments by which transcendental purposes are disclosed and fulfilled in our world, illustrating that God is directly present to us in daily life. Exodus 8:19 makes this claim directly. Referring to Moses' miracles before the Pharaoh and his staff, the Bible declares, "This is the finger of God."

Seung Ai Yang observes that of the 35 miracles ascribed to Jesus in the four Gospels, most fall into one of four categories: healings, exorcisms, resuscitations, and control of nature.[4] Of course, the line between the first two is difficult to confirm, as Capps insists; and the line between the last two may not exist, since raising the dead is an act of controlling nature. In this regard Brown discusses C. S. Lewis' Augustinianism in the matter of miracles.

> C. S. Lewis represented a return to a more Augustinian position with his definition of a miracle as "an interference with Nature by supernatural power" (*Miracles*, p. 15). This leaves open the question as to how nature has been interfered with. It gives recognition to the fact that God's working is ultimately a mystery. It allows for the fact that miracles are never seen directly. What is observed is a state of affairs before and after the event. Recognition of an event as a miracle is bound up with the wider view that one takes of reality, just as rejection of miracles is bound up with one's beliefs about the uniformities of nature.[5]

The Bible, of course, assumes a worldview in which the veil between the mundane and transcendent world is permeable. God and his agents seem to move back and forth through that screen rather readily. We do not need to adopt that worldview in order to wrestle with the issues of miracles, though we should not dispose of that worldview too readily either. Since we do not know a great deal about the transcendent world and the barrier that seems to exist between us and it, we should keep a mind of open wonder about any and all of the possibilities. Brown's emphasis is objective and useful.

> In their descriptions of Jesus' exorcisms, healings, and nature miracles the Gospels present the events either explicitly or implicitly as following His pronouncement of the word of God in the power of the Holy Spirit. Jesus acts and speaks with the authority of Yahweh Himself.
>   The tendency to treat the miracles of Jesus apart from His teaching and the course of His life has been encouraged by Christian piety, apologetic interests, and critical study. Piety has found encouragement and inspiration from reflection on individual miracles. Apologetics has tended to focus on the Gospel miracles as supernatural attestation of the divinity of Christ. Critical study has tended to prefer the teaching of Jesus to the miracles, and form criticism has seen the miracle stories as products of pious belief, produced by churches anxious to invest Jesus with the credentials of a divine man.[6]

Brown concludes that his miracles are an inherent part of his teaching and cannot be legitimately separated from it.

    Miracles, and therefore miracle workers, were fairly common in the Jewish and Greco-Roman world during and after Jesus' day. Two noted first-century CE miracle workers were Onias and Hanina ben Dosa, though it might be observed that their miracles were not associated with messianic claims, as generally Jesus' were. Miracles were standard healing practices at the medical centers of Asclepius at Epidaurus and Pergamum. Moreover the Egyptian Serapis held the same reputation. It was a popular endeavor of the History of Religions School of scholars, in the nineteenth and twentieth centuries, to demonstrate parallels between the biblical narratives and the miracle reports from the Hellenistic world in general. They were especially encouraged in this by the similarity between Luke 7:11–17, in which Jesus is described as raising the dead son of the widow at Nain, and the *Life of Apollonius* of Tyana iv:45, in which Apollonius restores to life a bride whose funeral he encountered at the city gate, and who had died just as she was to be married. Philostratus, who wrote the *Life of Apollonius*, expresses almost modern-day reservations as to whether Apollonius detected some spark of life or really raised a really dead person.

> Through the centuries critics of Christianity have repeatedly drawn atten-
> tion to what they conceived to be parallels between Jesus and Apollonius
> of Tyana, a Neo Pythagorean sage and wandering ascetic who lived in
> the first century and was credited with exorcistic and miraculous powers.
> Philostratus was commissioned by the Empress, Julia Domna, who was the
> wife of Septimius Severus, to write a *Life of Apollonius*. The circumstances
> and contents of the book have prompted the suggestion that Apollonius
> and his cult were fostered as a rival alternative to Christianity.[7]

In the September 2007 issue of *Discover, Science, Technology, and the Future,* Jeanne Lenzer published an article entitled "Citizen, Heal Thyself."[8] She de-clares that the sorts of miracles in the biblical narratives are happening all around us every day. John Matzke was 30 years old when informed that he had terminal melanoma with lung metastasis. The oncologist at the Veter-ans Administration hospital urged immediate treatment, despite the fact that patients with his condition have a 50 percent mortality within two and a half years after surgery. John chose to take 30 days to strengthen his body for the treatment. He spent much time walking in the mountains and forest, medi-tating, visualizing his healing cells killing the cancerous ones, and eating a healthy diet. When he returned to his physician the doctor expected to see two large lung lesions. Instead the radiographies showed a complete lack of any pathology. The physician said, "When John came back a month later, it was remarkable—the tumor on his chest x-ray was gone. Gone, gone, gone." He was given 18 months to live. He lived another 18 years. Then recurrence of the cancer in his brain killed him.

> Pinning down spontaneous remissions has been a little like chasing rain-
> bows. It's not even possible to say just how frequently such cases occur—
> estimates generally range from 1 in 60,000 to 1 in 100,000 patients. . . . But
> genuine miracles do exist, and throughout the history of medicine, physi-
> cians have recorded cases of spontaneous remission . . . not just cancer but
> conditions like aortic aneurysm, . . . Peyronie's disease, a deformity of the
> penis; and childhood cataracts.[9]

Researchers speculate that Matzke's immune system, reinforced by his change in lifestyle and psychospiritual address to his tumors, produced a healing effect. They noticed that during his month of meditation and healthy living his skin tumors were surrounded by white halo-like rings, indicating that the immune system was attacking the melanocytes, pigmented cells in the skin that give rise to the cancer.[10] Ever since 1700 or so a medical record has been developing indicating that certain serious infections such as erysipelas or those associated with streptococcus cure cancer by causing tumor regression. It was by following up on these cures that nature spontaneously induces that physicians were able to develop the chemotherapy that is used today. The medical statistics now available indicate that a surprisingly high number of patients are cured or significantly improved in health by both spontaneous remission and by assisting nature by inducing the infectious condition created by chemotherapy.

Lenzer reports the case of Alice Epstein, a brilliant academic diagnosed with kidney cancer in 1985. A month after the resection of her kidney, the cancer showed up in both lungs. Her life estimate at that time was three months.

> Epstein, who says she had a "cancer-prone personality," then turned to psychosynthesis, which she describes as a "combination of psychotherapy and spiritual therapy." It helped her overcome depression, difficulty expressing anger, and suppression of her own needs in order to please others—traits she and some psychologists believe are characteristic of the cancer-prone personality. Although she never received any medical or surgical treatment for the deadly cancer invading her lungs, six weeks after starting psychosynthesis, her tumors began to shrink. Within one year, they had disappeared without a trace. That was 22 years ago.[11]

Today Epstein is alive and well and 80 years of age.

The crucial points at stake here are as follows. First, given the right chance, the irrepressible life force in nature is able to induce spontaneous remission of horrible disorder in the physical organism of human beings. Second, the state of psychospirituality of that human person seems to have a great deal to do with the onset of illness and the effecting of cure. Third, a decisive shift in orientation in the psychospiritual world of that person seems to be the trigger that induces radical reorientation of the organic forces at play in the physiological organism, the human body. Focus upon the permission to be well and not sick, and focus upon the will to get well, is a high priority factor in mobilizing the power of our physiological organism to eliminate the deadly forces that work against the well-being of the person. It is clear that this works when the ill person determines to live and be well. One can confidently speculate that a directive to get well, given by an authority whom that the sick person respects as a healer, would be enough in some cases to trigger the will to empower the immune system to overcome the pathological and pathogenic condition in his or her body.

Lenzer concludes almost lyrically. "Although medical advances have dramatically improved outcomes in certain cancers . . . modern medicine has yet to come close to nature's handiwork in inexplicably producing spontaneous remission without apparent side effects for people like John Matzke and Alice Epstein, who have experienced the rarest hints of nature's healing mysteries."[12] The interesting question arising in the context of these reports of miraculous cures, combined with the focus of this volume upon the biblical narratives of miracles, is whether the miracle stories of the Bible were attempts to report similar literal histories of cured persons,[13] or described the imagination of the primitive missionary church at work in glorifying the attention-getting aspects of their memory of Jesus.[14]

NOTES

1. Donald Capps (2007), *Jesus the Village Psychiatrist*, Louisville: Westminster John Knox.

2. Howard Clark Kee (1993), Miracles, *The Oxford Guide to the Bible*, Bruce M. Metzger and Michael D. Coogan, eds., New York: Oxford University Press, 519–20.

3. Colin Brown (1986), Miracle, *The International Standard Bible Encyclopedia (ISBE)*, Fully Revised, vol. 3, Grand Rapids: Eerdmans, 371–81.

4. Seung Ai Yang (2000), Miracles, *Eerdmans Dictionary of the Bible*, David Noel Freedman, Allen C. Myers, and Astrid B. Beck, eds., Grand Rapids: Eerdmans, 903–4.

5. Brown (1986), 372–73, citing C. S. Lewis (1947), *Miracles: A Preliminary Study*, London: Geoffrey Bless, Ltd. and New York: Macmillan.

6. Ibid., 373.

7. Ibid., 377–78.

8. Jeanne Lenzer (2007), Citizen, Heal Thyself, *Discover: Science, Technology, and the Future*, September, 54–59, 73.

9. Ibid., 56.

10. Ibid., 56.

11. Ibid., 58.

12. Ibid., 73.

13. Charles Caldwell Ryrie (1984), *The Miracles of Our Lord*, New York: Nelson. See also Reginald H. Fuller (1963), *Interpreting the Miracles*, Philadelphia: Westminster.

14. Anton Fridrichsen (1972), *The Problem of Miracle in Primitive Christianity*, Minneapolis: Augsburg. See also Gerd Theissen (1983), *The Miracle Stories of the Early Christian Tradition*, Edinburgh: T&T Clark. Originally published in 1974 as *Urchristliche Wundergeschichten: Ein Beitrag zur formgeschichtlichen Erforschung der synoptischen Evangelien*, Gutersloh: Gutersloher Verlaghaus Gerd Mohn.

REFERENCES

Brown, Colin (1986), Miracle, *The International Standard Bible Encyclopedia (ISBE)*, Fully Revised, Vol. 3, 371–381, Grand Rapids: Eerdmans.

Capps, Donald (2007), *Jesus the Village Psychiatrist*, Louisville: Westminster John Knox.

Fridrichsen, Anton (1972), *The Problem of Miracle in Primitive Christianity*, Minneapolis: Augsburg.

Fuller, Reginald H. (1963), *Interpreting the Miracles*, Philadelphia: Westminster.

Kee, Howard Clark (1993), Miracles, *The Oxford Guide to The Bible*, Bruce M. Metzger and Michael D. Coogan, eds., 519–520, New York: Oxford University Press.

Lenzer, Jeanne (2007), Citizen, Heal Thyself, in *Discover: Science, Technology, and the Future*, September 2007, 54–59 and 73.

Lewis, C. S. (1947), *Miracles: A Preliminary Study*, London: Geoffrey Bless, and New York: Macmillan.

Ryrie, Charles Caldwell (1984), *The Miracles of Our Lord*, New York: Nelson.

Theissen, Gerd (1983), *The Miracle Stories of the Early Christian Tradition*, Francis McDonagh, trans., Edinburgh: T&T Clark. Originally published in 1974 as *Urchristliche Wundergeschichten: Ein Beitrag zur formgeschichtlichen Erforschung der synoptischen Evangelien*, Gutersloh: Gutersloher Verlaghaus Gerd Mohn.

Yang, Seung Ai (2000), Miracles, *Eerdmans Dictionary of the Bible*, David Noel Freedman, Allen C. Myers, and Astrid B. Beck, eds., 903–4, Grand Rapids: Eerdmans.

CHAPTER 2

Distorted Reality or Transitional Space? Biblical Miracle Stories in Psychoanalytic Perspective

Petri Merenlahti

In many ways faith in miracles exemplifies what traditional psychoanalysts think is wrong with religion. The psychoanalytic process is meant to improve the patient's psychic well-being by helping him or her to cope with reality on its own terms. To hope for a miracle to happen and change the way reality works is to reject this kind of growth and opt for fantasy, regression, and wishful thinking.

However, some psychoanalysts today take a more positive view of religion (Black 2006). They emphasize that the distinction between fantasy and reality is not always crystal clear and some fantasies can be beneficial to health. Together with art and other creative forms of human culture, religion allows for a particular merging of inner reality and external life, personal and objectively perceived meanings, so as to facilitate psychic growth and the building up of a capacity for interpersonal relationships. From this perspective, religious stories about miracles are not necessarily epitomes of regression. Even if they are not true in the objective sense, they may still carry psychological truth.

In this chapter, I will look at the biblical miracle stories as a case example. I will argue that the role they play in the biblical narrative displays both regressive and mature tendencies. On the one hand, they do recount and envision extraordinary acts of salvation by divine intervention. On the other hand, the narrative implies that the high season of such acts only lasted for a limited time, after which they became increasingly a thing of the mythical past. There will never be another Moses who will know God face to face. Jesus was taken up into heaven and will only return at the end of times.

Meanwhile, people will have to cope with the present reality, where miracles are rare and the divine presence is less tangible. In this sense, the narrative is encouraging its audience in the task of reality-acceptance.

Yet the tension between the two tendencies is never resolved completely. They should therefore not be seen as successive developmental phases but rather as oscillating positions that together characterize the biblical stance vis-à-vis the world.

AT ODDS WITH REALITY

According to the Letter to the Hebrews, "faith is the assurance of things hoped for, the conviction of things not seen" (11:1). Believers are dissidents towards common reality. They will not bow to the obvious, and they reserve the right to rely on other things than mere cold facts—even if this means being criticized for foolishness. As the apostle Paul puts it,

> God chose what is foolish in the world to shame the wise; God chose what is weak in the world to shame the strong; God chose what is low and despised in the world, things that are not, to reduce to nothing things that are. (1 Cor 1:27–28)

Now, Paul may well be demonstrating an ego defense mechanism known as *devaluation*, that is, he dismisses the frustration of being denied something by claiming that he did not care for it in the first place. Even in that case, his words contain remarkable subversive potential. Who decides by what standards individual people are to be considered wise or powerful or noble anyway? Sometimes reality, and social reality in particular, deserves to be challenged. This is one reason why there is demand for the kind of idealism that is the business of religion.

On the other hand, common reality has found strong supporters, too. They have accused religion of deliberate or instinctive self-deception.[1] According to Karl Marx's famous statement (Marx 1887), religion is the opium of the people.[2] The dream of a better world is a convenient painkiller: it helps the poor and the oppressed to put up with their lot.

Likewise for Sigmund Freud (1927, 1930), religious belief was essentially a pathology: in the religious worldview, infantile dependence and the demand for unlimited wish fulfillment survive into adult life as trust in the Heavenly Father's omnipotence. Religious myths and rituals correspond to obsessive thinking and behavior that are meant to repress unpleasant truths.

There are three unpleasant truths in particular, says Freud, that religions refuse to accept: that the only reward for morality will be civilized life on earth; that nature has no purpose; and that death will be the end. As all the three are fundamental truths about life, religion amounts to massive denial.

No psychologically mature person needs it, as he or she will be able to face reality as it is.

The biblical miracle stories are a case in point. They affirm the very same three ideas of which Freud thought people should let go.

First, they attest that history is all about justice. If the oppressed keep crying out for help long enough, God will take notice of them, as he did when the Israelites were Pharaoh's slaves in Egypt. The awesome wonders he displayed then signaled vindication to his people and judgment to their enemies. Similarly, Jesus' exorcisms in the New Testament confirm that the rule of Satan is over and the Day of Judgment is near. Soon the good will receive their reward, and the evil will be punished. If the present reality cannot deliver this promise, God will intervene to establish a new one.

Second, the biblical miracle stories encourage their audience to take God's acts personally. They imply that God gets involved because he cares for his own. Unwilling to have his chosen ones suffer any longer, he takes direct action, and reality will yield. So, when you see these extraordinary things taking place, you know that you are not insignificant. God's interventions are signs of his personal affection.

Moreover, last but not least, you will be saved. The whole point of negotiating reality is that you will not have to die. Paul writes to the Corinthians: "If for this life only we have hoped in Christ, we are of all people most to be pitied" (1 Cor 15:19). Indeed, Jesus did make the promise, in the Gospel of John: "Everyone who lives and believes in me will never die" (Jn 11:26). Death will not be the end.

MIRACLES EXPLAINED

So, Freud certainly had a problem with miracles, as did much of the psychoanalytic tradition after him. The same is true of the heritage of enlightened rationalism on the whole, including those enlightened rationalists who were willing to tolerate or even appreciate religion, once it was understood in a proper way. As the latter position characterizes the thinking of some contemporary psychoanalysts as well, it will be useful to take a brief look at the anatomy of the idea.

The eighteenth-century deists are a well-known case. They cherished the idea of a sensible natural religion that would stand for what they believed to be timeless spiritual values: faith in a benevolent creator and in the immortality of the soul, combined with high morals. Such religion would be in full harmony with scientific knowledge, and therefore not allow for miracles or any other kind of unreasonable superstition.

Today it is much easier than in the eighteenth century to reject religion altogether. It is now possible to conceive of life without a creator, and to explain mental and moral capacities in purely materialist terms. So there is no need to have a natural religion to make sense of the world. Yet the idea is not forgotten. Unlike what was predicted by many social scientists just a couple of decades ago, religion is not going extinct, although institutional religion continues to lose ground, especially in the global North (Berger 1999). Among Western educated people, there still seems to be demand for a *natural spirituality*, that will go together with modern values and the basic assumptions of the contemporary scientific worldview, and still be genuine spirituality. But what to do with those elements of religious tradition, such as the miracle stories of the Bible, that run counter to reason and experience?

Ever since the Enlightenment, there have been attempts for a rationalist solution. One popular approach was to argue that miracles were not really miracles. The Bible, although historically accurate, does not really mean what it says, or the biblical writers did not understand correctly what they heard or saw. So, when the Bible tells us that Jesus was walking on the sea, what he actually did was stroll on floating logs of wood. Or, when it says that darkness came over the land when Jesus died, this was because a massive sandstorm hid the sun, and so on: for every biblical miracle a natural explanation was to be found. The German nineteenth-century rationalist theologians became famous for their efforts in this field, and the name of H.E.G. Paulus in particular stood out among them (Paulus 1828; see Albert Schweitzer's account in Schweitzer 1906, 49–58).

This approach never turned out as a success, however. From a scholarly perspective, it is now a thing of the past, although in fiction, popular culture, and folklore, classic rationalist explanations of biblical miracles still flourish, and popular books presenting the natural causes of the biblical stories continue to be published (Humphreys 2003). In light of modern biblical criticism, not so much informed by rationalist arguments as by careful source criticism, the biblical stories are not direct eyewitness accounts but religious literature combining historical traditions, artistic creation, and folklore. There is therefore no need to explain every biblical account as historically possible.

Moreover, in their literary and religion-historical contexts, the biblical miracle stories hardly make sense except as stories about miracles. The biblical writers were not in the business to keep record of well-timed natural phenomena and furnish them with misguided explanations. Rather, they were to pass on, give expression to, and reshape genuine *religious* experiences and beliefs: what Moses or Jesus were believed to have been, done, and meant, and how this was integrated into experiences of the divine in the present. The same was true of Jesus himself. While we do not know too much about him with much certainty, we do know that he was not a naturalist philosopher preaching timeless moral truths. Most likely, he was a Jewish popular charismatic, a practicing healer and exorcist who, like many others in his time, waited for God's radical intervention in history (Theissen and Merz 1996). The problems we may have with calling anything supernatural were not his problems. What he and his followers believed made perfect sense in their historical and religious environment, although it may no more do so in ours.

This takes us to another solution, one that may have stood the test of time a little better. According to this solution, the biblical miracle stories are indeed about miracles, but their real meaning and value for our time lie on another level than that of historical truth. Modern history of ideas knows many versions of this approach, the roots of which go back to the allegorical exegesis of the ancient rabbis and the church fathers. They too thought the deepest meaning of the sacred text lay beneath the surface level and could only be grasped once one understood that the historical stories were in fact symbolic expressions of eternal spiritual truths. Like their modern colleagues, the rabbis and the church fathers were keen to apply this method to the texts they considered primitive (Smalley 1956, 2).

In the history of modern scholarship, a couple of key figures stand out for the influential way in which they reinterpreted the meaning of biblical miracles. The year 1835, "the revolutionary year of modern theology," saw the publication of the first volume of *The Life of Jesus* (*Das Leben Jesu, kritisch bearbeitet*) by David Friedrich Strauss. An eminent pupil of the philosopher Hegel, Strauss rejected both the belief in the supernatural and the rationalist attempts to discover the natural causes of the biblical stories. Clearly, he thought, the biblical writers recounted, as authentic narratives, stories that were at odds with nature and reason and therefore could not be historical. They could, however, have theological value as myths that communicated universal truths about the human spirit. For Strauss, those truths were happily congruent with Hegel's idealistic philosophy: in Christ, humanity became conscious of its true nature as absolute spirit.

One of the most important theological figures of the twentieth century, Rudolf Bultmann, introduced another famous program of demythologization (Bultmann 1933–65). He, too, considered the mythological language of the Bible severely outdated and therefore irrelevant to modern people. The answer was to reinterpret it so as to address the great existential questions of human life. While Strauss drew on Hegel, Bultmann's source of inspiration was Martin Heidegger's existentialist philosophy. For him, the real meaning of the Jewish and Christian scriptures, hidden under ancient mythological language, was to be found in how they related to the universal experience of the human condition.

Strauss and Bultmann were prime examples of progressive theologians running to the rescue of their religious tradition at a time when advanced scientific knowledge threatened to make it intellectually inadequate and ideologically irrelevant. Structurally, their solution was a standard one, known well from similar situations in the history of biblical interpretation, and the history of interpretation of sacred literature on the whole. The scriptures were to be interpreted symbolically as manifestations of some timeless truth.

The end result was a definition of biblical truth that conformed to the current scientific paradigm.

It is not unexpected that a similar approach to religious stories and traditions should occur within the guild of psychoanalysts. While Freud's blanket rejection of religion became the dominant psychoanalytic view for decades, not all of his colleagues shared this view, not even in the beginning. Since then, the Western intellectual climate has become more tolerant, if not towards all forms of religion, at least towards a spiritual dimension of life. Most importantly, the psychoanalytic method itself stands in close connection with the tradition of allegorical interpretation (cf. Frosh 2006, 216, quoting Ostow 1982, 8). Freud's very own oedipal interpretations of Christianity and Judaism assumed that the key to understanding biblical texts lay hidden beneath their surface level. Technically, then, it should be possible to neglect their supernaturalistic top layer and find other meanings that will not contradict the rationalist premises that psychoanalysis holds dear.

RETHINKING FANTASY

Since the mid-1980s, psychoanalytic interest in religion has grown steadily. Some commentators speak of "something of a flood" (Black 2006, 15). Numerous analysts, including Michael Eigen, Mark Epstein, James Jones, Sudhir Kakar, William Meissner, Paul Pryser, Ana-Maria Rizzuto, Jeffrey Rubin, and Neville Symington, have written on the topic, reconsidering the relationship between religion and psychoanalysis. Rejecting what they see as Freud's overly simplistic critique of religion, they suggest that some forms of religious belief and practice can support healthy psychological development. As a means of furnishing experienced reality, including one's experience of the self, with personal meaning, religion can help people in the task of reality-acceptance; quite unlike what Freud thought would be the case. This view seems to be gaining wider support, so that "overall among analysts today, there is a much greater openness to and acceptance of certain religious beliefs and practices than ever before" (Blass 2006, 23).

What happened? How is it possible to adopt an almost diametrically opposite position on religion from what was before, and still remain within the same psychoanalytic paradigm? It seems that two things made the difference: first, there was a new understanding of the sense of reality as a (or better, *the*) psychoanalytic criterion of psychic maturity; and, second, there was a new understanding of religion (cf. Blass 2006).

While the new psychoanalytic understanding of religion connects with the work of various theorists, it is probably D. W. Winnicott's ideas of transitional phenomena, transitional objects, and transitional experience that have made the most profound impact on how many analysts today perceive the relationship of religion, reality, and illusion. Special extensions of the self, transitional objects stand halfway between the subjective inner reality of the individual and the objectively perceived external reality or environment. Winnicott initially introduced these concepts with reference to a particular developmental sequence (Winnicott 1951); a typical example of a transitional object is a safety blanket or a soft toy that comes to be of special importance to the infant. Later, however, Winnicott expanded the idea into a broader vision of mental health and creativity. Giving birth to art and culture, transitional experience makes us able to connect our inner experience of the self with the world of other subjectivities (Winnicott 1971).

A key thing about the transitional phenomena is that their reality, outside fantasy, is not to be challenged. To ask if the teddy bear is *really* what the child conceives of it to be is to miss a point. The child is not lying or hallucinating. Instead, he or she is taking steps from subjective omnipotence, that is, the early, illusory experience of the world as created by the child's own wishes, to the actual, external world that exists on its own right, independently of the child. As the transition progresses and the child builds capacity for secure, trusted relationships with others in the external world, the transitional object ceases to perform this function and is left behind.

Similarly, the point of art and religion is not to make positive, verifiable statements of the external reality in the ordinary sense of the word. Rather, they constitute a protected realm for creative vision and play that is vital for our being in touch with ourselves and for our relatedness with others. The illusion of art and religion is not a way to escape or avoid painful reality, but "a vehicle to gain access to reality" (Black 2006, 14; Meissner 1984; cf. also Hopkins 1989, 239).

What Winnicott and other British *object-relations theorists* did was redefine the concept of illusion so that a new psychoanalytic understanding of religion became possible. They, of course, were not the only ones in the business. Even earlier, Melanie Klein had called into question Freud's clear-cut distinction between regressive fantasies and a mature sense of reality. Moreover, there are other instrumental cases as well. Heinz Kohut's self-psychology and especially his work on narcissism and idealization (Kohut 1971, 1984) is another good example.

For Freud, narcissism and idealization were infantile features to be outgrown. For Kohut, however, there was a positive side to them that remained relevant throughout one's entire life. In order to be well psychologically, people need to be able to feel that they, their love objects, and the communities to which they belong are special. This is not something dictated by the reality principle: objectively speaking, no part of reality is any more special, blessed, or meaningful than any other. Yet, such a feeling of worth is hardly delusional, either. It is rather something no one can live without: we need what Kohut called self-objects, special people, places, and things that help us sustain a sense of coherence and vitality. Religion provides for such experiences of positive idealization, as it assumes there is such a thing as the supreme good; that human beings are valuable and called to salvation; that all God's children are sisters and brothers to each other, and so on (cf. Jones 2002).

RETHINKING RELIGION?

The rehabilitation of illusion testifies to a shift of emphasis in the criteria of psychic maturity. Focus on interpersonal relatedness and self-experience has replaced oedipal notions of maturity in post-Freudian psychoanalysis. Illusion and fantasy are no more undesirable, by definition (cf. Blass 2006, 26–27).

Yet it is still illusion and fantasy we are talking about, and herein lies another key question regarding the new psychoanalysis of religion. Does the revised understanding of religion as an (positive) illusion not imply a new, normative idea of religion? A religion that would not make any claims to truth but rather regards its teachings and rituals as illusions, or illusion-generators, certainly sounds like a novelty.

Many analysts, who have adopted a positive understanding of religion with a Winnicottian twist, would readily admit that this indeed is the case: it is not religion on the whole but religion in the mature sense of the term that is compatible with psychoanalytic theory and practice (Blass 2006, 28–29). Some make a distinction, in the spirit of the deists, between natural religion(s) and revealed religions (see, for example, Wright 2006, 177, with reference to Symington 1993, 2006, 197). Many focus predominantly on traditions of mysticism, especially as they are featured in Eastern religions, and on Buddhism in particular, although often in a somewhat Westernized, meditation-oriented form (cf. Blass 2006, 29). Some even volunteer to cure pathologies of the spirit by means of analysis, to attain an even more refined form of religious practice and belief (Rubin 2006).

On the other hand, it is fair to say that there is also a growing awareness within psychoanalysis of the diversity of religious experience. If Freud did not realize that not all religion is the same, proreligion analysts have come to learn that no religious tradition should be idealized, either. Primitive and enlightened ideas and habits coexist in all quarters (cf. Black 2006, 5).

In any case, the new illusionist (re)definition of religion has met with strong criticism (Blass 2006; cf. Hood 1997). The key point of the critique is that such an ideal religion hardly exists in the real world. Would any true believer of any religious tradition consider his or her faith a mere meaningful illusion with no interest in actual truth? Rachel Blass (2006, 33) hits the mark, I think, when she quotes the theologian Hans Küng.

The man who believes . . . is primarily interested . . . in the reality itself. . . .
He wants to know whether and to what extent his faith is based on illusion

or on historical reality. Any faith based on illusion is not really faith but superstition. (Küng 1984, 418)

Even in the mystical traditions, the ineffable, and, in a sense, only that, is considered real. While art may indeed imitate reality and create independent worlds of pure imagination, religions do seem to make claims to truth about this reality, and sometimes about other realities as well. Should these claims turn out to be invalid or, for the present purposes, incompatible with the rationalist premises of psychoanalysis, this would make religion, from a psychoanalytic point of view, not only a purposeful illusion but a distortion of reality, very much like Freud said it would.

Freud did, in fact, note that a philosopher might view religion as a kind of fiction accepted as true for its practical significance (Freud 1927; Blass 2006, 31; Hood 1997, 53–54). However, he said, no serious believer would accept this. This seems to leave the original controversy between psychoanalysis and religion unresolved. When it comes down to it, both religion and psychoanalysis apply the same criterion to judge whether a particular belief is healthy or not: Is it the truth? In the words of the Second Letter of Peter:

> For we did not follow cleverly devised myths when we made known to you the power and coming of our Lord Jesus Christ, but we had been eyewitnesses of his majesty. (1:16)

Still, both religion and psychoanalysis should be allowed to change. Many a thing in contemporary religious thought would have been incomprehensible some hundred years ago, just as Freud would be surprised to learn what kinds of ideas and practices carry the name of psychoanalysis today. Although in the business of absolute, eternal truths, religions have hardly reached the end of their development, or the peak of their diversity, as systems of belief, sometimes reluctantly and often with a marked delay, they nevertheless keep adapting to what each time and culture finds possible to accept as true. This is precisely because they are interested in reality. If the material reality should become too narrow for them, they will turn to other spiritual, philosophical, or psychological realities for more living space. This is nothing new under the sun: ancient allegorists like Philo and Origen did it, when they taught that awkward-looking passages of the Hebrew scriptures must be understood as symbolic expressions of Platonic or Christian doctrines. So did modern theologians like Strauss and Bultmann, although for them truth was Hegel and Heidegger. While they may represent a small intellectual elite rather than the common believer, they still succeeded in laying the basis for the entire systems of medieval biblical interpretation and modern liberal Protestantism, respectively; not to mention the impact of those early Christian intellectuals who concluded that their Christ was not only a Jewish prince but also the Greek *logos*, the ruling principle of the universe, incarnate.

So, perhaps the psychoanalytic mystics, too, are up to something, when they ask if religious stories can carry psychological truth. It is with this question in mind that I will now turn to the Bible and its treatment of miracles and the supernatural.

THE FANTASTIC GOD

At first sight, it seems that Freud was right. The biblical God is fantastic in the fullest sense of the word. The awesome signs and wonders he displays promise the restoration of the original state of "primary narcissism": his loved ones will want no more. Their desire for protection, love, and worth will be satisfied. He has chosen them out of all the peoples on earth to be his people, his treasured possession. He will take them to a land flowing with milk and honey, and there they will eat their fill. Their friends will be blessed and their enemies will be cursed. Their souls will enjoy the calm and quiet of the weaned child (as in Ps 131:2).

Even in an utter catastrophe, the idealized image of God survives. The dominant interpretation of history in the Hebrew Bible is that the destruction of Jerusalem in the year 587 BCE was not a sign of God's failure, but it was God's premeditated punishment of his chosen people. That he failed to protect them was their own fault: they broke the covenant with him by worshipping idols and neglecting justice. This, of course, is a textbook example of securing a good object by means of creating a bad self-image. The object-relations theorist W.R.D. Fairbairn framed it in explicitly religious terms: "It is better to be a sinner in a world ruled by God than to live in a world ruled by the Devil" (Fairbairn 1943, 66).

Like Father, like Son: a successful healer and miracle-worker, Jesus has constant access to sources of nourishment and well-being. He encourages his followers to model themselves after little children, and he serves them like an ideal mother, indeed, so intensely that he has almost no room to move about or time to rest and eat. He neglects conventional social boundaries that would rather have satisfaction postponed: he will not wait until the Sabbath is over or his hands are clean to feed and heal people. Not surprisingly, people keep coming to him, while his enemies, the established religious authorities, become so jealous they could kill.

So, the infantile aspect is arguably there, even if the divine parental figure smacks more of a preoedipal, omnipresent mother than an idealized omnipotent father. The picture shows features of illusion: fantasy is incorporated in the representation of reality as God's presence breaks into history in an unparalleled way.

In their wider narrative context, the biblical miracles build up to *epiphany*. In the Exodus narrative, which establishes the covenant between God and Israel and is in many ways the heart of the Hebrew Bible, God's signs and wonders against Pharaoh make known to Israel his might. The revelation culminates in the apparitions on Mount Sinai and the giving of the Law. God descends on earth and speaks to Moses face to face.

Likewise, in the New Testament gospels, reports of signs, wonders, and fulfilled prophesies confirm that we are witnessing an epiphany: "we have seen his glory, the glory as of a father's unique son" (Jn 1:14). The miracle stories verify Jesus' true status: "these [signs] are written so that you may come to believe that Jesus is the Messiah, the Son of God" (Jn 20:31). The audience should take after the characters in the story, who, astounded at what they see, ask, "Who then is this?" (Mk 4:41), and conclude, "Truly this man was God's Son!" (Mt 27:54; Mk 15:39). Make no mistake: the savior became flesh and lived among us.

THE DISAPPEARING GOD

However, fantasy seems to be only one part of the story. Epiphany is not the end but a beginning. As both Jack Miles (1995) and Richard Elliot Friedman (1995) have pointed out, the Hebrew Bible tells the story of a disappearing God. The Almighty gradually leaves the earth and finds a new residence in heaven. Likewise, the Gospels are literature of renunciation: Jesus' followers need to accept that he must go away. The mythic Galilean spring is to be transformed into reality as we now have it, uncompromising and nonnegotiable. What results is a twofold coming-of-age story. On the one hand, God finds his proper place and role as a transcendent, otherworldly being. On the other hand, people are expected to cope with reality that involves frustration and suffering.

In the opening narratives of Genesis, God and humanity are simultaneously present in one space. It takes no special revelation to bring them together. Neither party has to leave its own reality to enter the reality of the other. In mythical Paradise, God's world and the world of the humans are truly one.

In the world of the patriarchs, too, God is still very much like a human character. He enters and leaves the stage, approaches people and engages in conversation with them without special notice, in a matter-of-fact style. No cloud of smoke is necessary, no extraordinary light phenomena, or burying your face between your knees. The coming of the God of Abraham, Isaac, and Jacob is no news, and if he needs people to know his will, he will tell them in person. It is only with Moses that changes crawl in. The God he meets is much more than ever before a *"mysterium tremendum,"* to quote Rudolph Otto's (1917) classic definition of the holy. The revelations of this God are mystical and exceptional, and no ordinary person may know what he truly looks like: "for no one shall see my face (glory) and live" (Ex 33:20).

The hidden God reveals himself by hiding, in a burning bush, in a pillar of cloud or a pillar of fire, inside the curtain of the tent of meeting, or on a cloud-covered mountaintop with thunder and lightning and a blast of a trumpet. Moses alone may know him, even though he cannot know God's essence, his full nature; so it is his lot to act as a mediator between God and his people.

Assisted by Moses, God makes the necessary preparations for his departure to heaven. He wants to make sure he will be remembered when he is gone, and he insists that each generation will be reminded of him:

> When your children ask you in time to come, "What is the meaning of the decrees and the statutes and the ordinances that the Lord our God has commanded you?" then you shall say to your children, "We were Pharaoh's slaves in Egypt, but the Lord brought us out of Egypt with a mighty hand. The Lord displayed before our eyes great and awesome signs and wonders against Egypt, against Pharaoh and all his household. He brought us out from there in order to bring us in, to give us the land that he promised on oath to our ancestors. Then the Lord commanded us to observe all these statutes, to fear the Lord our God, for our lasting good, so as to keep us alive, as is now the case. If we diligently observe this entire commandment before the Lord our God, as he has commanded us, we will be in the right. (Dt 6:20–25)

Israel's rescue from Egypt is something to remember. Yet it is the law that enables God to retire from service, when his people embark on a new life in the promised land. From now on the Law is the medium of God's presence. Its directions guide people to responsible living now that God himself is no more there to give personal advice. And indeed,

> Never since has there arisen a prophet in Israel like Moses, whom the Lord knew face to face. (Dt 34:10)

Once the Torah, the Law of Moses, established itself as the supreme authority of the Jewish religion, there was no way God could come back. The Talmud tells the story of a Rabbi Joshua, who refused to take into account a voice from heaven in a debate of the law (Bava Metziah 59b; see Visotzky 1991, 51–55, for an entertaining treatment of the story). The point he made was that the law "is not in heaven" (Dt 30:12). Since God has tasked his people to observe it, he has no right to intervene in its interpretation. Upon hearing Rabbi Joshua's words, God smiled and said, "My children have outwitted me."

According to traditional Jewish thinking, God's prophetic Spirit has left the world for good. In the time of the patriarchs, all righteous people had it. When the Israelites fell to idolatry and worshipped the golden calf, it was limited to few: prophets, high priests, and kings. With the death of the last writing prophets, Haggai, Zechariah, and Malachi, it was quenched alto-gether, due to the sins of the people. Since then, the best you could hope to hear was a remote echo of God's voice from heaven, a poor substitute, as the story of Rabbi Joshua so aptly illustrates (see Jeremias 1970, 80–82).

In the New Testament, however, the Spirit makes a flamboyant return. It descends like a dove from heaven on Jesus in his baptism. After all these years, God is here again, truly in the flesh, as John the evangelist is so keen to emphasize.

Yet he is not here to stay, not even this time. The Gospels are stories of bereavement, with the community of Jesus' followers in the leading role. The believers will need to grow stronger and more independent, so that they may survive after Jesus has returned to his Father in heaven. The original fantasy of God's all-encompassing presence must be transformed into a desire to-wards an absent God and an acceptance of reality.

The beginning of Jesus' career is a dream come true. The sick are healed, the crippled and maimed are made whole, the dead are raised, and the poor have good news brought to them. Jesus embodies the promise of absolute sat-isfaction: "Whoever comes to me will never be hungry, and whoever believes in me will never be thirsty" (Jn 6:35).

Soon it will turn out, however, that following Jesus is no key to happiness. The gate is narrow and the road is hard that leads to life (Mt 7:14). There is no resurrection without suffering and death. This is a difficult lesson for Jesus' disciples to learn, as they are quite fond of their original fantasy of un-limited personal wish-fulfillment. Although corrected by Jesus, the fantasy keeps returning, as fantasies do. The disciples argue with one another about who is the greatest (Mk 9:33–37; Lk 9:46–48) and pursue leading positions in the coming kingdom of God (Mt 20:20–28; Mk 10:35–45). This claim to power, comfort and security, however, is precisely what they need to abandon. Jesus' followers are not to lord it over other people, but rather to be slaves of all. This makes them vulnerable to persecution, suffering, and even death. Jesus himself is destined to suffer and to die at the hands of his enemies.

The news about the necessity of suffering traumatizes the disciples, and they will not take in the message. In the famous scene in Caesarea Philippi, Peter rebukes Jesus: "God forbid it, Lord! This must never happen to you!" (Mt 16:22). Yet the message keeps repeating itself, as traumas do: on the road to Jerusalem, Jesus predicts his passion and death three times.

The story that began as a clean-cut fantasy is gradually transformed into a story about the necessity of a loss. The disciples witness Jesus to be wounded and dying, to go away and turn into symbols. Feeding miracles will be replaced by the bread and wine of the Eucharist, and Jesus' care for his own survives in their own capacity to love: "Just as I have loved you, you also should love one another" (Jn 13:34). This is how life is going to be in God's absence, between the magnificent days of the past and the numinous future world to come. The illusion of fulfillment in the present gives way to a long-ing for what once was and for what has not yet arrived.

Jesus' ascension to heaven, where his Father has taken up residence al-ready, marks the end of a mythical era. All the fantastic things that were possible when he was here are now irrevocably things of the past. From now on, that time will be a lost golden age, a paradisiacal island in history, an ideal to which there is no access from our present and hopelessly imperfect world. Encased in the story of the mythic Galilean spring, the ideal survives along-side the reality that is now allowed to follow its own, natural rules.[3]

THE "GOOD-ENOUGH" GOD

So, there is a peculiar dialectics of infantile fantasy and mature realism running through the biblical narrative. The latter element culminates in God's gradual exit from this world on the one hand, and in his appearance in the form of a vulnerable human being on the other. The same God who at one point was prepared to take on reality and make all things well for his children is now encouraging them to bear with the toil and trouble of their earthly life. The good God, who would never fail to fill the needs of his little ones, turns out to be a good-enough God, who provides a secure framework for their acceptance of reality, very much like Winnicott thought a good-enough mother would do, another term he coined for psychoanalytic use.[4]

Yet the two elements do not make one coherent story of maturation and growth. In Winnicott's words, "the task of reality-acceptance is never com-pleted" (Winnicott 1951, 217). Instead of constant progress, there is a con-tinuing struggle between two conflicting interests, namely, the resolve of the heart to have what it desires, and the call of reality to be recognized in its full severity. As a result, God is inclined to return from heaven whenever the existing patterns of religious thought, such as apocalypticism or certain forms of charismatic Christianity, make it possible.

For the serpent-handling Pentecostals, the biblical reality of Mark 16:17–18 is fully intact even today, and their case is not as extraordinary as it may seem. What makes them exceptional is not so much the principle but the ex-treme way in which they put it to a test. It was never an option for Christians to turn back time and pretend that the return of the prophetic Spirit never happened. As promised by Jesus, the Holy Spirit came and took his place in the world, which enables the Christian churches to assert God's continuing presence in their midst. The more concretely they take it, the more relevant it makes any tension between the biblical (mythical) truth and the present (experiential) reality. What was possible then should be possible now as well. If this does not seem to be the case, which reality will yield?

Moreover, Jesus said he would come back, which brings in a further ele-ment of instability. Time and again apocalyptic movements seize the hope that his return is at hand; and the same happens to Jews who wait for the Messiah and to Muslims who wait for the Mahdi. Sometimes they even believe he has actually arrived, for example in the figure of some charismatic religious person. Although Jesus warns against this in the gospels (Mt 24:23–24; Mk 13:21–22; Lk 21:8), it is bound to happen over and over again. The idea of a divine revelation is a risky one: once God has proven his ability to appear to people, he is known to have that capacity, even if he was said to have retired for good. At the moment he first made himself known on earth, heavens were torn apart, and sealing them off again has turned out to be difficult.

Perhaps this is good: perhaps the realms of illusion and reality cannot and should not be kept too far apart. Fantasy, transitional phenomena, and idealized self-objects are believed to be vital for human health. Maybe the biblical fantasy would be too weak to fly, if it was strictly a thing of the mythical past or a mere dream in the distant future.

However, the higher the tension, the greater the risk. There is no return to the kind of supernaturalism that was characteristic of the biblical times. Faith in miracles cannot replace empirical science as the basis of medical treatment. That the end times are here is a feasible working assumption for a limited time only; after that, it becomes denial. If a person today tells us that Jesus is alive and well and calls her every day on a magic telephone, we probably should not speak of illusion at all but psychosis.

There is more at stake than the simple question of truth or self-deception. An essential feature of mature reality-acceptance is the ability to tolerate ambiguity, to accept that even the best of the things we hold dear can only be good-enough. As long as we live in this world, God will not be there to fill all our needs. If we cannot comply with this, the consequences can be grave. To protect an idealized image of an all-satisfying God, we need to repress any negative feelings we may have about our religious life. Typically, we will project them onto others, each onto his or her favorite enemy, or introject them back into ourselves, blaming ourselves for not being worthy of the good things we have. This kind of behavior is characteristic of religious extremists. The absolute perfection of their beliefs is something they will not contest. Whatever frustration it may make them feel, they transform that feeling into guilt, or develop paranoia to explain why they should feel worried.

THE COMPASSIONATE GOD

A key dynamic of early human development, the challenge of accepting reality, reemerges and intensifies in times of crises. Denial is a standard first response to a major personal loss, and acceptance is where a successful process of grief work is supposed to end.

The biblical storyline, of course, rambles from one major crisis to another. The expulsion from Paradise is no small loss, and the End of the World and the Last Judgment sound critical enough. Between these two cosmic mega-crises there are plenty of minor catastrophes: the Flood, the slavery in Egypt, the destruction of Jerusalem, the Babylonian Captivity, the scandal of Jesus' death, the failure of the Christian mission among the Jews, and Jesus' delayed return. At the individual level, too, the biblical characters go through tribulations that put their faith to a test. The patriarchs must leave home for an unknown destination. Jesus' followers are to leave house, wife, brothers, parents, and children for the sake of God's kingdom. The identity of the biblical God takes form through a series of crisis narratives. He is the one who hears cries for help, comes over, gives consolation, helps us through, restores hope, and encourages action.

But what sort of a counselor, or therapist, will a Savior God make? Will he lead people to acceptance, or is he rather encouraging futile, unrealistic hope? Drawing on Walter Brueggemann's work on the biblical psalm of lament (Brueggemann 1977), Donald Capps (1981) has made an informative structural comparison between the psalm of lament and the classic Kübler-Ross model of grief work (see Kübler-Ross 1969). The two have marked similarities. They both provide a structure for recovery from a personal or communal loss. They also allow expression of anger. However, whereas according to the Kübler-Ross model the fifth and final stage of grief is acceptance, the typical lament concludes with an assurance of God's help and a vow to praise him for what he has done on the suppliant's behalf. From the perspective of realism, this is the critical point. Not only do we receive the good at the hand of God, but also the bad. Does an over-optimistic reliance on divine intervention not border on denial?

On the other hand, there is a variant of the same lament form that involves a less simplistic position. In the books of Isaiah, Hosea, and Jeremiah, a new version of the lament emerges. In "The Lament of God" God himself bemoans the afflictions he must bring on his people due to their transgressions. This reversal of roles opens a view to yet another development in the characterization of the biblical God. The intervening God, who used to reward the faithful with oxen and sheep and slay the wicked with famine and plague, is joined by and gradually gives way to a compassionate God, a source of hope rather than retaliation. While the compassionate God will not necessarily step in and rescue his servant from "the arrow that flies by day or the pestilence that stalks in darkness" (as in Ps 91:5–6), he will pity the desolate and "weep with those who weep" (Rom 12:15b).

In the Christian grand narrative, the compassionate God goes so far as to empty himself of his divinity altogether, "taking the form of a slave, being born in human likeness" (Phil 2:7), to share human pain and vulnerability. It is true that he will later resume his power in full, "so that at the name of Jesus every knee should bend, in heaven and on earth and under the earth" (Phil 2:10); inside the compassionate Son of God, the not-so-compassionate apocalyptic Son of Man remains dormant, waiting for the appropriate moment to return. That moment, however, is now pushed far over the edge of the present reality, to the numinous world to come. Meanwhile, the compassionate God will be happy to make his sun rise on the evil and the good, and to send rain on the righteous and the unrighteous (Mt 5:45).

The compassionate God's long experience of humans seems to have refined his character. The trigger-happy world policeman has grown into a keen listener. The original promise of a timely and decisive intervention on behalf of the righteous has lost credibility, as injustice, unfairness, and misery abound in the world. At the same time, however, the claim that God understands what people go through and feels sympathy for them gains new weight. Great wonders are replaced with silent appreciation and assurance of worth: no matter how life may treat people, they are still of immense value to God, more so than sparrows, ravens, or lilies, which are not insignificant, either (cf. Mt 6:25–34; 10:29–31; Lk 12:6–7, 22–31).

In a sense, the compassionate God has paid the price of becoming more real. He is considerably smaller than the old intervening God was, and he has essentially left the business of miracles. Yet he has the advantage of being commensurate with the present reality and therefore not being rejected by it. He has grown to accept, for the time being, the reality he is said to have created, and reality is willing to tolerate him in return, as a matter of faith.

CONCLUSION

From a psychoanalytic point of view, the Bible displays not one but many strategies of coping (or not) with historical and existential crises. Judged on the grounds of whether they support reality-acceptance, some of these are healthier and more mature than others. Some of them seem primitive, while others have obviously taken some time to take form. They do not, however, represent successive stages of development but rather complementary positions. It is not unusual for them to coexist even if there are apparent contradictions between them.

It seems clear that the Bible contains fantasy, infantilism, and wishful thinking. Faith in miracles can become a way of rejecting reality and clinging to primary narcissism. On the other hand, there are biblical themes and traditions that, implicitly or explicitly, challenge infantile religious thinking as a barrier to spiritual growth. Both the Hebrew Bible and the Christian New Testament introduce the idea that God's direct involvement in reality increasingly belongs to the mythical past and to the eschatological future, whereas the present reality, between the biblical story time and the future *eschaton* (end time), is something with which people need to cope on their own. In Judaism, the supreme role of the law as the people's self-managed guide to life makes this particularly clear. In Christianity, the presence of the Holy Spirit in the world leaves more room for God to move in personally, yet the anticipated fruits of the spirit, self-restraint, ethical excellence, and concern for the well-being of others (see Gal 5:22–26), hardly count as narcissistic fantasy.

While Freud's rejection of religion became the dominant view in the psychoanalytic movement, many analysts today are tolerant or even appreciative towards religious beliefs and practices. However, their idea of religion as beneficial illusion has met with criticism, as it seems incompatible with the way most religious believers understand their faith. Yet it is hardly disconnected from contemporary (Western) religious experience. On the contrary, it seems to be linked to a general rise of interest in mysticism in its many forms: Zen Buddhist, Hindu, Jewish Cabbalistic, Christian Charismatic, Islamic Sufi.

It is not surprising that the mystical idea of God should have appeal among Western educated people, including, and especially, psychoanalysts. If traditional God-images, including the biblical portrayal(s) of God, are merely illusions hiding rather than revealing the true nature of the ineffable God, then there is no need to worry about their scientifically or morally questionable features. Besides, the evasive God of the mystics is so much like the treasured unconscious of the analysts (cf. Bomford 2006, 256): never to be exposed, he only appears "in the mirror, dimly" (1 Cor 13:12).

NOTES

1. This is the core idea expressed in Deuteronomist theology, which is suggested to have motivated the final redaction of the so-called Deuteronomic History Work (Dt, Joshua, Jud, 1–2 Sam, 1–2 Kg) in the Hebrew Bible. The theory of the Deuteronomic History Work and the ideology behind it originated with the publication of Martin Noth's *Überlieferungsgeschichtliche Studien* in 1943.

2. In his *Introduction to a Critique of the Hegelian Philosophy of Right, Karl Marx and Friedrich Engel's Collected Works*, Vol. 3, London: Lawrence and Wishard, 1987, p. 175, Karl Marx wrote, "Religion is the sign of the oppressed creature, the feelings of a heartless world, just as it is the spirit of unspiritual conditions. It is the opium of the people."

3. The emphasis on Jesus's ministry as a bygone golden age when things were different from now—not only in terms of supernatural influence, but also as it comes to the social radicalism of the early Jesus movement as opposed to the more bourgeois lifestyle of the later church—is particularly characteristic of Luke (see Robinson 1986, 108–109; Robinson is here building on Hans Conzelmann's classic work, *Die Mitte der Zeit* [1954]).

4. See also Brooke Hopkins's Winnicottian account of the story of Jesus (Hopkins 1989). In Hopkins's interpretation, based on Winnicott's concept of object usage, Jesus' survival of human wickedness into a new, eternal life in resurrection corresponds to the baby's experience that the mother survives the "ruthless" way the baby uses her as an object for his own pleasure. The growing sense of the durability of the mother as a love-object leads the baby to understand that she is a real other who

exists independently of the baby's inner feelings and sensations. A similar sense of the durability of the other is essential in all our love-relationships—and finds an illustration in what Hopkins calls "the resurrection myth."

REFERENCES

Berger, P. L., ed. (1999), *The Desecularization of the World: Resurgent Religion and World Politics*, Washington, DC: Ethics and Public Policy Center.

Black, D. M. (2006), Introduction, in *Psychoanalysis and Religion in the 21st Century: Competitors or Collaborators?* D. M. Black, ed., 1–20, The New Library of Psychoanalysis, London and New York: Routledge,.

Black, D. M., ed. (2006), *Psychoanalysis and Religion in the 21st Century: Competitors or Collaborators?* The New Library of Psychoanalysis, London and New York: Routledge. Published in association with The Institute of Psychoanalysis, London, England.

Blass, R. B. (2006), Beyond Illusion: Psychoanalysis and the Question of Religious Truth, in *Psychoanalysis and Religion in the 21st Century: Competitors or Collaborators?* D. M. Black, ed., 23–43, The New Library of Psychoanalysis, London and New York: Routledge.

Bomford, R. (2006), A Simple Question? in *Psychoanalysis and Religion in the 21st Century: Competitors or Collaborators?* D. M. Black, ed., 252–69, The New Library of Psychoanalysis, London and New York: Routledge.

Brueggemann, Walter (1977), The Formfulness of Grief, *Interpretation* 31, 263–75.

Bultmann, Rudolph (1933–65), *Glauben und Verstehen: Gesammelte Aufsätze*, Vols. 1–4. Tübingen: Mohr. Reprinted in 1954, 1968, 1960, 1975, Tubingen: Mohr-Siebeck.

Capps, Donald (1981), *Biblical Approaches to Pastoral Counseling*, Philadelphia: Westminster.

Conzelmann, Hans (1954), *Die Mitte der Zeit: Studien zur Theologie des Lukas, Beiträge zur historischen Theologie (BHT)* 17. Tübingen: Mohr Siebeck.

Fairbairn, W.R.D. (1943), Repression and the Return of Bad Objects, in W.R.D. Fairbairn, *Psychoanalytic Studies of the Personality*, 59–81, London: Tavistock. Republished in 1952, London: Tavistock.

Freud, Sigmund (1927), *The Future of an Illusion, The Standard Edition of the Complete Psychological Works of Sigmund Freud*, J. Strachey, ed. and trans., Vol. 21, 1–56, London: The Hogarth Press and The Institute of Psychoanalysis. Reprinted by publisher in 1961.

Freud, Sigmund (1930), *Civilization and Its Discontents, The Standard Edition of the Complete Psychological Works of Sigmund Freud*, J. Strachey, ed. and trans., Vol. 21, 57–145. London: The Hogarth Press and The Institute of Psychoanalysis. Reprinted by publisher in 1961.

Friedman, R. E. (1995), *The Hidden Face of God*, New York: HarperCollins.

Frosh, S. (2006), Psychoanalysis and Judaism in his *Psychoanalysis and Religion in the 21st Century: Competitors or Collaborators?*, D. M. Black, ed., 205–22, London and New York: Routledge.

Hood, Ralph W., Jr. (1997), Psychoanalysis and Fundamentalism: A Lesson from Feminist Critiques of Freud, in *Religion, Society, and Psychoanalysis: Readings in*

Contemporary Theory, J. L. Jacobs and Donald Capps, eds., 42–67, Boulder: Westview Press.

Hopkins, B. (1989), Jesus and Object Use: A Winnicottian Account of the Resurrection Myth, in *Freud and Freudians on Religion: A Reader*, Donald Capps, ed., 230–40, New Haven and London: Yale University Press. Reprinted by publishers in 2001.

Humphreys, C. J. (2003), *The Miracles of Exodus: A Scientist's Discovery of the Extraordinary Natural Causes of the Biblical Stories*, London and New York: Continuum.

Jeremias, Joachim (1970), *New Testament Theology, The Proclamation of Jesus*, J. Bowden, trans., London: SCM Press. Republished in 1971, New York: Charles Scribner's Sons.

Jones, J. W. (2002), *Terror and Transformation: The Ambiguity of Religion in Psychoanalytic Perspective*, Hove: Brunner-Routledge.

Kohut, Heinz (1971), *The Analysis of the Self: A Systematic Approach to the Psychoanalytic Treatment of Narcissistic Personality Disorders, The Psychoanalytic Study of the Child Monograph Series* 4, New York: International Universities Press.

Kohut, Heinz (1984), *How Does Analysis Cure?* Chicago: University of Chicago Press.

Kübler-Ross, Elizabeth (1969), *On Death and Dying*, New York: Macmillan.

Küng, Hans (1974), *On Being a Christian*, E. Quinn, trans., New York: Image Books. Reprinted by publisher in 1984.

Marx, Karl (1970), *Critique of Hegel's Philosophy of Right*, A. Jolin and J. O'Malley, trans., *Cambridge Studies in the History and Theory of Politics*, Cambridge: Cambridge University Press. Originally published (1887), *Critique of the Hegelian Philosophy of Right, Karl Marx and Frederick Engels Collected Works*, Vol. 3, London: Lawrence and Wishard.

Meissner, W. W. (1984), *Psychoanalysis and Religious Experience*, New Haven and London: Yale University Press.

Miles, Jack (1995), *God: A Biography*, New York: Alfred A. Knopf.

Noth, Martin (1943), *Überlieferungsgeschichtliche Studien*, Halle (Saale): Max Niemeyer Verlag.

Ostow, M. (1982), *Judaism and Psychoanalysis*, New York: KTAV.

Otto, Rudolph (1917), *The Idea of the Holy: An Inquiry into the Non-Rational Factor in the Idea of the Divine and Its Relation to the Rational*, J. W. Harvey, trans., London: Oxford University Press. Republished by Oxford University Press in 1990.

Paulus, H.E.G. (1828), *Das Leben Jesu als Grundlage einer reinen Geschichte des Urchristentums*, 2 volumes, Heidelberg: C. F. Winter.

Robinson, James M. (1986), Gospels as Narrative, in *The Bible and the Narrative Tradition*, F. McConnell, ed., 97–112, New York and Oxford: Oxford University Press.

Rubin, J. R. (2006), Psychoanalysis and Spirituality, in *Psychoanalysis and Religion in the 21st Century: Competitors or Collaborators?* D. M. Black, ed., 132–53, London and New York: Routledge.

Schweitzer, Albert (1906), *Geschichte der Leben-Jesu-Forschung*, Tübingen: Mohr-Siebeck. Reprinted in 1951.

Smalley, B. (1952), *The Study of the Bible in the Middle Ages*, Oxford: Blackwell.

Strauss, David F. (1835–1836), *Das Leben Jesu kritisch bearbeitet 1–2*, Tübingen: C. F. Osiander.

Symington, N. (1993), Is Psychoanalysis a Religion? in *Is Psychoanalysis Another Religion: Contemporary Essays on Spirit, Faith and Morality in Psychoanalysis*, I. Ward, ed., 49–56, London: Freud Museum.

Symington, N. (2006), Religion: The Guarantor of Civilization, in *Psychoanalysis and Religion in the 21st Century: Competitors or Collaborators?* D. M. Black, ed., 191–201, London and New York: Routledge.

Theissen, Gerd, and A. Merz (1996), *The Historical Jesus: A Comprehensive Guide*, J. Bowden, trans., London: SCM Press. Reissued by the publisher in 1998.

Visotzky, B. L. (1991), *Reading the Book: Making the Bible a Timeless Text*, New York: Schocken Books, 1996.

Winnicott, David W. (1951), Transitional Objects and Transitional Phenomena, in *Freud and Freudians on Religion: A Reader*, Donald Capps, ed., 211–19, New Haven and London: Yale University Press. Reissued by the publisher in 2001.

Winnicott, David W. (1971), *Playing and Reality*, London: Tavistock.

Wright, K. (2006), Preverbial Experience and the Intuition of the Sacred, in *Psychoanalysis and Religion in the 21st Century: Competitors or Collaborators?* D. M. Black, ed., 173–90, London and New York: Routledge.

CHAPTER 3

Jesus and Miracles in Historical, Biblical, and Psychological Perspective

Wayne G. Rollins

Thomas Jefferson was a Deist who believed that Jesus was a great moral thinker—rather like Jefferson himself, only better. He assembled his own version of the Gospels, slicing out everything miraculous with a razor.

—*Richard Brookhiser*

A miracle is the violation of mathematical, divine, immutable, eternal laws. By this very statement, a miracle is a contradiction in terms. A law cannot be immutable and violable at the same time. . . . God cannot do anything without reason; so what reason could make him temporarily disfigure his own handiwork?

—*Voltaire*

Miracles are not contrary to nature, but only contrary to what we know about nature.

—*Augustine*

There are only two ways to live your life. One is as though nothing is a miracle. The other is as if everything is.

—*Dan Wakefield*

When Thomas Jefferson deleted everything miraculous from his version of the Gospels, he might have exercised more caution had he realized that the word *miracle,* as he understood it, does not appear in the original Greek or Hebrew. For him, and Voltaire, the word *miracle* denoted a violation of eternal, immutable laws of nature and nature's God. Augustine, in the fourth century, had already dented the armor of that conception with his observation that miracles are not violations of natural law, but violations of what we know of natural law. Biblical authors would agree. When biblical authors write of a miraculous event like Jesus walking on water, the healing of a blind man, or the descent of manna from heaven, they use language that expresses the meaning implied in the original meaning of the Latin word *miraculum*, derived from the root, *mira*—wonder and awe.

In his book, *Healing in the New Testament: Insights from Medical and Mediterranean Anthropology*, John J. Pilch (2000), a New Testament scholar with expertise in medical anthropology, argues that in approaching stories of healing, miracles, and cures, in cultures far removed from our own, one must adopt a cross-cultural approach that acknowledges the difference between *emic* and *etic* perspectives. Pilch writes:

> Generally speaking, *emic* is the native view, the perspective from within any system under study, the insiders' views. The *emic* view includes the shared ideology and perceptions of phenomena by members of a given society. Thus, natives in Matthew's community apparently recognized an illness that they called moonstruck (Mt 4.24; 17.15). This is the *emic* perspective. English translators routinely render this as epileptic, representing the translator's *etic* perspective. Both perspectives are an integral part of the discipline of cross-cultural studies. (Pilch 2000, 153; italics added)

Our purpose in this chapter is to examine the New Testament miracle stories in historical, biblical, and psychological perspective: (1) the historical perspective, aimed at *emic* assessment, describes the environment of miracles, healings, and healers commonplace in the Greco-Roman and Judaic worlds of the Gospels; (2) the biblical perspective, aimed also at *emic* assessment, refers to appreciation of the different types of miracle stories in the biblical text, the language used to speak of miracles, what biblical writers were attempting to communicate with these stories, and how these stories would have functioned in the mind of a first-century audience in the nascent Judaeo-Christian cultus; and (3) the psychological perspective, returning to a contemporary *etic* view, will examine analogues to the miracles of Jesus in twentieth and twenty-first century perspective.

THE HISTORICAL PERSPECTIVE

Howard Clark Kee reminds us in his 1986 book, *Medicine, Miracle, and Magic in New Testament Times*, that the healing techniques of medicine, miracle, and magic are not unique to the New Testament. They are indigenous to human society. In fact, their appearance in the New Testament is fundamentally a function of their ubiquitous presence in first-century Greco-Roman and Jewish culture. Kee provides a thumbnail sketch of the differences among the three:

Medicine is a method of diagnosis of human ailments and prescription for them based on a combination of theory about and observation of the body, its functions and malfunctions. Miracle embodies the claim that healing can be accomplished through appeal to, and subsequent action by the gods, either directly or through a chosen intermediary agent. Magic is a technique, through word or act, by which a desired end is achieved, whether that end lies in the solution to the seeker's problem or in damage to the enemy who has caused the problem. (Kee 1986, 3)

The difference in the three forms of healing are evident in the three theories concerning the cause and cure of illness. "These include the theory that human difficulties are the work of demons, for which exorcism is the appropriate cure; or that they are the results of a magical curse, for which counter-magic must be invoked; or that they are functional disorders of the body, which call for medical diagnosis and a prescribed remedy" (Kee 3–4).

Surprisingly, medicine, as opposed to miracles and magic, was not the healing agency of preference for many. Pliny the Elder (23–79 CE) in his *Natural History* voices a suspicion about physicians, shared by many. He denigrates the growing numbers of physicians whose healing protocol has displaced the authentic, tried and true folk remedies found "in the kitchen garden," where herbal remedies provided a fitting cure for every ailment known to human or animal (26.21.5; Kee 1986, 5–7). Pliny expresses disgust over the fortunes these charlatan physicians have accrued with their excessive charges, concocted procedures, and diagnoses. He cites a particularly odious example in a certain Asclepiades, who had turned to medicine only after failing to earn a decent living as a rhetorician (Kee, 5). Pliny does concede the excellence of the medical standards laid down by the great physician, Hippocrates (460–350 BCE), but adds to his list of complaints the tendency of physicians to attribute their healings to the work of the gods in order to "lend an aura of sanctity to their enterprise" (Kee, 6).

A hint of this same disdain for physicians is captured in Mark's Gospel, telling of a woman who comes to Jesus with a 12-year history of a "flow of blood." Mark tells us she "had suffered much under many physicians, and had spent all that she had, and was no better but rather grew worse" (Mk 5:26).

THE GRECO-ROMAN CONTEXT

Though various routes to healing were available in the Empire, often vending on the same street, the most admired and popularly sought after were the shrines and temples associated with the Egyptian deity Isis and the Greek god Asclepius, whose sanctuaries were havens for the ill, fountains of healing.

By the first century, the cult of Isis had spread to Rome, the British Isles, the Eastern Mediterranean, and Western Europe. The most common mode of cure was incubation, sleeping in the temple precinct. Diodorus Siculus describes the setting. A supplicant, often disappointed with physicians, spent the night awaiting a healing dream.

> Standing above the sick in their sleep she [Isis] gives aid for their diseases and works remarkable cures upon such as submit themselves to her; and many who have been despaired of by their physicians because of the difficult nature of their malady are restored to health by her, while numbers who have altogether lost the use of their eyes or of some other part of the body, whenever they turn for help to this goddess are restored to their previous condition. (Diodorus Siculus, *Library of History*, 1.25.5; Kee 1986, 68)

A second source of healing, also known across the Empire, was Asclepius (Latin: Aesculapius) whose primary shrine was at Epidaurus in the Peloponnesus in Greece. As with Isis, the many shrines and temples were the equivalent of hospitals. They consisted of large halls for the sick to recline, rest, and await the powers of healing to work during their sleep. The shrine at Epidaurus was known for its dogs and snakes that would quietly visit the incubants sleeping on the temple grounds, licking the wounded part of the body. The ailments listed in the testimonies at Epidaurus include "facial and mouth injuries, dumbness, kidney and gall stones, extended pregnancies, leeches, baldness, dropsy, tumors, lice, worms, headaches, tuberculosis, disfigured limbs, wounds from weapons and blindness" (Kee 1986, 70). Cripples were reported to walk again; mutes regained speech; the blind recovered sight. Testimonial symbols of cured parts, sometimes wrought in silver and gold, were exhibited in the shrine of Epidaurus as Pausanias (II.xxvii.3) and Strabo (VIII.374) attest (McCasland 1962, 400; Lohse 1976, 226–27).

In addition to the care and cure associated with the shrines of Isis and Asclepius, Asia Minor produced one of the most widely recounted healers in the first century, Apollonius of Tyana, an itinerant philosopher who healed the sick and exorcised the demonized. His story was recorded in mid-third century by Philostratus under the patronage of Julia, the wife of the Emperor Septimius. In fact, it is speculated that the publication of the *Life of Apollonius* may have been supported by imperial Rome in order to counter the growing popular interest in the Christian cultus and the healing it offered.

As an indication of the popular image of healers, Apollonius is reported to have had the gift of understanding a foreign language without studying it, and of telepathic ability to see events far removed in time or space from the present. He is said to have cured a boy bitten by a dog and to have exorcised the daughter of a woman who was demonized by the ghost of the woman's husband, who had become outraged over her having remarried so quickly after his death (Kee 1986, 84–86). On one occasion Apollonius, lecturing in Athens, was interrupted by a young man, known for a dissolute life, who broke out in boisterous laughter. Apollonius announced to the man that he was possessed of an evil spirit. Philostratus tells us:

> He actually was possessed, without being aware of it. He laughed when no one else laughed, wept without cause, and sang and talked to himself. The people thought that his licentious youth was to blame for this, but the truth is that he was being guided by an evil demon, and he appeared, in his impiety, as drunken. Now when Apollonius looked at him still more steadily and wrathfully, the demon cried out, like a person who is being branded or otherwise tortured, and swore that he would leave the youth and never again attack a man. But when Apollonius angrily addressed him, as an angry master might address a shamelessly wicked servant, and commanded him to come forth visibly, he cried, "I will throw down yonder statue," and pointed to a statue in the king's portico. Then the statue started moving and fell over. What fear and wonder! Who could describe it all! But the young man rubbed his eyes like someone just awakening, looked toward the sun, and was embarrassed because all eyes turned toward him. From that time on he no longer appeared wild and unrestrained as previously, but his healthy nature appeared, as though he had been treated by medicines. (Philostratus, *Life of Apollonius* IV.20; Lohse 1976, 227–28)

Healing stories were also told of prominent figures with special powers, in this instance, with a parallel to the Gospel stories. In his history of the emperor Vespasian, Suetonius reports the emperor's trip to Alexandria shortly after he was instated, only to be asked to moisten the eyes of a blind beggar with his saliva, and to touch the leg of a lame man with his heel, resulting in the cure of both (Suetonius' *Vespasian*, vii; Lohse 1976, 227; see Jesus' use of spittle in Mk 8:23; Jn 9:6).

THE JUDAIC CONTEXT

Though Judaism in the first century lacked the shrines associated with Isis and Asclepius, its sacred literature and popular memory were awash in miraculous events associated with prominent Old Testament figures: Moses, Aaron, Joshua, Elijah, and Elisha. Moses had precipitated a path through the Red Sea (Ex 14:21–25), brought forth water from a rock (Ex 17:1–7), set up a healing bronze serpent in the wilderness (Nm 21:9), and competed magically with the wise men and sorcerers in Pharaoh's court (Ex 7:8–13). Joshua had made the sun stand still (Jo 10:12–14). Jonah survived three days in a "whale" (Jon 1:17). Elijah had raised a youngster from the dead (1 Kgs 17:17–24), saved a widow and her son from starvation with a self-refilling jar of meal and cruse of oil (1 Kgs 17: 8–16), and had ascended to heaven in a fiery chariot (2 Kgs 2:11). Elisha had caused an axe-head to float on water (2 Kgs 6:5–7), had resuscitated the Shunammite's deceased son (2 Kgs

4:11–37), and had cured a Syrian king of leprosy (2 Kgs 5:1–14). Shadrach, Meschach, and Abednego had been delivered from the fiery furnace, and Sarah, Rachel, and Hannah had been cured of their barrenness. The biblical miracle stories had even been expanded in the Dead Sea Scrolls in the Genesis Apocryphon from Qumran Cave 1, which reports Abram engaged in laying on of hands and prayer to cure a Pharaoh of an affliction caused by an evil spirit (Fitzmyer 1991, 60).

Beyond first-century Judaic consciousness of the miraculous past, is an active tradition of healers, miracle workers, and exorcists. The New Testament, in fact, makes reference to the commonplace reality of exorcism in first-century Judaism (Mt 12:27).

Within Judaism, stories were told of miraculous cures and events associated with individuals whose virtue produced special powers. Some of the tales bear resemblance to Gospel stories in the New Testament. The *Babylonian Talmud* recounts a seafaring tale reminiscent of the calming of the storm in Mark 4:35–41. The key figure is Rabban Gamaliel II, a scholar-teacher, who found himself aboard ship when the storm struck. Fearing that it was punishment for his collaboration with an opposing rabbi, Eliezer b. Hyrcanus, with whom he should never have in good conscience collaborated, Gamaliel turned to God in prayer, explaining that his collaboration was motivated not by pride but by his desire for harmony in Israel. We are told that when the prayer was completed, the sea calmed (*Babylonian Talmud*, Baba Mezia 59b. See Lohse 1976, 179).

Exorcisms were also known in the Judaic tradition, as noted by Josephus, who recounts the expulsion of a demon in the Emperor Vespasian's presence by a certain Eleazar.

He [Eleazar] held under the nose of the possessed man a ring in which was enclosed a root. . . . He had the sick man smell it, and thus drew the evil spirit of him through his nose. The possessed man immediately collapsed, and Eleazar then adjured the spirit, by pronouncing the name of Solomon . . . [commanding the spirit] never to return to the man. (Josephus, *Jewish Antiquities* VIII 46–49)

In the postlude, Eleazar, whose exorcism leaves some in doubt, performs another wonder to prove his power over the spirit. He sets up a vessel filled with water and commands the spirit when it leaves the possessed man to upset the vessel, in order to demonstrate to the gathering that it had really left. Josephus tells us, "This in fact happened and thus Solomon's wisdom and knowledge became known" (Lohse 1976, 180).

Two figures stand out in Talmudic and Mishnaic literature as models of charismatic Hasidim, devout men with remarkable powers, who stood in the tradition of Elijah, whose prophetic powers could cause rain (1 Kgs 17:1). In their piety, their prayer, their confidence in the Almighty, their seemingly miraculous powers, and their lives of renunciation, they bear resemblance to certain aspects of Gospel records about Jesus. Both "were venerated as a holy Hasid so close to God that his prayer exhibited miraculous efficiency" (Vermes 2001, 254).

The first is a rabbi from the first century BCE, named Honi the Circle Maker, who was famous for the power of his prayer to bring much-needed rain to his people. Mishnah Taanit 3:8 relates the story:

> Once Honi the Circle-Drawer was asked: "Pray that it may rain." He answered "Go and bring in the Passover ovens [made of dried clay] that they may not become soft." He prayed but it did not rain. What did he do? He drew a circle and stood in it and said to God, "Lord of the world, Thy children have turned to me because I am like a son of the house before Thee. I swear by Thy great name that I will not move from here until Thou hast mercy on Thy children." Drops of rain fell. "I have not asked for this," he said, "but for rain to fill the cisterns, the pits and rock-cavities." There came a cloud-burst. "I have not prayed for this but for a rain of goodwill, blessing and grace." Then it rained steadily until the Israelites were compelled to flee from Jerusalem to the Temple Mount. (Vermes, 255)

Josephus tells us of the circumstances of Honi's death, following the pattern of a prophet. He was stoned to death by Hyrcanus II when he refused to collaborate in Hyrcanus' plot to depose Hyracanus' brother, the high priest, Aristobulus II.

The second is a first-century CE figure, a rabbinic counterpart to Jesus, who lived in the first half of the first century. He was a Galilean rabbi named Hanina ben Dosa. He was born a dozen miles north of the city of Nazareth, and became a pupil of Johanan ben Zakkai, one of the founders of rabbinic Judaism. Rabbi ben Dosa was portrayed in the Mishnah as a saintly man with thaumaturgic powers, whose personal life was marked by humility, unworldliness, and stoic frugality (Vermes, 259–63). One story relates how his prayers led to the cure of one of ben Zakkai's sons. Another healing was telepathic, taking place at a distance, with the healing of the son of the patriarch Gamaliel II. Though far from the lad, Hanina ben Dosa assured Gamaliel that his son had been cured, a fact attested to subsequently by Gamaliel's servants. Popular lore also recounts his ability to make the rain cease and to endow common vinegar that had mistakenly been poured into a lamp with the properties of lamp oil that burned all the next day (Yarushalmi Berakot v. 9d).

The story is also told of a lizard biting ben Dosa. He was so engrossed in his prayers he barely noticed. The Mishna Berakhot 5.1 had dictated that if a man is at prayer, even a snake wound around his leg should not deter him. When Hanina ben Dosa's disciples expressed concern, they found the lizard dead, leading to the rumor that animals biting ben Dosa did so at their peril. "Woe to the man whom a lizard bites, and woe to the lizard that bites R. Hanina ben Dosa!" (Yarushalmi Berakot v. 9a).

Geza Vermes proposes that Hanina ben Dosa was rabbinic Judaism's most prominent wonder-worker whose death marked the end of the era of the "men of deeds." Jesus of Nazareth, he observes, "as healer and exorcist . . . is perfectly at home in Hasidic company" (Mishna Sotah 9.15; Vermes, 258, 269).

THE BIBLICAL PERSPECTIVE

Howard Clark Kee concludes in his 1986 book, *Medicine, Miracle and Magic in the New Testament*, that healing is "a central factor in primitive Christianity, and was so from the beginning of the movement. It is not a later addendum to the tradition, introduced in order to make Jesus more appealing to the Hellenistic world, but was a major feature of the Jesus tradition from the outset" (Kee 1986, 124). That it was true of Jesus is affirmed by the fact that all Gospel sources (Mk, Mt, Lk, Q, and Jn) attest to the miraculous as a prominent feature of his ministry.

Our goal in this section is to adopt an *emic* approach (Pilch 2000, 153) in examining the New Testament healing stories of Jesus, which seeks to examine healing and the miraculous from the perspective of the original New Testament audience. We will examine (1) the terminology and protological thinking employed to describe these so-called miraculous events, (2) the four types of miracle stories (healings, exorcisms, resuscitations, and nature miracles), and (3) the rhetorical function of the miracles stories within the earliest Christian communities.

TERMINOLOGY AND PROTOLOGICAL THINKING

The Greek of the New Testament uses six words to refer to miraculous events, none of which means miracle in the sense Thomas Jefferson or Voltaire understood it, namely as violation of natural law. One is the word *ergon* (a word), connoting something produced with remarkable effect. A second is *paradoxa* (Lk 5:26), a counter-intuitive, inexplicable happening. The third is *dynamis* (power), an event that has achieved a powerful outcome. Fourth is *thaumasia*,wonders or marvels (Mt 21:15), the rough equivalent of the Latin *miraculum*, having nothing to do with the notion of a violation of natural law. Fifth and sixth are a recurring word combination rooted in its matching pair in the Old Testament, translated "signs (*semeia*) and wonders (*terata*)," appearing frequently in Hebrew as *'ôt* and *môpet*, as for example in the Exodus saga (Ex 7:3, Dt 4:34), referring to events that signify something beyond themselves.

It is important to recognize that in describing these events, the Gospel authors and their communities resort to protological or primary thinking, native to their time. For example they attribute illness to demons or diagnose an epileptic as being moonstruck (Mt 17:14; Fitzmyer 1991, 59). Protological thinking is at work in the description of techniques Jesus uses to heal, putting his finger in the ear of a deaf man with a speech impediment, then spitting and touching his tongue (Mk 7:33–34), or by spitting on the eyes of a blind man and laying his hands upon him (Mk 8:23), or by uttering an Aramaic word, *Ephphatha* (be opened) (Mk 7:34), echoing the magical-sounding Hebrew incantations of Jewish healers of the period.[1] Jesus' healings can be effected with a touch (Mk 1:31; Lk 5:12–25; Lk 13:11–13; Mt 9:27–30), or by seeming telepathy, at a distance, as with a centurion's slave (Mt 8:5–13), the daughter of the Syrophoenician woman (Mt 15:22–28), and the royal official's son (Jn 4:46–54). On occasion the Gospel authors add folkloric additions to the stories, for example, reporting a demonized herd of pigs jumping over a cliff into the sea in a locale (Gadara) more than five miles from the water (Fitzmyer 1991, 58).

FOUR TYPES OF MIRACLE STORIES

The gospel records cite four types of miracle stories: healings, exorcisms, resuscitations, and nature miracles.

Healing stories, along with exorcism, constitute one-fifth of all the stories about Jesus in the synoptic Gospels (Kee 1986, 1). In an unusual scene, when John the Baptist sends his disciples to inquire of Jesus whether he is "the one to come or whether they should look for another," Jesus replies in a way that suggests he regards what he is about to share as the most distinctive aspect of his ministry: "Go tell John what you have seen and heard: the blind receive their sight, the lame walk, lepers are cleansed, and the deaf hear, and the dead are raised up, the poor have good news preached to them with" (Lk 7:22).

A glossary of Jesus' healings in the Gospels include a demonized madman from Gadara (Mk 5:1–20), a paralytic (Mk 2:1–12), a man with a "withered" hand (Mt 12:9–13), a woman bent over for 18 years (Lk 13:10–13), a woman with an issue of blood for 12 years, who had spent her fortune on physicians to no avail (Mk 5:25–34), Peter's fevered mother-in-law (Mk 1:30–31), an official's son near death with a fever (Jn 4:47–53), the blind beggar, Bartimaeus (Mk 10:46–52), a man with dropsy (Lk 14:1–4), and a young boy with epileptic convulsions (Mk 9:14–29).

Exegetical study of the Gospel accounts of the healing stories makes plain that for the Gospel authors, the main point of a miracle story is not the miracle itself, but the truth(s) to which it points. Two examples will suffice.

A first example is an opening scene in Mark's gospel (1:21–27), that describes Jesus confronting a man with an "unclean spirit" in the synagogue at

Capernaum. When Jesus commands the demon "to come out of him," Mark tell us that the onlookers respond with the words, "What is this? A new teaching! With authority he commands even the unclean spirits." A Christological leitmotif of Mark's Gospel is Jesus' authority (*exousia*). Chapter after chapter, Mark's objective is to spell out the authority of Jesus—over demoniacs, over tax collectors and sinners who had been excluded by the ritual requirements of the law, over the sea, over disease, over ritual traditions of the Pharisees, over nature, and eventually over the temple, symbolized with the rending of the temple veil.

A second example is the tale of Jesus healing a man with a withered hand (Mk 3:1–6). The telling point of the story is not the cure itself, but that it took place on the Sabbath, challenging a law that prefers compliance to mercy, and introducing a new teaching that "the Sabbath was made for man, not man for the Sabbath" (Mk 2:27–28).

The healings and exorcisms exercise a religious-subversive function within the storytelling tradition of early Christianity, portraying Jesus' acts of healing as acts of protest against the policies and practice of the first-century cultus. Jesus heals on the Sabbath, contrary to religious law (Mk 3:1–6); he assumes the prerogative of the religious hierarchy by forgiving the sin he construed to be the cause of an illness (Mk 2:1–12); he healed the religiously marginalized—tax-collectors (Lk 19:1–10), a Greek, a Syrophoenician woman (Mk 7:24–30), a demonized man from Gerasa who lived in the ritually unclean haunts of a pagan cemetery (Mk 5:1–20), a leper, regarded as ritually unclean (Mark 1:40–45), and a ritually unclean menstruating woman (Mk 5:25–34; Kee 1986, 78–79).

Exorcism is rooted in the sociocultural conviction that illness is caused by demons and is played out in socially conventional patterns of demoniac behavior. Demon-possession and exorcism were standard features of first-century Palestinian, biblical, and Greco-Roman culture.

The New Testament mentions demons 90 times, sometimes referring to them as unclean spirits (Mk 3:30) or evil spirits (Lk 7:21). The lords of the demons are also mentioned, Beelzebul (Mt. 16:24) and Satan (Mk 3:23). Luke, both in his Gospel and in Acts, assumes the presence of demons and spirits as a feature of everyday life (e.g., Lk 8:2; 13:16; 22:3; Acts 16:16–18).

The Gospels never imply that Jesus alone had the power to exorcise. It was a widely practiced art. The Gospels imply that Jesus acknowledges exorcists among his rivals: Jesus tells them, "If I cast out demons by Beelzebul, by whom do your sons cast them out?" We sometimes hear of itinerant exorcists casting out demons in the name of Jesus (Mt 7:22; Acts 19:13–14).

The Gospels indicate that Jesus' religious rivals acknowledged that he was competent as an exorcist (Mk 3:22). It is also clear that he trained and commissioned his disciples in the art of exorcism (Mt 10:8; Mk 3:15; 6:13).

When the disciples are sent out on mission, they return glowing: "Lord, even the demons are subject to us in your name" (Lk 10:17).

Demons are widely acknowledged in the culture at large. The Dead Sea Qumran covenanters had composed hymns against the demons with psalms of exorcism and antidemonic incantations (Martinez 1994, 371–78). In the Magical Greek Papyri we read of encounters between the demon-possessed and exorcists in language that resembles verbal exchanges between demoniacs and healers in the Gospels. Mark 1:24 reads, "I know who you are." The Papyri Graeca Magicae VIII.13 reads, "I know you, Hermes, who you are and whence you came." In Mark 5:7 we hear, "I adjure you by God." The Papyri Graecae Magicae XXXvi.189–90 reads, "I adjure you by the great name Ablanatha."

What meaning did the first Christians find in these stories of exorcism? A key is found in Luke's report of a statement of Jesus: "If it is by the finger of God that I cast out demons, then the kingdom of God has come upon you" (Lk 11:19–20). For a first-century Gospel audience the stories of Jesus' authority over demons, and therefore over disease, represented the collapse and unseating of the demonic powers, a theme that will be played out on a much larger screen with the writing of the Book of Revelation during the persecution in the reign of Domitian, 81–96 CE. This same eschatological image of the dispossessing of the demonic is a theme in the Dead Sea Scrolls (1QS 3:24–25; 4:200–22; 1 QH 3:18; 1 QM 1:10–11). Thus, exorcism connotes personal healing but also a corporate social healing in which the oppressive power of principalities and powers are in the process of being brought down.

The incipient collapse of the demonic world powers may be hinted in Mark's elaborate version of the story of the Gadarene demoniac (Mk 5:1–20). When Jesus asks the demoniac, "What is your name?" he replies, "My name is Legion, for we are many." In the mind of first-century Christians the word Legion (rendered as a recognizable Latin word, transliterated in the Greek text) would ring with associations of another kind of "being possessed," in view of the presumed setting of Mark's Gospel shortly after the brutal Neronic persecution of Christians in the winter of 64–65 CE.

Resuscitations constitute the smallest class of miracle stories. There are three of them: the raising of the daughter of Jairus, ruler of the synagogue (Mt 9:18–25), the raising of the widow's son at the village of Nain (Lk 7:11–15), and the raising of Lazarus, brother of Mary and Martha (Jn 11).

No story of being brought back to life from the dead could be thought of in the early church without reference to the resurrection of Jesus and to the general doctrine of final resurrection of the dead that originated in Pharisaic thought. For the early Christian cultus, the three resuscitation tales reflected the conviction that the age of resurrection and the messianic return were breaking in. The most dramatic and extravagant expression of this conviction is found in Matthew 27:51–53, with the news that at the death of Jesus, tombs were opened and bodies of the saints who had fallen asleep were raised and had been seen in Jerusalem. The age of resurrection was dawning.

Beyond this echo of resurrection, these stories also propagated fundamental convictions about Jesus.

The central rhetorical point in the story of Jairus' daughter resides in the phrase, repeated three times, that Jairus was "one of the rulers of the synagogue." Within the apologetic pattern of Mark's Gospel, forged in the growing tension within the earliest church between traditional Jews and Christian Jews, the story announces that a synagogue leader is among those who have recognized the new life that Jesus brings.

The second story, of the widow's son at Nain, derives theological power in its transparent parallel to Old Testament accounts of the life of Elijah. Why Elijah? The Old Testament stories about Elijah gained popularity in the early church as parallels were discerned between Jesus and Elijah. 1 Kings 17:8–24 tells of Elijah's visit at God's command to a poverty-stricken widow, who discovers, with Elijah as her guest, that her jar of meal is miraculously replenished, and subsequently, that her son, who suddenly dies, is brought back to life by Elijah. In the story of the widow at Nain, the Early Christians saw a "return" of Elijah at a time within Judaism when Elijah's messianic return was expected (Mal 4:5–6) and when speculation abounded on whether John the Baptist (Mt 11:11–15) or Jesus might be his reincarnation.

The third resuscitation story, the raising of Lazarus, constitutes an entire chapter in the Gospel according to John. It serves a dual purpose theologically. The first is to promulgate the Christological confession that Jesus is the true resurrection and life (Jn 11:25). The second is to see the story of Lazarus' resurrection in the first half of John's Gospel as a typological anticipation of the resurrection of Jesus in the second half.

In all, these stories affirm the evidence of new life that has been infused individually and communally into the community by the presence of the man Jesus, *Elijah redivivus*, who resuscitates the dead.

Nature miracles in the New Testament put the greatest strain on credibility of any of the miracle narratives. There are six of them: the story of Jesus calming the storm, the walking on the water, two stories of Jesus feeding people in the wilderness, the horticultural oddity of Jesus cursing the fig tree, and the coin found in the fish's mouth.

I came to appreciate the difference between an *etic* and *emic* reading of the nature miracles in my reaction to an altar painting in a church I attended over the course of a decade. It was a wall-size Renaissance-style fresco of the Matthean account of Peter beginning to sink in the waves, reaching out to Jesus for help as he was coming toward him, walking on the water. My post-Enlightenment, academic response was a sense of disdain, born of disappointment, that any contemporary church would install a nature miracle as its centerpiece of faith. Within a decade, however, my *etic* opposition to the painting began to change as I began to consider what the early church, or for that matter, what members in that congregation, might have seen in that painting as they contemplated it week after week.

From a contemporary critical, *etic* perspective, the nature miracles fall into the genre of legend or prodigy. But for the biblical authors and their first audience, they functioned as mythos or homily, inviting hearers to consider their meaning for daily existence. Ironically, the nature miracles, as stunning as they are in their meta-rational extravagance, point beyond the miracle itself to the rhetorical message seated in the story.

The story of the calming of the sea (Mk 4:35–41) recounts Jesus' rebuking the fierce wind of a storm on the Sea of Galilee and inducing a magical calm in a scenario which only minutes before had struck fear in the disciples. As is often the case in this genre, the point of the story for the Gospel author is found in the last verse. In this case it reads, "Who then is this, that even sea and wind obey him?"

Within the context of a first-century Jewish-Christian congregation, an answer is found in a psalm that provides a mirror image of the tale:

> Some went down to the sea in ships,
> Doing business on the great waters;
> They saw the deeds of the Lord,
> His wondrous works in the deep.
> For he commanded, and raised the stormy wind,
> Which lifted up the waves of the sea.
> They mounted up to heaven, they went down to the depths . . .
> They reeled and staggered like drunken men,
> And were at their wits' end.
> Then they cried to the Lord in their trouble,
> And he delivered them from their distress;
> He made the storm be still,
> And the waves of the sea were hushed. (Ps 107:23–29)

Who is it that sea and wind obey? For the early Christians it was YHWH, the God of the Exodus, now present in the Lord Jesus as his word and spiritual presence were seen to calm the troubled seas on which they rode.

The story of Jesus walking on the water (Mk 6:45–52), in similar fashion, contains several lines that highlight meanings implicit in the text for early Christian ears. The first is the utterance of Jesus to the disciples in their terror as they see him approaching their boat, walking on the water: "Take heart. It is I. Have no fear." At the heart of this statement, both for the disciples in the boat and for the listeners in the congregation hearing the story, is the highly symbolic phrase, "It is I," which in the Greek text, can be construed simply as "I am." Early Christians would have instantaneously recognized the "I AM" as the name that God disclosed to Moses at Mt. Sinai: "Say

this to the people of Israel, I AM has sent me to you" (Ex 3:14).[2] The phrase
I AM appears scores of times in Hebrew scriptures as the shorthand symbol
for the God of the Exodus.[3] It appears 26 times in the Gospel of John on the
lips of Jesus (e.g. I AM the bread of life; I AM the good shepherd, etc.) as a way
to express Jesus' presumed sense of transparency to the I AM at work in him,
implying that the one whose powers parted the Red Sea is again working
powerfully in their midst, making his "path through the waters":

> The crash of thy thunder was in the whirlwind.
> Thy lightnings lighted up the world
> The earth trembled and shook.
> Thy way was through the sea,
> Thy path through the great waters,
> Yet thy footprints were unseen,
> Thou dist lead thy people like a flock
> By the hand of Moses and Aaron. (Ps 77:18–20)

A second flashpoint of meaning lies in the incorrigibly cryptic last line of
the story, which reads: "They (the disciples) were utterly astounded for they
did not understand about the loaves, but their hearts were hardened" (Mk
6:52). No line in the New Testament can better demonstrate the fact that the
Gospel authors have planted special meanings between the lines for the readers to find. No line in the Gospels is more hermeneutically challenging.

The most likely explanation of this cryptic statement about the loaves
is found in an odd interlude about "bread" in Mark 8:14–21. Jesus asks the
disciples, "When I broke the five loaves for the five thousand, how many
baskets full of broken pieces did you take up?" The answer the disciples offer,
correctly, is "Twelve." The question is repeated concerning the feeding to the
four thousand and the answer is "Seven." After they answer, Jesus says with
puzzling abruptness, "Do you not yet understand?" And the answer to this
question for most readers is, "No."

But one thing is clear. For Mark the meaning of this episode (and the
story of the walking on the water) resides in the significance of the numbers, two sets of them. The first set is a combination of 5 (thousand) and
12. The second is a combination of 4 (thousand) and 7. Commentators have
suggested that the first set could be symbolic of Judaism (five books of Torah
and twelve tribes), and the second symbolic of Pythagorean (i.e., gentile)
interest (the virtues of the numbers 4 and 7). A compelling case can be made
that the two sets of numeric symbols represent the transition of Jesus' ministry, so conspicuous in Mark, from a Judaic (5 and 12) to a gentile (4 and 7)
context. The transition is conspicuous in Mark's geographical-theological
scheme in chapters 1 to 8, which show Jesus taking his ministry from Judaic
(3:7) to gentile territory (7:26–31). Though this solution is necessarily tentative, there is nothing tentative in the judgment that the numbers symbolism

of the loaves is on Mark's mind and that he wants you to seek out its meaning if you are to understand the larger significance of Jesus walking on the water.

The two stories of feeding the multitudes, feeding the five thousand (Mk 6:30–44) and feeding the four thousand (8:1–10) also provide hermeneutical clues to their meaning. One needs only to read them aloud to pick up the flashpoint in the language that would spark a connection in the cultic memory bank of the Gospel's first audience.

In the introductory statement of the first feeding, Jesus invites the disciples and the townspeople to a "wilderness" place (often incorrectly translated "lonely" place; Mk 6:31), evoking the memory of wilderness as a place where the wandering people of Israel "saw" God and where they received bread, the manna in the wilderness. In this wilderness Jesus distributes the loaves, using a sequence of words: he "blesses," "breaks" and "gives." Eight chapters later with the institution of the Lord's Supper the same sequence of words appears: "he blessed and broke it and gave it to them" (14:22).

The nature miracle stories of the feeding in the wilderness are less focused on the miraculous multiplication of the loaves, than on the typological repetition of YHWH's feedings in the wilderness: in the time of Moses, in the life of Jesus, and now, in the life of the Markan readers as they celebrate the Eucharist within the wilderness of their own time.

A fifth, in some ways the oddest of the nature miracles, is the story of Jesus cursing the fig tree, a tale that Matthew tells in two stages, sandwiched around the story of Jesus driving the money changers out of the temple (Mt 12:12–14, 20–25). The reader steeped in the prophetic literature of the Hebrew Bible will soon see the point.

The fig tree story is told at the outset of a face-off between Jesus and temple Judaism, beginning in Mark 11:11 with the note: "And he entered Jerusalem, and went into the temple, and when he had looked around at everything, as it was already late, he went out to Bethany with the twelve." What may sound to the modern reader as a gratuitous travel note, the reader of Mark's Gospel will recognize as a battle-cry between Jesus and the temple as a symbol of a religious system that had lost its way and from which the early church was gradually dissociating itself. The theme of Jesus' opposition to temple Judaism is played out in the stories immediately following the fig tree episode. The first is a series of Jesus' encounters with chief priests and scribes (11:27), with Pharisees and Herodians (12:13), and with Sadducees (12:18) and scribes (12:28). In each case Jesus confounds them in debate over central religious and political issues in the life of Mark's church. The sequence continues with the Little Apocalypse in Mark 13, predicting that not one stone of the temple will be left upon another. It concludes with the stark announcement following the crucifixion, that the curtain of the temple has been torn in two, from top to bottom.

How does the fig tree story relate to this? A clue is to be found in the prophet Micah's protesting the corruption of the temple hierarchy with the words: "Woe is Me! For I have become as when the summer fruit has been gathered . . . there is no cluster to eat; no first-ripe fig which my soul desires." The fig tree for Micah is a symbol of the religious bankruptcy of the temple system in his own time. Luke's version of the story makes the same point. Luke chooses to omit the story of the cursing of the fig tree, but replaces it with a parable that tells of a fig tree that will be cut down if it continues to be fruitless.

The sixth nature miracle is the most amusing. Matthew 17:24−27 recounts the story of Peter asking Jesus about the legitimacy and financial feasibility of paying the half-shekel temple tax, a point on which Peter had been pressed by the tax collectors. Jesus responds to Peter with a rejection of the tax in principle, but adds this witty counsel: "But so as not to give offense to them, go to the sea and cast a hook, and take the first fish that comes up, and when you open its mouth you will find a shekel; take that and give it to them for me and for yourself."

Jesus' response raises the question whether Peter in fact did go fishing to find the coin, or whether Jesus' response was a political witticism, counseling compromise but at the same time providing assurance that the funds will appear somehow in God's grace, even miraculously. If the latter, the story no longer belongs in the nature miracle category and constitutes one of the most explicitly political statements in the collection of Jesus' sayings. If the former, it remains to be determined whether Peter caught the coin-bearing fish, a likelihood that I found extremely remote, that is, until I read a British morning paper one day in 1970, while on sabbatical leave in Cambridge, England. It reported that a young man had caught a fish with a first-century Roman coin in its gullet. The moral? Even the most preposterous biblical legend might have a grain of a dimly remembered historical truth at its core. In any event, from the standpoint of the earliest hearers of the tale, the message would have been clear. Christians wrestling with the question of paying the half-shekel temple tax should refuse in principle, but in the spirit of political compromise, pay the tax, with the assuring footnote that "the Lord will provide."

PSYCHOLOGICAL PERSPECTIVE

Having examined the miracle stories from an *emic* perspective, we turn now to the *etic* task of reflecting on them from a psychological perspective, restricting our observations to the first two types of miracle story, healings and exorcisms.[4]

Though we are far too removed to offer precise reconstructions of what transpired behind these stories, we can make observations about the psychodynamics operative within the stories themselves, noting that in each case the healing rests on a therapeutic exchange between two persons.

Within the spectrum of fields that constitutes the discipline of psychology, the group that has emerged under the aegis of the psychoanalytic tradition, including cognitive psychology, developmental psychology, object relations theory, family systems theory, and the like, seems most capable, with their diagnostic and prescriptive protocols, to illumine the therapeutic transaction between a healer and the diseased.

These diagnostic and therapeutic protocols include the heuristic concepts of neurosis and psychosis, of introversion and extraversion, of defense mechanism, projection, transference, dissociation, sublimation, repression, displacement, reaction formation, introjection, rationalization, obsessive compulsive disorder, inflation, substitution, cognitive dissonance, posttraumatic stress disorder, multiple personality disorder—all of which have been employed to date by biblical scholars and psychologists in analyzing the nature and habits of the human psyche at work in biblical stories, as well as in the processes of creating and interpreting biblical texts (see Ellens and Rollins 2004; Rollins 1999; Rollins and Kille 2007).

A number of commentators offer helpful preliminary observations on the psychology of healings and exorcisms. For example, in speaking of the protological thinking at work in biblical descriptions of exorcisms, Bible scholar Joseph Fitzmyer, S.J., writes: "Persons afflicted with what we would call today mental disturbances were regarded as possessed, because observers were unable to analyze or diagnose properly the causes of the maladies in question" (Fitzmyer 1991, 59). Pastoral counselor Morton Kelsey comments that many illnesses are the "result of psychogenic rather than physical causes." He cites the cases of hysterical blindness, muteness, or paralysis that he believes lie behind the conditions of the blind, dumb, and paralytic healed by Jesus. The "hysterical person can copy reliably nearly any disease syndrome," Kelsey writes. "There is little organic damage, only the unconscious idea that one cannot use that particular organ—an idea so deep that the person is literally unable to do so, while hysterical patients can be suggested out of this state or tricked in various ways to reveal the psychic cause of the problem, still they are genuinely ill and cannot just snap out of it" (Kelsey 1995, 59). *The Diagnostic and Statistical Manual of Mental Disorders* confirms instances of paralysis and motoric immobility as a function of catatonic disorders (American Psychological Association 2000, 293).

One of the miracle stories that serves as a case study for psychological commentary is the exorcism of the Gerasene demoniac in Mark 5:1–20. It has attracted extensive psychological commentary because of its elaborate interpersonal detail. The commentary illustrates the richness of insight forthcoming from a variety of psychological and psychosocial perspectives that lay bare the dynamics at work in this account, especially when considered within the setting of Roman-occupied Judea in the first century CE.

The story is told in three episodes. The first tells of Jesus meeting a man with an unclean spirit who lived in the tombs. No one could bind him. Even when bound, he broke the fetters and chains to pieces. He wandered night and day among the tombs, crying out and bruising himself with stones. When Jesus saw him he ran and bowed down before Jesus, crying aloud: "What have you to do with me? I adjure you by God, do not torment me." "For Jesus had said to him, 'Come out of the man, you unclean spirit!'" When Jesus asked him his name, he replied, "My name is Legion, for we are many." A great herd of swine was feeding on the hillside. The demoniac begged Jesus, "Send us to the swine, let us enter them." Jesus complied, and two thousand pigs rushed down the bank into the sea and drowned.

The second episode takes place in the city to which the herdsmen, who had witnessed the event, went with the tale. People came out to the tombs see what had happened, and found Jesus and the demoniac sitting there. The demoniac was clothed and in his right mind. In seeing this sight the crowd was filled with fear. They begged Jesus to depart from their neighborhood.

The third episode describes Jesus getting into the boat to leave, when the man who had been possessed with demons begged that he might be with him. Jesus refuses: "Go home to your friends, and tell them how much the Lord has done for you, and how he has had mercy on you."

Some commentators have made observations on the nature of the demoniac's illness in terms of a contemporary psychological reading of Mark's description. Hankoff (1992) sees in the story the earmarks of Multiple Personality Disorder, created by a "dissociation, which works by splitting off unbearable feelings, images and thoughts that create psychological overload," leading to the acting out of these feelings with no conscious memory of his bizarre, self-destructive behavior (Hankoff 1992, 8; Ludwig 2006, 5).

Robert Leslie sees the demoniac's illness as the symptomatology of a person who had become ill because of a sense of having been robbed of his dignity. The result is behavior that expresses "anger turned in against himself. Angry at himself, at war with himself, he feels only the conflict of the unresolved forces struggling within his make up and loses sight of the essential unity that dignity implies" (Leslie 2007, 214).

Paul Hollenbach offers an insightful commentary on the phenomenon of the demoniac from a social-psychological perspective. "The Gerasene's possession is both disease and cure. . . . His very madness permitted him to do in a socially acceptable manner what he could not do as sane, namely express his total hostility to the Romans; he did this by identifying the Roman legions with demons. His possession was thus at once both the result of oppression and an expression of his resistance to it" (Hollenbach 1981, 581).

In his comprehensive analysis of the story of the Gerasene demoniac, Michael Willett Newheart (2004) introduces the work of Rene Girard (1986) on scapegoating, spelling out the ways in which a three-way relationship combines to create a small society of pathological interaction, consisting of a *demoniac*, of the *society* that excludes him and tries to chain him, and of a *Roman occupation government* that allows no protest other than that which may come in a disguised form from a demoniac (Newheart 2004, 70–78).

Other commentators have focused their observations on the psychodynamics of exorcism that transpire between Jesus and the demoniac. Carroll Wise (1954) recounts the story of Harry Stack Sullivan, a skilled psychiatrist at work with a schizophrenic patient during a staff presentation. The doctor making the presentation was unable to evoke any response or communication from the patient. With a "shrug of futility" he deferred to Harry Stack Sullivan:

> Sullivan's first move was to edge his chair just a little closer to that of the patient and to lean forward so that he could look directly at the patient in a very friendly, warm manner. To the amazement of all, the patient responded to every question and comment that was made by Dr. Sullivan. For half an hour or more they conversed together, seemingly oblivious to the fact that there was any one else in the room. (Leslie 2007, 216; Wise 1954, 57)

Leslie comments that such radical change in behavior demonstrates an observation of Victor Frankl: "even the manifestations of psychosis conceal a real spiritual person, unassailable by mental disease. Only the possibility of communication with the outside world and of self-expression are inhibited by the disease; the nucleus of man remains indestructible." The schizophrenic, as well as the manic-depressive, has a remnant of freedom with which he can confront his illness and realize himself, not only in spite of it but because of it (Frankl 1965, 98; Leslie 2007, 217).

With respect to episode three, Jesus' departure and the healed man's request to go with him, Wilhelm Wuellner and Robert Leslie draw on a book by James Dittes, *When the People Say No*, making the point that people who at times oppose us, do so to our own benefit by leading us to a new level of responsibility. "Like any good counselor who recognizes an unhealthy dependency, Jesus sent the man back home to his friends . . . to be . . . integrated," which in effect called for "an active program on the man's own part of taking the initiative" for his own continued health. Furthermore, in commending to the man that he tell his friends "how much the Lord has done for you, and how he has had mercy on you," Jesus invites a cognitive shift in the healed man. This develops in him conscious recognition of life as a context of mercy that sustains him (Wuellner and Leslie 1984, 36; Dittes 1979).

The story of the Gerasene demoniac is an example of one of the primary postulates of the NT, that healing was a primary objective of the ministry of the historical Jesus, and that this healing was the function of a transaction between the healer and the healed, lending credence to the contention of analytical psychologist Carl Jung that "Religions are psychotherapeutic systems in the truest sense of the word" (Jung 1963, vol. 10, par. 367).

NOTES

1. A typical example is found in the Paris Magical Papyrus, dating from 300 C.E.: "For those possessed by daemons, an approved charm by Pibechis. Take oil, make from unripe olives, together with the plan mastigia and lotus pith, and boil it with marjoram saying: 'Joel, Ossarthiomi, Emori, Theochipsoith, Sithemeoch, Sothe, Joe, Mimipsothiooph, Phersothi, Aeeioyo, etc.' ... Write this phylactery upon a little sheet of tin: 'Jaeo, Abraothioch, Phtha, Mesentiniao. ...' And hang it round the sufferer: it is of every demon a thing to be trembled at" (Barrett, 34).

2. The verb *I am* in Hebrew is from the same root as the name YAHWEH (Jehovah in the King James Bible), which means "He who causes things to come into being."

3. Its significance in the Hebrew scriptures is epitomized in Isaiah 52:6: "Therefore my people shall know my name; therefore in that day they shall know that it is I who speak; here I AM." See, also, for example, Isaiah 43:10, 11, 13, 225; 51:12; Exodus 12:12; 14:4, 18; 15:26.

4. Despite the protological thinking that often colors the biblical accounts of healings and exorcisms, the healings and exorcisms belong to the genre of first-century historical writing, whereas the second two classes of miracle story, resuscitations and nature miracles, fall within the genre of legend, that is, events with possible vestiges of historical truth that have been exaggerated for apologetic effect.

REFERENCES

American Psychological Association (2000), *Diagnostic and Statistical Manual of Mental Disorders*, 4th edition, Washington, DC: American Psychological Association

Barrett, C. K., ed. (1989), *The New Testament Background: Selected Documents*, revised and expanded edition, San Francisco: Harper & Row.

Dittes, James (1979), *When the People Say No*, New York: Harper & Row.

Ellens, J. Harold, ed. (2004), *The Destructive Power of Religion: Violence in Judaism, Christianity, and Islam*, Westport, CT: Praeger.

Ellens, J. H., and W. G. Rollins, eds. (2004), *Psychology and the Bible: A New Way to Read the Scriptures*, Westport, CT: Praeger.

Fitzmyer, Joseph A. (1991), How Are the Gospel Accounts of Jesus' Miracles to be Understood? In *A Christological Catechism: New Testament Answers*, revised and expanded edition, 56–62, New York: Paulist.

Frankl, Victor (1965), *Existence and Values: Foundations of Logotherapy*, Unpublished manuscript.

Girard, Rene (1986), *The Scapegoat*, Baltimore and London: Johns Hopkins University Press.

Hankoff, L. D. (1992), Religious Healing in First-Century Christianity, *The Journal of Psychohistory* 19 (4), 387–408.

Hollenbach, P. W. (1981), Jesus, Demoniacs, and Public Authorities: A Socio-Historical Study, *Journal of the American Academy of Religion* 99, 567–88.

Jung, Carl G. (1963), *Memories, Dreams, Reflections,* R. Winston and C. Winston, trans., New York: Vintage Books.

Kee, Howard C. (1986), *Medicine, Miracle and Magic in the New Testament Times,* Cambridge: Cambridge University Press.

Kelsey, Morton T. (1995), *Healing Christianity,* Minneapolis: Augsburg.

Leslie, R. (2007), The Gerasene Demoniac, in *Psychological Insight into the Bible: Texts and Readings,* W. G. Rollins and D. A. Kille, eds., 214–19, Grand Rapids: Eerdmans.

Lohse, E. (1976), *The New Testament Environment,* J. E. Steely, trans., Nashville: Abingdon.

Ludwig, M. B. (2006), *The Healing of Jesus and the Early Church,* unpublished paper, Hartford Seminary.

Martinez, Florentino G. (1994), *The Dead Sea Scrolls Translated,* New York: E. J. Brill.

McCasland, S. V. (1962), Miracle, *The Interpreter's Dictionary of the Bible (IDB),* G. A. Buttrick, ed., Vol. K–Q, 392–402, New York and Nashville: Abingdon.

Newheart, Michael W. (2004), *My Name Is Legion: The Story and Soul of the Gerasene Demoniac,* Collegeville, MN: Liturgical Press.

Pilch, J. J. (2000), *Healing in the New Testament: Insights from Medical and Mediterranean Anthropology,* Minneapolis: Fortress.

Rollins, Wayne G. (1999), *Soul and Psyche: The Bible in Psychological Perspective,* Minneapolis: Fortress.

Rollins, Wayne G., and D. Andrew Kille, eds. (2007), *Psychological Insight into the Bible: Texts and Readings,* Grand Rapids: Eerdmans.

Strachey, J. (1953–74), *The Standard Edition of the Complete Psychological Works of Sigmund Freud,* London: Hogarth Press and the Institute of Psychoanalysis.

Vermes, Geza (2001), *The Changing Faces of Jesus,* New York: Penguin Putnam.

Wise, Carroll A. (1954), Psychiatric interview of Harry Stack Sullivan, *Pastoral Psychology* 5, 8 (November), 39–46.

Wuellner, W. H., and R. C. Leslie (1984), *The Surprising Gospel: Intriguing Psychological Insights from the New Testament,* Nashville: Abingdon.

CHAPTER 4

Miracles in the Old Testament

Antti Laato

The aim of this chapter is to orient the modern reader on how to read the Old Testament (OT), and understand the miracles that are recounted in those ancient Hebrew scriptures. I shall describe ancient Near Eastern speculative thought and the way the semantic fields of the Hebrew terms for miracles were connected with it. Then I shall discuss how certain explanations in modern science are useful models for the so-called miracles, but also how scientific methods are limited.

SPECULATIVE THOUGHT OF ANCIENT MAN

There is a fundamental difference between our modern culture and its scientific preconditions on the one hand, and the intellectual and speculative thought of ancient man, on the other. Therefore, we can understand miracle stories in the OT only if we have an idea about this distinction. In fact the concept of miracle should be regarded as a post-OT idea. There are no good equivalents of the concept of miracle in OT Hebrew. Nevertheless, we have different Hebrew terms that have been used to characterize certain extraordinary features in the OT stories. How can we explain this lack of the term *miracle* in Hebrew?

Frankfort and Frankfort edited an interesting study on the speculative thought of ancient man.[1] Their study "attempts to underpin the chaos of experience so that it may reveal the features of a structure: order, coherence, and meaning" (3). They argued that ancient man had only one mode of expression: personal. They understood reality as personal but other, the you out there; and "the gods, as personifications of power among other things, fulfill early man's need for reasons that explain the phenomenal world" (17). The distinction between an ancient and modern man could be demonstrated, for example, by the reaction of each to the collapse of a house in which people are killed. The modern man seeks causal reasons for this accident. He could come to the conclusion that termites have destroyed the wood and finally led to the fatal accident. The ancient man was less interested in these causal reasons. He wanted to know why the people living in the house died. His interest was less in cause and effect and more in meaning and purpose. Why do gods or divine powers want to kill such people?

The expression of reality as personal other (you) led to various myths that tried to explain what was going on in nature and human life. Everything that happened in reality was an action and a reflection of the personal other. The language of myth was an attempt to capture the actions of the personal other in an understandable form. The language of myth opened the mind of the ancient man to miracles. The myth of divine powers behind the mysterious otherness of things helped explain the extraordinary events that are beyond human control. This explains well why the boundary between miracle and ordinary natural event was not very opaque, indeed, it was permeable. Rain was always an expression of the mysterious other. The myth of Baal, for example, was an attempt to explain how the storm god, Baal, is responsible for this event. If the rain did not come in time, this mysterious other had some personal reasons to postpone it.

This being the case, we can say that ancient man lived in miracles. He could see every day how the mysterious other in various natural phenomena appeared and produced events that were beyond human control and comprehension. Such an ancient Near Eastern mythic background is a necessary precondition to understanding the Hebrew concepts used in the OT to speak about miracles or rather extraordinary events.

THE CONCEPT OF MIRACLE IN
THE HEBREW LANGUAGE

The Hebrew language contains five different terms that can be connected with the concept of miracle. These terms are connected with the mighty acts of God in history. One of the most important terms is the feminine plural form of the adjective *great: gedolot*. The basic meaning of this plural form is mighty acts, or something similar. The adjective *great* is often connected with Yahweh and his mighty deeds in the OT. According to Mosis there are two roots for the theological tradition of Yahweh's greatness: (1) the Zion tradition, which is expressed in Psalms and in such expressions as "Great is Yahweh"; and (2) historical experiences.[2] In particular, historical experiences are important in this connection because the mighty acts of Yahweh are regarded as milestones in the history of Israel, indicating that God will take care of his people even in the unknown future.

A typical example of the mighty acts of God is marvelous events he is described as performing in the Land of Egypt. Therefore we read, for example (Dt 10:21): "[H]e is your God, who performed for you those *great and awesome wonders* that you saw with your own eyes."[3] In Psalm 106:21 the people are accused of forgetting the God "who had done *great things* in Egypt." The great acts of God indicate that there are no other gods who can be compared with him: "Your righteousness reaches to the skies, O God, you who have done *great things*. Who, O God, is like you?" (Ps 71:19). Among the great things that God is reported to have done are not only historical events but also natural phenomena. Job 37 describes how God is behind all natural phenomena. In verses 5–6 it is said: "God's voice thunders in marvelous ways; he does *great things* beyond our understanding. He says to the snow, 'Fall upon the earth,' and to the rain shower, 'Be a mighty downpour.'" This passage of Job corroborates well our introductory remarks of ancient Near Eastern speculative thoughts: God's mighty acts in nature are beyond human understanding or human efforts. God does not only perform great acts for his people but even his revenge can be great. Ezekiel 25:17 refers to Yahweh's great revenges against Philistia.

The term, great deeds (*gedolot*) has also been used for the miracles performed by Elisha. Thus we read (2 Kgs 8:4), "The king was talking to Gehazi, the servant of the man of God, and he had said: 'Tell me about all the *great things* Elisha has done.'" Elisha could do great things; and the people could do great sins. Thus, for example, the prophet Ezekiel accused his people of doing "utterly detestable things," that is, great things of an evil nature. This expression appears three times in Ezekiel 8 (verses 6, 13 and 15) and indicates well how the term, *great things* emphasizes events and phenomena that are extraordinary in some sense, but do not necessarily fit in well with our category of the miracle.

As indicated above, in Deuteronomy 10:21 and Psalm 106:21, *great things* is used to describe the great things God performed in Egypt. In the Exodus story itself, as well as in Deuteronomy, the Hebrew term for *sign* (*'ot*) is used frequently to describe those mighty acts and plagues against the Egyptians. According to Exodus 10:1–2, "The Lord said to Moses, 'Go to Pharaoh, for I have hardened his heart and the hearts of his officials so that I may perform these miraculous signs of mine among them, that you may tell your children and grandchildren how I dealt harshly with the Egyptians and how I performed my *signs* among them, and that you may know that I am the Lord.'" In Exodus 7:3 the Hebrew word *'ot* (sign) is used together with another Hebrew word, *mopet*, portent,[4] "But I will harden Pharaoh's heart . . . though I multiply my signs and portents in the land of Egypt." Deuteronomy 6:22 connects the adjective *great* with *sign:* "Before our eyes the Lord sent miraculous signs and *portents*—great and terrible—upon Egypt and Pharaoh and his whole household." It is worth noting that the adjective *great* is connected with *signs* and *portents* in numerous other OT texts speaking about the mighty acts of God.[5]

Words for signs and wonders are often used in parallel and then the reference is to extraordinary things or events, as in Exodus 7:3. But *sign* can also be prophetic as in 1 Samuel 2:34: "And what happens to your two sons, Hophni and Phinehas, will be a *sign* to you—they will both die on the same day." In a similar way Samuel predicted some signs to Saul that would take place so that Saul could be sure that God would be with him (1 Sam 10:7, 9). According to Deuteronomy 13:1–2, the false prophet can do signs and wonders and exhort the people to worship other gods than Yahweh: "If a prophet, or one who foretells by dreams, appears among you and announces to you a miraculous sign or portent, and if the sign or portent of which he has spoken takes place, and he says, 'Let us follow other gods,' gods you have not known, 'and let us worship them.'"

While the terms *'ot* and *mopet* do not exclude the aspect of wonder or miracle, their basic meaning is sign. Sun and moon are signs for festivals, days, and years (Gen 1:14). Circumcision is a sign for the covenant God established with Abraham (Gen 17:11). The birth of the child can also be a sign (Is 7:11, 14). Sometimes it has been emphasized that the sign in Isaiah 7:14 refers to an extraordinary birth like the virgin birth. Even though such a reading cannot be categorically excluded it is clear that such an interpretation in Isaiah 7:14 is not necessary. The woman referred to in this verse is a young woman (*'almah*) who is not necessarily a virgin (translated with *parthenos* in the Septuagint). For example, in Isaiah 37:30 (cf. 2 Kgs 19:29) the prophet Isaiah gives a sign of salvation to Hezekiah that refers to ordinary events: "This will be the sign for you, O Hezekiah: This year you will eat what grows by itself, and the second year what springs from that. But in the third year sow and reap, plant vineyards and eat their fruit." On the other hand, in Isaiah 37:7–8 (cf. 2 Kgs 20:8–9) sign refers to an extraordinary natural phenomenon: "'This is the Lord's sign to you that the Lord will do what he has promised: I will make the shadow cast by the sun go back the ten steps it has gone down on the stairway of Ahaz.' So the sunlight went back the ten steps it had gone down."

The prophet himself and his symbolic action can also be a sign for the coming event that Yahweh will realize. Therefore Isaiah was exhorted to walk naked: "Then the Lord said, 'Just as my servant Isaiah has gone stripped and barefoot for three years, as a *sign* and *portent* against Egypt and Cush, so the king of Assyria will lead away stripped and barefoot the Egyptian captives and Cushite exiles, young and old, with buttocks bared—to Egypt's shame'" (Is 20:3–4). In a similar way both the prophet and his disciples are signs and portents in Israel for the message of Isaiah that will be realized (Is 8:18). Also Ezekiel himself became a sign to the people (Ez 24:24, 27). According to Zechariah 3:8 the high priest Joshua and his colleagues are "men of *portent*" of the coming of the Messiah, the Branch: "Listen, O high priest Joshua and your associates seated before you, who are men symbolic of things to come: I am going to bring my servant, the Branch."

Psalm 74 is a lamentation of the people who have experienced the destruction of the enemy. In verse 4 it is noted how the enemy has set up their signs of victory: "Your foes roared in the place where you met with us; they set up their standards as *signs*." In this distress the people lament that they have no *signs* that is, prophetic visions, that could give them hope: "We are given no miraculous signs; no prophets are left, and none of us knows how long this will be" (Ps 74:9).

The term *sign* (*'ot*) can also be used to denote the covenant between Yahweh and the people. In Ezekiel 20:12 the Sabbath is a sign of the covenant: "Also I gave them my Sabbaths as a *sign* between us, so they would know that I the Lord made them holy" (so also Ez 20:20). Beside *signs* and *wonders* we should also mention the Hebrew word *nes*, often used for *standard, banner, signal,* or *sign*, which could be stood up in the battle or as a pole for the copper snake (Num 21:8–9).[6] But even this word could be used in the OT figuratively and its meaning in that case was similar to *signs* and *wonders*. According to Numbers 26:10, "the earth opened its mouth and swallowed them along with Korah, whose followers died when the fire devoured the 250 men. And they served as a *warning sign*." Even a person can be a banner. In Isaiah 11:10 the reference is made to the Root of Jesse, that is, the Messiah who will stand as banner for the peoples: "In that day the Root of Jesse will stand as a *banner* for the peoples; the nations will rally to him, and his place of rest will be glorious." Specifically, in Isaiah 40–55 the word for *banner* is used a decisive historical event where the people and the exiles are gathered (Is 49:22; 62:10). In later Hebrew and Aramaic as well as in rabbinical Hebrew, *nes* (banner) began to denote *sign, wonder,* and *providential* event.[7]

Finally there are the Hebrew verb *pl'* and the related words *pele'* and *nifla'ot* (only in plural). Concerning the meaning of the verb *pl'* Conrad writes that "the texts all deal with extraordinary phenomena, transcending the power of human knowledge and imagination."[8] Thus these Hebrew words refer to things that are *beyond one's power, difficult, extraordinary, or wonderful. Nifla'ot* is used in the OT almost always as substantive wonderful acts or mighty acts. Job experienced (10:16) that God was against him and acted inexplicably against him: "If I hold my head high, you stalk me like a lion and again *display your awesome power* against me."

The Hebrew word *pele'* designates an extraordinary thing or event, which has often been translated with the English word, *wonder*. Typical is the expression about God who "performs *wonder(s)*."[9] For example, in Exodus 15:11 the reference is made to the Exodus from Egypt and the mighty acts of God in the Reed Sea (so also in Ps 78:12):[10] "Who among the gods is like you, O Lord? Who is like you–majestic in holiness, awesome in glory, *working wonders*."

The semantic field of *pele'* does not restrict it to *wonders*. For example, Isaiah 29:14 uses the word to describe unpredictable political events that Yahweh will realize in Judah (cf. Hab 2:5–8): "Therefore once more I will astound these people with wonder upon wonder; the wisdom of the wise will perish, the intelligence of the intelligent will vanish." Isaiah 9:6 calls the coming righteous Davidic ruler with various names and one of them is Wonderful Counselor (*pele' yo'ets*). These throne names in Isaiah 9:6 are connected with the Assyrian (and Babylonian) throne titles.[11]

Psalm 119:129–30 calls Yahweh's instructions wonderful, which can give understanding: "Your statutes are wonderful; therefore I obey them. The unfolding of your words gives light; it gives understanding to the simple." In a corresponding way *nifla'ot* is used for the Torah: "Open my eyes that I may see *wonderful things* in your law" (Ps 119:18); "Let me understand the teaching of your precepts; then I will meditate on your *wonders*" (Ps 119:27).

David can express that Jonathan's love and friendship toward him was extraordinary: "I grieve for you, Jonathan my brother; you were very dear to me. Your love for me was wonderful, more wonderful than that of women" (2 Sam 1:26).

The Hebrew word *nifla'ot* is used when Yahweh's deliverance from Egypt is described. Thus we read in Exodus 3:20: "So I will stretch out my hand and strike the Egyptians with all the wonders that I will perform among them." In Psalm 106 reference is made to the same event: "When our fathers were in Egypt, they gave no thought to your miracles; they did not remember your many kindnesses, and they rebelled by the sea, the Reed Sea. . . . They forgot the God who saved them, who had done great things in Egypt, miracles in the land of Ham, and awesome deeds by the Red Sea" (Ps 106:7, 22).

The expression *do mighty acts* appears often in the OT when it speaks about God.[12] Another common expression is to *tell mighty acts of God*, which emphasizes often God's mighty acts in history that the people should commemorate.[13] Psalm 107 is a thanksgiving hymn in which the great acts (*nifla'ot*) of Yahweh are commemorated. It contains four repetitions of the expression: "Let them give thanks to the Lord for his unfailing love and his wonderful deeds for humankind" (Ps 107:8, 15, 21, 31).

This survey has shown how the mighty acts of God are connected; in particular, the events of the Exodus from Egypt. We have also seen that there are several linguistic and thematic parallels between God's mighty acts in creation and in history. This gives us reason to study this connection in detail.

MIGHTY ACTS OF GOD IN CREATION AND IN HISTORY

In the light of our introductory remarks it would be reasonable to assume that ancient speculative thought plays an important role in the description of the historical events in the Hebrew tradition. The divine personal, you or other, is evident both in nature/creation and in historical events.

One of the most influential studies in understanding the history and religious ideas in early Israel is Frank Moore Cross' *Canaanite Myth and Hebrew Epic*. He argues that the mythical language of the Canaanite myth of Baal's victory over chaos powers in creation was transformed to describe in early Hebrew epic how Yahweh managed to help his people in history. In the Canaanite myth, gods promised Baal a palace if he could destroy the powers of chaos and establish harmony. Baal struggled against *Yammu* (Chaos, Sea) and later against *Mot* (Death) and managed to establish harmony. He was granted the palace "which is his sanctuary where he is worshiped."[14] Exodus 15 follows this same theme by describing the crisis, the political chaos that threatens the existence of Israel, and can be presented as follows:[15]

Combat victory and theophany of Divine Warrior (vv 1–12)
Salvation of the Israelites (vv 13–16a)
Building of the sanctuary and procession (16b–17)
Manifestation of Yahweh's universal reign (18)

Yahweh will appear and struggle against the enemies of Israel and establish his people in the land of Canaan. The sanctuary is established for Yahweh. Cross demonstrates in different ways that this connection functions well in the early poetic texts where the Divine Warrior is described.[16] The themes of creation, in which the god struggles against the powers of chaos, were historicized in the early Hebrew epic. They indicate Israelite understanding of God who intervenes in historical events. Cross showed that this mythical pattern of the coming of Yahweh to help his people has lived in Hebrew epic and Israelite theology and has been used also in very late eschatological texts.[17]

Cross' analysis explains well the theological emphasis in the OT, according to which Yahweh is the Lord of creation and history. In particular, the Book of Isaiah takes up this connection. In his massive commentary on Isaiah 1–39, Hans Wildberger has analyzed some key texts that connect Yahweh's mighty acts in creation and history. One good example is Isaiah 17:12–14:[18]

Oh, the raging of many nations
they rage like the raging sea!
Oh, the uproar of the peoples
they roar like the roaring of great waters!
Although the peoples roar like the roar of surging waters,
when he rebukes them they flee far away,
driven before the wind like chaff on the hills,
like tumbleweeds before a gale.
In the evening, sudden terror!

before the morning, they are gone!
This is the portion of those who loot us,
the lot of those who plunder us.

Wildberger connects this passage to the Zion tradition, which is presented
in Psalms 46, 48, and 76, among others. Nations are compared with raging chaotic waters that threaten the existence of the inhabitants of Jerusalem; but Yahweh will rebuke these waters and they will suddenly disappear. Similar texts
in Isaiah 1–39, in which enemies are compared with chaotic powers attacking
Jerusalem, are Isaiah 8:5–10 and 29:1–8, among others. I have contended elsewhere that these texts are closely connected with the story of Sennacherib's
invasion of Judah (Is 36–37; cf. 2 Kgs 18–19).[19] Sennacherib attempted to conquer Jerusalem but was stopped by mighty acts of God when the Assyrian
army, according to 2 Kings 19:35, was destroyed by the angel of Yahweh.

There is a very useful analysis of how the language of creation is used to
describe Yahweh's salvation acts in history. It is in C. Stuhlmueller's work
Creative Redemption in Deutero-Isaiah.[20] He has shown how the typical Hebrew
vocabulary of creation motifs has been used in the texts that describe the redemption of Israel from the Babylonian exile: The "idea of creation served
to enhance many features of the prophet's concept of redemption, transform-
ing it into an *exceptionally wondrous* redemptive act, performed with personal
concern by Yahweh for his chosen people, bringing them unexpectedly out
of exile, into a new and unprecedented life of peace and abundance, with re-
percussions even upon the cosmos and world inhabitants."[21] A good example
is Isaiah 51:9–16. I have quoted this text below and added square brackets
some explanations in order to emphasize how creation, Yahweh's mighty
acts in history, and the coming salvation from the Babylonian captivity are
connected with each other.

[Yahweh has beaten Rahab, the symbol of the powers of chaos, in creation]

9. Awake, awake! Clothe yourself with strength,
O arm of the Lord.
Awake, as in days gone by,
as in generations of old.
Was it not you who cut Rahab to pieces,
who pierced that monster through?

[Yahweh has saved his people from slavery in Egypt]

10. Was it not you who dried up
the sea, the waters of the great deep.
Who made a road in the depths of the sea
so that the redeemed might cross over?

[Yahweh will redeem his people from Babylonia]

11. The ransomed of the Lord will return;
they will enter Zion with singing.
Everlasting joy will crown their heads;
gladness and joy will overtake them,
and sorrow and sighing will flee away.

[The Lord of creation comforts the exiles]

12. I, even I, am he who comforts you;
who are you that you fear mortal men,
The sons of men, who are but grass,
13. that you forget the Lord your Maker,
who stretched out the heavens
and laid the foundations of the earth,
that you live in constant terror every day
because of the wrath of the oppressor,
who is bent on your destruction;
for where is the wrath of the oppressor?

[The exiles will be set free by the Lord who governs the powers of chaos]

14. The cowering prisoners will soon be set free;
they will not die in their dungeon,
nor will they lack bread.
15. For I am the Lord your God,
who churns up the sea so that its waves roar—
the Lord Almighty is his name.
16. I have put my words in your mouth
and covered you with the shadow of my hand.
I who set the heavens in place,
who laid the foundations of the earth,
and who says to Zion,
"You are my people."

The cursory reading of Isaiah 40–55 reveals that themes of creation and redemption of Israel are intertwined. The Lord of the creation is the Lord of history. The Lord who could execute mighty acts in creation can perform similar wonderful acts in history. Isaiah 43:9–13 presents us the following scenario.

All the nations gather together
and the peoples assemble.
Which of them foretold this
and proclaimed to us the former things?

Let them bring in their witnesses to prove they were right,
so that others may hear and say, "It is true."
"You are my witnesses," declares the Lord,
"and my servant whom I have chosen,
so that you may know and believe me
and understand that I am he.
Before me no god was formed,
nor will there be one after me.
I, even I, am the Lord,
and apart from me there is no savior.
I have revealed and saved and proclaimed—
I, and not some foreign god among you.
You are my witnesses," declares the Lord, "that I am God.
Yes, and from ancient days I am he.
No one can deliver out of my hand.
When I act, who can reverse it?"

The text seems to be dependent on the Babylonian creation-epic, *Enuma Elish*, according to which the creation was a process in which various gods came into existence.[22] However, the text in Isaiah 43 emphasizes that no other gods have been before Yahweh or appear after him (in the process of creation). Therefore, Yahweh is the only one who can save his people from the Babylonian exile.

The idea of Yahweh's coming to help his people continued in postbiblical apocalyptic literature. In his study, *Dawn of Apocalyptic*, Paul Hanson contended that many texts in Trito-Isaiah (Is 56–66) and Deutero-Zechariah are connected with this old idea about Yahweh's kingship in creation. In the postexilic period this theme was developed further and it was used to describe how Yahweh will help his loyal servants against established and godless government in the land of Judea.[23]

HISTORICAL CREDO

Our analysis has shown that Yahwism was deeply rooted in a belief that God acts in history. This explains well the so-called historical credos in the OT. The basic analysis of these credos was made by Gerhard von Rad.[24] His massive work on the theology of the OT is based on this idea. God is no philosophical idea but a God whose mighty acts can be seen in creation and history.[25] The OT contains several historical credos in which Yahweh's mighty acts in history have been listed. Von Rad began his analysis with the historical credo in Deuteronomy 26:5–9. The one who brings first fruits and tithes to Jerusalem should recite the following credo:

Then you shall declare before the Lord your God: "My father was a wandering Aramean, and he went down into Egypt with a few people and lived there and became a great nation, powerful and numerous. But the Egyptians mistreated us and made us suffer, putting us to hard labor. Then we cried out to the Lord, the God of our fathers, and the Lord heard our voice and saw our misery, toil and oppression. So the Lord brought us out of Egypt with a *mighty hand and an outstretched arm*, with *great terror* and with miraculous *signs and portents*. He brought us to this place and gave us this land, a land flowing with milk and honey; and now I bring the first-fruits of the soil that you, O Lord, have given me."

This credo uses typical terms for the mighty acts of God and indicates that Yahweh-belief is belief in God who intervenes in history with mighty and wonderful acts. There are several other texts where similar historical surveys of Israel have been presented.[26] Such historical credos structure the history of Israel and emphasize that Yahweh has governed its course with his mighty acts. Therefore, it is also understandable why the actions of Yahweh in history are a constitutional element in OT theology. Horst Dietrich Preuss formulated a thesis that Yahweh-belief has always been belief in God who will also act in the future.[27] The constitutional element in Yahwism is openness to the possibility of mighty and wonderful acts. This background helps us to understand the New Testament (NT) stories about the miracles of Jesus. They are not loans from the Hellenistic world but intimately connected with the OT and the Jewish milieu.[28]

MIRACLE WORKERS

We have seen that, according to the OT, Yahweh has power to do mighty acts in creation and history. Therefore also a man who is close to God and becomes part of the divine sphere can perform wonders. Moses is capable of wonderful acts in Egypt because God has given this power to him, as we can read in Exodus 7:1: "Then the Lord said to Moses, 'See, I have made you like God to Pharaoh, and your brother Aaron will be your prophet.'"

Problems of magic became actual in this connection. In the story of Exodus the Egyptian magicians could perform miracles similar to the miracles of Moses. Moses ordered Aaron's staff to become a snake and Exodus 7:8–13 tells us that even Egyptian magicians could do the same. It is worth noting that the present form of the OT contains critical attitudes toward divination and magic.[29] One reason for the rise of this criticism is that mighty acts of God have become the constitutional basis for the Israelite religion and, therefore, no new magical tricks or wonders can change this basis. We have already seen that Deuteronomy 13:1–3 warns the people that no extraordinary acts would lead it away from its God: "If a prophet, or one who foretells by dreams, appears among you and announces to you a miraculous sign or wonder, and if the sign or wonder of which he has spoken takes place, and he says, 'Let us follow other gods,' gods you have not known, 'and let us worship them,' you must not listen to the words of that prophet or dreamer. The Lord your God is testing you to find out whether you love him with all your heart and with all your soul." This warning indicates well how the religious reality was understood in Deuteronomy and subsequently also in the present form of the OT. All kinds of extraordinary acts and events can take place but they cannot change or nullify the mighty acts of God in history, which constitute the existence of Israel and guide the people to live according to instructions of God given through Moses.

CONFUSED MODERN READER

When a modern reader studies the OT he may be readily confused as to how to interpret texts about the mighty power of Yahweh, manifest in producing wonderful acts in history. I have attempted to level the path to understanding this problem in the context of the ancient Near Eastern speculative thought that lies behind the OT. Clearly, it is impossible to choose any restricted scientific approach in studying the narratives that report the biblical miracles. Our choice options are limited and simple. First, we must simply understand the fundamental attitudes toward reality that prevailed at the time the narratives were crafted. Second, we cannot avoid reductionism when we employ scientific methodologies that are bent upon trying to prove whether some extraordinary events have actually taken place.

The use of such compartmentalized methods of verification imply that a scholar wants to seek some natural explanation for the extraordinary act in the text. After all, in terms of scientific philosophy it is impossible to conclude, by methods of scientific verifiability, that a miracle has occurred. If such a result would be achieved then other scholars could replicate the examination and come to the same conclusion. If that were possible the object of examination would not be a miracle.

Therefore, in scientific analysis the fundamental question is not whether a miracle has occurred, but rather whether we can discern a responsible way to approach the story of miracle. If we aim to give a scientific answer then we have simply decided to find relevant natural clarifications to the outcome of the story of miracle. A third option is, of course, that modern scholars consider scientific and verifiable methods as *restricted* approaches to understanding phenomena that are described as miraculous. In that case scientific analysis can attempt to give useful information about the story of the miracle without proposing to explode the story or afford us a final answer regarding the reality behind the story of the miracle.

When a modern scholar begins to study an OT miracle text he or she usually takes into consideration the following three methodological viewpoints that concern the transmission of the text:[30]

1. With the aid of textual criticism he studies the Hebrew text and ancient translations in order to establish as accurate and reliable a version as possible. Copyists can have caused various inaccuracies or intentional modifications in the text, though it is always surprising how well the biblical texts have been transmitted over the centuries.[31]

2. Literary and redaction (editorial) critical analysis is an attempt to discuss in which way the story has been reworked. For example, scholars agree that the Elijah and Elisha stories in the present form of the Deuteronomistic History[32] are based on earlier traditions. By carefully analyzing these stories in 1 and 2 Kings it is possible to detect which parts have been reworked by Deuteronomistic redactor(s) or editors. With the aid of literary and redactional analysis it is possible to come closer to older literary cores behind the present form of the OT text.[33] For example, in the biblical story of the mysterious setback of the Assyrian army at Jerusalem (2 Kgs 18–19 = Is 36–37) I argued that 2 Kings 18:14–16 consists of an independent source that should be separated from 2 Kings 18:13, 17–19:38 (= Is 36–37) because it had been added later by a different editor.[34]

3. Finally a scholar has the option of dealing with possible oral traditions behind the transmission process of the OT texts. In the case of the Elijah and Elisha stories it is necessary to discuss whether these two story-cycles have been transmitted together or whether they were two separate stories that finally were modified and edited into the Deuteronomistic History.

   After having established the transmission process of the biblical text the scholar relates the evidence of different literary strata to other available methods.

4. Form historical analysis of phrasing, sentences, and sections of the story aims to discuss which kind of text we are reading. For example, the literary form of the letter is different than a novel. Scientific articles with footnotes differ from newspaper articles, and so on. Every literary form in the OT has also its own typical features. For example, 2 Kings 18:14–16 is a typical annalistic account that apparently originates from royal archives of Jerusalem; while 2 Kings 18:13, 17–19:38 (= Is 36–37) is composed of two stories circulated among the people. These considerations help the modern scholar to evaluate his sources when he makes an historical synthesis.

5. Tradition history is a method used to study the cultural, religious, and ideological background of the text. For example, 2 Kings 18:13, 17–19:38 (= Is 36–37) is possible to connect with Zion theology such as is presented in Psalms 46, 48, and 76, for example. These psalms deal with the attacks of nations against Zion and the way the Lord of creation, Yahweh, will rebuke these enemies and save his city. This same theme is visible also in many texts of Isaiah 1–39 (8:5–10; 17:12–14; 30:27–33; 31:4–9; 33) and gives the scholarly orientation in which the spiritual and theological atmosphere 2 Kings 18:13, 17–19:38 (= Is 36–37) has been composed.

6. The historical situation or setting of the text aims to detect all available historical information that can be acquired. In the case of 2 Kings 18:13, 17–19:38 it is possible to date the Assyrian invasion in Judah in 701 BC. We

have Sennacherib's own inscriptions related to this event as an independent source outside of the Bible. Sennacherib tells us that he was victorious and humiliated Hezekiah. The Greek historian, Herodotos (Book II, 141), preserved this story as he heard it from Egyptian priests, who recorded in their archives the mystical setback of the Assyrian army. The famous Lachish Reliefs found in the palace of Sennacherib in Niniveh depict how the Assyrian army besieged and overtook the city. Finally, we have also archaeological evidence that shows the total destruction of the cities of Judah in that year, 701.

All these methodological options give the modern scholar a better possibility of evaluating which kind of story we have in the Bible, when the biblical record recounts an extraordinary event or miracle, to use our modern term. If the scholar wants to continue and attempts to explain such an extraordinary event he must find good scientific solutions for the miracle. In case he succeeds, the phenomenon no longer can be characterized as a miracle because natural scientific causes have been discovered to explain it.

EXAMPLES OF SCIENTIFIC ATTEMPTS
TO *PROVE* A MIRACLE

The modern scholar who examines the story of a miracle attempts to find a relevant explanation to it by seeking cause-and-effect relations in it. An illustrative example could be the 10 plagues in Exodus and the way these events have been interpreted in the OT. The modern scholar can illumine the story of the 10 plagues by seeking possible prototypes in the ancient Near East. For example, he finds that even Egyptian sources (*The Admonitions of Ipuwer*) record that at certain times under certain circumstances the River Nile turned to blood.[35] Assuming that there is some real natural phenomenon behind this transformation of the river to blood, the scholar may present a theory that could explain the order of these plagues. Greta Hort has written an interesting article in which she presents the following natural theory for the plagues. Hort's theory is very detailed and I shall briefly summarize its main ideas.[36]

Heavy rains in the highlands of Ethiopia caused the tropical red earth in the basin of the Blue Nile and Atbara to be discharged into the river. This turned the water red. The Nile seemed to be turned to blood (first plague in July–August). A consequence was that oxygen decreased and great amounts of fish died. When fish did not eat the tadpoles, many frogs appeared (second plague in September–October). Unusual flooding and dead fish became a good breeding ground for insects, which can explain mosquitoes (third plague in October–November) and bloodsucking flies (fourth plague). The disease of cattle can be explained as having been caused by bacteria that multiplied in the dead fish and in the fly stings on the cattle (fifth plague). The inflammation or anthrax was caused by flies that transmitted this disease to human beings (sixth plague). In this way Hort could explain the six first plagues as natural consequences of the unusual high flooding of the Nile.

The plagues of hailstorms (seventh plague between November and March) and locusts (eighth plague in February–March) can easily be explained as frequent natural events in Egypt. So also the case of darkness (ninth plague in March), which is caused regularly by sandstorms called *khamsin*. Assuming that this chain of natural catastrophes followed each other in the land of Egypt, we can well imagine that it was understood as divine intervening. In this way the modern scholar may find relevant scientific explanation for the *miracles* recounted in the Book of Exodus. The result of this kind of scientific analysis is the explosion of the miracle narrative. In point of fact, in such a case, there were no miracles, namely, events contrary to natural laws.

Another example of the way to give a natural explanation to a miracle narrative is that regarding the mysterious destruction of the Assyrian army (2 Kgs 19:35). "That night the angel of the Lord went out and put to death a hundred and eighty-five thousand men in the Assyrian camp. When the people got up the next morning—there were all the dead bodies!" After having studied Sennacherib's inscriptions I conclude that they seem to follow the principle detected also in other Assyrian annals. All setbacks have been played down. Herodotos' story is another witness to the mysterious setback of the Assyrian army, and is independent of both the biblical narrative and Sennacherib's reports. Herodotos tells that field mice destroyed the weapons of the Assyrian soldiers. The mice-motif is probably connected to the god, Apollos Smintheus, that was responsible for the bubonic plagues.[37] In a corresponding way the angel motif has been used in the OT as referring to the bubonic plague (2 Sam 24). It is my view of the events of 701 BC in Judah that the Assyrian army was victorious, as indicated in 2 Kings 18:14−16, and Sennacherib's inscriptions; but that it was forced to stop its military invasion because of the bubonic plague.[38]

These examples give a good indication of how scholars can analyze wisely and accurately some of the biblical stories of miracles. On the other hand, it is clear that scholars do not always want to give a scientific explanation. One reason may be that they do not regard restricted scientific viewpoints to be good enough to solve the problem of some miracles described in the biblical text; or that they see that our present knowledge does not yet allow us to understand completely the dynamics of a given reported miracle. The American philosopher and the "father of semiotics," Charles Sanders Peirce, formulated this in a nice way:[39]

> If, walking in a garden on a dark night, you were suddenly to hear the voice of your sister crying to you to rescue her from a villain, would you stop to reason out the metaphysical question of whether it were possible for one

mind to cause material waves of sound and for another mind to perceive them? If you did, the problem might probably occupy the remainder of your days. In the same way, if a man undergoes any religious experience and hears the call of his Savior, for him to halt till he has adjusted a philosophical difficulty would seem to be an analogous sort of thing, whether you call it stupid or whether you call it disgusting. If on the other hand, a man has had no religious experience, then any religion not an affectation is as yet impossible for him; and the only worthy course is to wait quietly till such experience comes. No amount of speculation can take the place of experience.

NOTES

1. H. Frankfort and H. A. Frankfort, eds. (1977), *The Intellectual Adventure of Ancient Man: An Essay on Speculative Thought in the Ancient Near East*, Chicago: Chicago University Press.

2. See R. Mosis in *Theological Dictionary of the Old Testament (TDOT)* 2, 406–412.

3. I follow the New International Version translation if I do not interpret the text otherwise.

4. S. Wagner notes in his article concerning *môp't* (*TDOT* 8, 174–81) that 19 of 36 passages where the Hebrew word appears "occur in an immediate or, in a few instances, indirect connection with the Exodus event" (175). In a similar way F. J. Helfmeyer, in his article *'ôth* (*TDOT* 1, 167–88) asserts that the Hebrew word *'ôt* appears often in the contexts of Exodus events.

5. See, e.g., Job 24:17; Ps 78:43; 105:27; Neh 9:10.

6. According to H. J. Fabry (*TDOT* 9, 436–42), the secular use of *n's* remains speculative because the word is not mentioned in any of the Old Testament descriptions of battle. It is also worth noting that in the Qumran War Scroll (1QM) the Hebrew word *'ôt* denotes "military standard" and not *n's*. Cf. also Ps 74:4, quoted above.

7. See the meaning of *nes* in David J. A. Clines (2001), *The Dictionary of Classical Hebrew*, Sheffield: Sheffield Academic Press, 5:697. Concerning the late Hebrew and Aramaic texts see K. Beyer (1984), *Die aramäischen Texte vom Toten Meer*, Göttingen: Vandenhoeck und Ruprecht, 637; concerning the rabbinical Hebrew see M. Jastrow (2004), *Dictionary of the Targumim, Talmud Bavli, Talmud Yerushalmi and Midrashic Literature*, Judaica Treasury, 914–15; R. Rengstorff, Teras, *Theological Dictionary of the New Testament (TDNT)*, 8:113–26, especially 123–24; Y. Zakovitch, Miracle, *Anchor Bible Dictionary (ABD)* 4, 845–856, especially 845.

8. See J. Conrad, *pele'*, *Theological Dictionary of the Old Testament (TDOT)* 11, 533–46; quotation is from p. 534.

9. Ex 15:11; Is 25:1; Ps 77:14; 78:12; 88:10, 12.

10. The Hebrew expression *yam sûf* (Ex 10:19; 13:8; 15:4–22; 23:31; Ps 106:22) means the Reed Sea. In the Septuagint the name was translated *thalassa erythra* and through that term the translation Red Sea was established in many biblical translations.

11. See A. Carlson (1974), The Anti-Assyrian Character of the Oracle in Is IX:1–6, *Vetus Testamentus (VT)* 24, 130–35; A. Laato (1988), *Who Is Immanuel? The Rise and the Foundering of Isaiah's Messianic Expectations*, Turku: Åbo Akademi Förlag, 192–94.

12. See Ex 34:10; Jo 3:5; Jer 21:2; Ps 72:18; 78:4; 86:10; 98:1; 105:5; cf. also Ps 107:24.

13. See, e.g., Jgs 6:13; Ps 9:2; 26:7; Ps 71:17 [the verb *higgîd*]; 75:2; 96:3.

14. See this Baal myth, e.g., in J.C.L. Gibson (1978), *Canaanite Myths and Legends*, Edinburgh: Clark, 2–19, 37–81.

15. Frank M. Cross (1973), *Canaanite Myths and Hebrew Epic: Essays in the History of the Religion of Israel*, Cambridge: Harvard University Press, 112–44; Paul D. Hanson (1989), *The Dawn of Apocalyptic: The Historical and Sociological Roots of Jewish Apocalyptic Eschatology*, Philadelphia: Fortress, 300–303.

16. See Dt 33:2–3, 26–29; Jgs 5; and Ps 29, 77–78, 114.

17. Cross, *Canaanite Myths*, 144.

18. H. Wildberger (1978–82), *Jesaja 1–12*; *Jesaja 13–27*; *Jesaja 28–39*, *Biblischer Kommentar Altes Testament* X/1–3; Neukirchen-Vluyn: Neukirchener Verlag, especially *Jesaja 13–27*, 664–77.

19. Antti Laato (1998), *"About Zion I Will Not Be Silent!": The Book of Isaiah as an Ideological Unity*, *Coniectanea Biblica, Old Testament Series* 44, Stockholm: Almqvist and Wiksell International, especially 102–17.

20. C. Stuhlmueller (1970), *Creative Redemption in Deutero-Isaiah*, *Analecta Biblica* (AB) 43; Rome: Biblical Institute Press.

21. Ibid., 233. Italics are Stuhlmueller's.

22. See the Babylonian creation epic Enuma Elish in Stephanie Dalley (1992), *Myths from Mesopotamia: Creation, The Flood, Gilgamesh and Others*, Oxford: Oxford University Press, 228–77.

23. See the study by Hanson, *The Dawn of Apocalyptic*.

24. Gerhard Von Rad (1961), Das Formgeschichtliche Problem des Hexateuch, in *Gesammelte Studien zum Alten Testament (GSAT)*, Munich: Kaiser Verlag, 9–86.

25. Gerhard Von Rad (1982, 1984), *Theologie des Alten Testaments*, Band I–II, Munich: Kaiser Verlag.

26. See, e.g., Job 24:2–13; 1 Sam 12:8; Ps 78; 105; 136:1–26; Neh 9:6–14. It is worth noting that even these passages contain Hebrew terminology that refers to the mighty acts of God.

27. H. D. Preuss (1968), *Jahweglaube und Zukunftserwartung*, Stuttgart: Kohlhammer.

28. See Erkki Koskenniemi's contributions in this volume as well as his two main studies in this area: Erkki Koskenniemi (1994), *Apollonius von Tyana in der neutestamentlichen Exegese*, *Wissenschaftliche Uuntersuchungen zum Neuen Testament (WUNT)* II, 61, Tübingen: Mohr-Siebeck; Erkki Koskenniemi (2005), *The Old Testament Miracle-Workers in Early Judaism*, *WUNT* II, 206, Tübingen: Mohr-Siebeck.

29. See, e.g., Ex 22:17; Dt 18:10; Mi 5:11; Mal 3:5. A good survey of how magic and divination was practiced in ancient Palestine and Syria is Ann Jeffers (1996), *Magic and Divination in Ancient Palestine and Syria, Studies in the History and Culture of the Ancient Near East* 8, Leiden: Brill.

30. A good presentation of exegetical methods is O. H. Steck (1996), *Old Testament Exegesis: A Guide to the Methodology*, Atlanta: Scholars Press.

31. A good presentation of different textual evidences to the Old Testament is Emmanuel Tov (2001), *Textual Criticism of the Hebrew Bible*, Minneapolis: Fortress.

32. Scholars have established that Deuteronomy, Joshua, Judges, 1–2 Samuel, and 1–2 Kings consist of coherent historical work in which similar vocabulary, style, and theology have been used. They call this work Deuteronomistic History. This historical

74 Religious and Spiritual Events

work received its final form during the exile in the sixth century, but it contains earlier traditions that have been adopted, modified, and redacted.

33. The traditional German-style literary and redaction-critical method aimed to establish very accurately the wordings of earlier literary sources. However, I am skeptical regarding this proposal because we have the ability to follow the literary transmission of certain texts in the ancient Near East. These empirical models show that later editors could also make changes in the wordings of earlier texts. See J. H. Tigay (1982), *The Evolution of the Gilgamesh Epic*, Philadelphia: University of Pennsylvania Press; J. H. Tigay, ed. (1988), *Empirical Models for Biblical Criticism*, Philadelphia: University of Pennsylvania Press; H. J. Tertel (1994), *Text and Transmission: An Empirical Model for the Literary Development of Old Testament Narratives, Beiheft den Zeitschrift zur Alttestamentliche Wissenschaft (BZAW)* 221, Berlin: de Gruyter; Antti Laato (1996), *History and Ideology in the Old Testament Prophetic Literature: A Semiotic Approach to the Reconstruction of the Proclamation of the Historical Prophets, Coniectanea Biblica, Old Testament Series* 41; Stockholm: Almqvist and Wiksell International, 62–147.

34. Antti Laato (1995), The Assyrian Propaganda and the Historical Falsifications in the Royal Inscriptions of Sennacherib, *Vetus Testamentus (VT)* 45, 198–226. In fact, even in 2 Kings 18:13, 17–19:38 (cf. Isa 36–37) it is possible to detect two parallel stories.

35. See this text in James B. Pritchard, ed. (1955), *Ancient Near Eastern Texts Relating to the Old Testament*, Princeton: Princeton University Press, 441.

36. Greta Hort (1957), The Plagues of Egypt, *Zeitschrift zur Alttestamentliche Wissenschaft (ZAW)* 69, 84–103; Greta Hort (1958), *ZAW* 70, 48–59.

37. See, e.g., Bürchner (1927), Sminthe, Sminthos, *Paulys Real-Encyclopädie der classischen Altertumwissenschaft (PRECAW)* 2. Reihe III/1, Stuttgart, cols 724–25. The name Smintheus is etymologically derived from the Greek word *mus* (mouse).

38. Antti Laato, The Assyrian Propaganda, 198–226.

39. Charles Hartshorne and P. Weiss, eds. (1931–1935), *Collected Papers of Charles Sanders Peirce*, vols. 1–6; Arthur W. Burks, ed., vols. 7–8, Cambridge, Mass.: Harvard University Press. Reissued by the publisher in 1958. Quoting is from vol. 1.655. Peirce has also interesting philosophical discussions about God and his existence. D. R. Anderson (1995), has emphasized that religion is an important part of Peirce's philosophy even though scholars often have downplayed this aspect and regarded his transcendentalism as "cultured bacilli" in his worldview; *Strands of System: The Philosophy of Charles Peirce*, West Lafayette: Purdue University Press, vii.

REFERENCES

Beyer, K. (1984), *Die aramäischen Texte vom Toten Meer*, Göttingen: Vandenhoeck und Ruprecht.

Bürchner, L. (1927), Sminthe, Sminthos, in *Paulys Real-Encyclopädie der classischen Altertumwissenschaft* 2. Reihe III/1 Stuttgart, cols 724–25.

Carlson, A. (1974), The Anti-Assyrian Character of the Oracle in Is IX:1–6, *Vetus Testamentum (VT)* 24, 130–35.

Clines, David J. A. (2001), *The Dictionary of Classical Hebrew (DCH)*, Sheffield: Sheffield Academic Press.

Conrad, J. (2001), *Pele', Theological Dictionary of the Old Testament (TDOT)* 11, 533–46.

Cross, F. M. (1973), *Canaanite Myths and Hebrew Epic: Essays in the History of the Religion of Israel*, Cambridge: Harvard University Press.

Dalley, Stephanie (1992), *Myths from Mesopotamia: Creation, the Flood, Gilgamesh and Others*, Oxford: Oxford University Press.

Fabry, H. J. (1998), *n's Theological Dictionary of the Old Testament* 9, 436–42.

Frankfort, H. and H. A. Frankfort, eds. (1977), *The Intellectual Adventure of Ancient Man. An Essay on Speculative Thought in the Ancient Near East*, Chicago: Chicago University Press.

Gibson, J.C.L. (1978), *Canaanite Myths and Legends*, Edinburgh: T&T Clark.

Hanson, Paul D. (1989), *The Dawn of Apocalyptic. The Historical and Sociological Roots of Jewish Apocalyptic Eschatology*, Philadelphia: Fortress.

Helfmeyer, F. J. (1997), *'ôth, Theological Dictionary of the Old Testament (TDOT)* 1, 167–88.

Hort, Greta (1957–58), The Plagues of Egypt, *Zeitschrift für Alttestamentliche Wisssenschaft (ZAW)* 69, 84–103; *ZAW* 70, 48–59.

Jastrow, M. (2004), *Dictionary of the Targumim, Talmud Bavli, Talmud Yerushalmi and Midrashic Literature*, Judaica Treasury.

Jeffers, Ann (1996), *Magic and Divination in Ancient Palestine and Syria*, Leiden: Brill.

Koskenniemi, Erkki (1994), *Apollonius von Tyana in der neutestamentlichen Exegese*, Tübingen: Mohr-Siebeck.

Koskenniemi, Erkki (2005), *The Old Testament Miracle-Workers in Early Judaism*, Tübingen: Mohr-Siebeck.

Laato, Antti (1988), *Who Is Immanuel? The Rise and the Foundering of Isaiah's Messianic Expectations*, Turku: Åbo Akademi Förlag.

Laato, Antti (1995), The Assyrian Propaganda and the Historical Falsifications in the Royal Inscriptions of Sennacherib, *Vetus Testamentus (VT)* 45, 198–226.

Laato, Antti (1996), *History and Ideology in the Old Testament Prophetic Literature: A Semiotic Approach to the Reconstruction of the Proclamation of the Historical Prophets*, Stockholm: Almqvist and Wiksell International.

Laato, Antti (1998), *"About Zion I Will Not Be Silent!": The Book of Isaiah as an Ideological Unity*, Stockholm: Almqvist and Wiksell International.

Mosis, R. (1999), *Theological Dictionary of the Old Testament* 2, 406–12.

Peirce, Charles Sanders, C. Hartshorne, and P. Weiss, (eds.) (1931–1935, 1958), *Collected Papers of Charles Sanders Peirce*, vols. 1–6; Arthur W. Burks, ed., vols. 7–8, Cambridge, MA: Harvard University Press.

Preuss, H. D. (1968), *Jahweglaube und Zukunftserwartung*, Stuttgart: Kohlhammer.

Pritchard, J. B., ed. (1955), *Ancient Near Eastern Texts Relating to the Old Testament*, Princeton: Princeton University Press.

Rengstorff, R (1972), *Teras, Theological Dictionary of the New Testament (TDNT)* 8, 113–26.

Steck, O. H. (1995), *Old Testament Exegesis: A Guide to the Methodology*, Atlanta: Scholars Press.

Stuhlmueller, C. (1970), *Creative Redemption in Deutero-Isaiah*, Rome: Biblical Institute.

Tertel, H. J. (1994), *Text and Transmission: An Empirical Model for the Literary Development of Old Testament Narratives*, Berlin: de Gruyter.

Tigay, J. H. (1982), *The Evolution of the Gilgamesh Epic*, Philadelphia: University of Pennsylvania Press.

Tigay, J. H., ed. (1988), *Empirical Models for Biblical Criticism*, Philadelphia: University of Pennsylvania Press.

Tov, E. (2001), *Textual Criticism of the Hebrew Bible*, Minneapolis: Fortress.

Wagner, S. (1997), *môp?t, Theological Dictionary of the Old Testament* 8, 174–181.

von Rad, Gerhard (1961), Das formgeschichtliche Problem des Hexateuch, in *Gesammelte Studien zum Alten Testament*, Munich: Kaiser.

von Rad, Gerhard (1982, 1984), *Theologie des Alten Testaments. Band I–II*, Munich: Kaiser.

Wildberger, H. (1978-82), *Jesaja 1–12; Jesaja 13–27; Jesaja 28–39*, Neukirchen-Vluyn: Neukirchener Verlag.

Zakovitch, Y. (1992), Miracle, *Anchor Bible Dictionary (ABD)* 4, 845–56.

CHAPTER 5

OLD TESTAMENT FIGURES
AS MIRACLE WORKERS

Erkki Koskenniemi

Religio-historical investigation has carefully observed the contacts between the Greco-Roman miracle tradition and the New Testament (NT). Simultaneously, the rich Jewish tradition was too often overlooked.[1] This tradition included historical persons, like Theudas or the "Egyptian," but also the later reputation of the great figures of scripture. Later generations eagerly retold biblical stories, always changing more or less the original by adding, omitting, or modifying the biblical narrative. Thus it is a fascinating task to study exactly what was retained and what omitted, or what new material or perspective was introduced to the stories. This is the impact of the study of the "Rewritten Bible," or more precisely here, the study of rewritten biblical stories.[2] The investigation of the narrative tradition tells how and when new details were added to the reputation of the biblical figures. When the question of miracles is asked, markedly new traits are seen in the later traditions. I have investigated all Jewish texts retelling the Old Testament (OT) miracles diachronically in my book *The Old Testament Miracle-Workers in Early Judaism*. In this article I will briefly present the most important biblical figures who were treated as miracle workers in the later tradition.

ABRAHAM

The biblical material on Abraham includes nothing that a modern reader could define as miracles. However, the later tradition eagerly retold the stories and partly reshaped the figure of the father of the nation. In this tradition, Abraham was considered invincible, and sometimes he also performed miracles. Jews were known as great astrologers in classical antiquity. Some Jewish teachers rigorously rejected astrology as magic, but others proudly accepted it, and Abraham especially was presented as the father of all astrologers. The only biblical starting point was Genesis 15:5, which informs us merely that God showed Abraham the stars of heaven; but this was enough for people who were willing to present him as a master of all astrological knowledge. Artapanus, an Egyptian Jew, wrote a romantic, historical work, *Concerning the Jews*, that is preserved only in fragments; but in his work many biblical figures were reshaped as astrologers, especially Abraham.

Genesis tells us how God miraculously protected and saved Sarah, who had been taken from Abraham and led to Pharaoh's house. In the Jewish tradition, Abraham, who is a powerless man in the scripture, receives a more important role. The fragments from Qumran (*Genesis Apocryphon*, 20) inform us that Abraham prayed that the ruler must be punished, and tell us how God sent a spirit who tormented the king during two years such that no Egyptian was able to help him. The Pharaoh gave Sarah back, and Abraham was willing to help: he prayed for the king and laid his hands upon his head, and the spirit was banished from him. Perhaps this story helped people to make Abraham an exorcist, who expelled bird-like demons (cf. Gen. 15:11), as in the *Book of Jubilees* (11.11–13) and in the *Apocalypse of Abraham* (13.4–14). In this role, he certainly acted as patron of Jewish exorcists: what Abraham did could not be wrong.

MOSES

Although almost all the biblical stories were retold by ancient Jewish teachers, the stories about Moses received a special status. We hardly can imagine how minutely Jews studied these stories, finding both urgent problems and new solutions that are both rather alien to a modern reader's perspective.[3] This especially is true of the stories with miraculous elements. The later tradition reflects the ideas of the retellers. The stories of Moses' childhood and youth were retold and the miraculous traits were exaggerated. Moses' birth was foretold, he was born circumcised, and his capacity to learn was extraordinary.[4]

Both Philo and Josephus seem to have believed that God taught Moses to perform miracles in the theophany at Horeb, so that he could repeat them at will. Indeed, he needed these skills, because the Jewish tradition often retold in rich colors the meeting with Egyptian opponents. The opponents are interpreted as priests (Artapanus, Josephus), sorcerers (Jubilees, Philo), physicians (Artapanus), or bad philosophers (Philo): All these variants mean that the biblical story is used to attack a new front; the ancient scholars did not always distinguish sharply between their own time and the biblical era, but mostly used the biblical material to attack opponents of their own days. The tradition gave names to Moses' opponents (Jannes and Jambres),[5] and had here the evidence that miracles could also be performed by people hating God: some miracles were allowed and were done by God's will, some were not, but were caused by evil spirits.

All the Jewish writers known to me retold the plagues in Egypt (Ex 7:14–12:36) freely. The roles of God and Moses vary greatly. Sometimes, as in Wisdom 17, it is only God who performed miracles, but sometimes God is hardly mentioned, and Moses gains more importance. The writers change the order, omit some plagues or combine them with others, as Artapanus does (Fr. 3.27–33), and embellish the original with many interesting details. If they do not interpret the plagues allegorically, as Philo often does, they may describe the catastrophe in a way that adds new details, such as the gnats of Exodus 8:16–18. Sometimes the retelling simply exaggerates them, as when Josephus claims that the greater part of the Egyptians died from the wounds (Ex 9:8–12; *Antiquities* 2.304). Many details, like the unnatural darkness (Ex 10:21–29), were soon adopted by Christian writers like Melito of Sardes, and became a part of the Christian tradition.

Hardly any modern Bible reader is able to repeat in accurate order all the details of the events at the Red Sea (Ex 13:17–14:31), and all early Jewish versions deviate from the biblical original. The tradition treats Israel's overwhelming victory over the Egyptians freely and in rich colors. Ezekiel the Tragedian, for example, puts everything in the form of a classical Greek tragedy, imitating the famous *Persians* of Aeschylus. The narrative tradition, like Philo but especially *Biblical Antiquities* of Pseudo-Philo, knew that Israel was divided: some tribes were willing to surrender, others willing to fight (10.3). Of course, the number of drowned Egyptians was given variously, sometimes a million (Ezekiel the Tragedian, v. 203), sometimes (Josephus) in precise numbers of infantry, chariots, and horsemen (*Antiquities* 2.324). These events were never forgotten in Judaism: the Passover was always present in Israel, and the hymns celebrating the great miracle never ceased.

The Christian tradition has always used the journey from Egypt to Canaan in ethical instruction (cf. 1 Cor 10), but Jewish scholars had long before paved the way for such applications of the Exodus and the triumphal and redemptive metaphor that it became. For Philo especially, the escape from Egypt and the trials on the way meant, allegorically, that the soul must leave pleasures and go through much arduous labor to freedom. This kind of escape meant, according to him, that a human being becomes as divine as possible through the ordeal. The model is openly Platonic.[6] But all the biblical stories lived in literal interpretation, too, and with new details. The miracles of manna, the water from the rock, the mutiny of Korah and his sons (or did the sons join their father?),[7] Israel's punishment by snakes, and the miraculous help through the bronze snake were, like all biblical miracles, retold in early Jewish tradition. They attest to the way in which the concept of miracle was alive in Judaism.

Moses' death meant a puzzling problem for early Jewish teachers. On the one hand, the Torah says that he died. On the other, "Moses" tells about his own death in the Torah. Moreover, Deuteronomy 34:1–8 first tells about the death and burial of Moses, and then informs us that he was "a hundred and twenty years old when he died, yet his eyes were not weak nor his strength diminished." These two details allowed different speculations about the end of his earthly life. Some thought that he did not die *at all*. Moses died and did not die, in the tradition. These various versions were to some degree compatible with and perhaps reflective of Greco-Roman mythology. Josephus depicts Moses as disappearing like Aeneas or Romulus (*Antiquities* 4.326). However, one is reminded that similar stories were told in the scripture about Enoch and Elijah.

Like Abraham, the father of the nation, Moses, the law-giver, was always present in early Judaism. The scripture often tells about Moses' great deeds, which meant that his miracles were retold and reshaped for centuries, first among Jews and then among Christians, as well.

JOSHUA

In most cases, the scripture tells about miracles of God, and although human beings may act as his helpers, it is usually clear that the great deeds are not their work but God's. Werner Kahl developed a useful tool that leads scholars to ask for the role of the human beings.[8] This role is clearly a subject of variation in the later tradition. When God led Israel to Canaan, he and not Joshua performed the great miracles, namely, stopped the Jordan (Jo 3:1–5:1) and destroyed the walls of Jericho (Jo 5:13–6:27). Already here, Joshua acted as God's helper and as a superb leader of the nation. Moreover, he was able to stop the sun with his prayer (Jo 10:8–14). But Joshua understandably may receive a stronger role as miracle worker in the later tradition.

The militant Joshua was, however, a person who divided opinions in later traditions. Ben Sira could still refer to his deeds freely (Sir 46:1–8), but he was a problematic figure for people who had to deal with foreign overlords in Israel. Josephus heavily abridges the stories of Joshua, and certainly not emphasize his militant miracles (*Antiquities* 5.17–61). However, there were others who took the opposite direction. Joshua, the spirit-filled and militant leader of the nation, was highly esteemed by everyone who was waiting for God's help against overlords. This part of the tradition is preserved only in fragments, but it illumines the distinctively Jewish element in miracle stories. Miracles and God's help in the sacred history belong together with the hope for a useable future. The eschatological hope waited for another man like Joshua. This thought is attested in the fragments the last Jewish rebels left behind in Masada during the Jewish war.[9] Understandably, Josephus and other authors collaborating with Romans were not emphasizing the material that had stimulated, for example, Theudas and the "Egyptian."[10]

SAMSON

Samson, the spirit-filled judge (Jgs 13–16), was simultaneously a problem and an inspiration for early Jewish teachers. On the one hand, he was not an ideal model for later Jews; his sexual morals and his affair with Delilah, the Philistine woman, were not compatible with the ideals with which Jewish teachers were inclined to inspire their followers. We happen to have a Jewish sermon that explains how Samson, the man of God, could lose the spirit and be beaten by his enemies. The reason was, of course, that his errors gave Satan an opportunity to destroy his power.[11]

On the other hand, Samson was clearly a man of God. The spirit moving him around and his extraordinary physical power made him useful for everyone who supported brutal violence against the opponents of Israel. Pseudo-Philo, in his *Biblical Antiquities*, retells these stories, expanding them and emphasizing the violence (42–43). Josephus, of course, shows that after the Jewish war he had learned his lesson. He had no more interest in spirit-filled men who mixed religion with militant violence. A careful investigation of Josephus' text shows that the role of the divine spirit is removed from the stories (*Antiquities* 5.276–316). Sometimes, retelling biblical stories meant a quarrel about the heritage of Judaism. Josephus, who had promised that he did not add or omit anything (*Antiquities* 1.17) in his accounts of the history of his people, nonetheless, took part in this quarrel through additions, omissions, and changes.

DAVID

The biblical David did nothing that we would call a miracle. However, the scripture tells us something which could be and indeed was useful for the retellers of later generations. It is told that an evil spirit tormented Saul, and that David was sought to relieve his problems with playing music (1 Sam 16:14–23). This was enough for later Jewish exorcists. Pseudo-Philo expands the story by rendering the psalm David sang. In this psalm, David exactly tells the cosmological origin of the demons and threatens the spirit with a harsh punishment (60.1–3).

The psalm added by Pseudo-Philo resembles hymns in Qumran (esp. 11Q11) and attest that Jews attempted to ward off evil spirits with help of biblical and more or less reworked Psalms inside as well as outside of the walls of Qumran. In this tradition, the decisive element seemed to have been the cosmological knowledge. An exorcist who was able to describe the cosmological order got the upper hand over evil spirits. God created the world and set here his order, and it is not allowed that any spirit should violate it by assaulting God's people. On the other hand, the *Book of Jubilees* (10) boldly says that the reason why there are demons in the world is that it is their mission to assault all nations except Israel and lead them astray.

ELIJAH

The biblical Elijah (1 Kgs 17–2 Kings 2) caused enthusiasm and problems similar to the ambivalence felt regarding Joshua. Elijah, who did numerous miracles in scripture, was the zealous prophet who fearlessly stood before kings, attacked the false prophets, and killed hundreds of them. He called fire from heaven to destroy his enemies, and finally he left this world in a fiery chariot. Malachi promised that Elijah the prophet would return to this world to complete a new mission given by God.

Ben Sira could still celebrate Elijah freely without political reservations (48:1–11). At least in the times of *Biblical Antiquities* of Pseudo-Philo (48.1) he was even identified with Phinehas, another zealous servant of God (Num 25:6–15). The man who was expected to return had returned already once and saved Israel. This identification attests how closely miracles were connected with politics. Josephus, of course, treated Elijah with caution and did not emphasize his political fervor (*Antiquities* 8.319–9.28). However, the power of the biblical stories prevented him from completely removing Elijah's political import.

ELISHA

Unlike his teacher, Elijah (1 Kgs 19–2 Kgs 13), Elisha never found a marked reputation in early Judaism as a leader. Of course, the stories of his miracles were noted (cf. Sir. 48:12–16) and Josephus was clearly fond of him (cf. *Antiquities* 8.535–s9.180). However, in the scripture Elisha rarely played a political role, which means that he was never a favorite of later militant miracle-workers. However, not all miracles needed political importance. Some of them happened in the ordinary circles of daily life. It is precisely here that Elisha's miracles could be imitated. Healings, feedings, resuscitations of dead people; surprisingly many of Elisha's miracles were repeated in Jesus' activity.

ISAIAH

Sometimes the rewriting of the scripture narratives already begins within the OT, itself. A good example of that is what the Hebrew Bible (OT) says about the miracles of Isaiah, namely the healing of the king Hezekiah. The story is reported with a prominent role for the agency of the prophet in the similar narratives of 2 Kings 18:13–20:11 and Isaiah 36:1–38:22; but in 2 Chronicles 32 the prophet's role has been almost totally forgotten. Ben Sira, for his part, gives a role back to Isaiah and expands it (48:20–25). It was now Isaiah who turned the sun back and prolonged the king's life. Taken separately, the lines in Ben Sira attribute a very strong role to the prophet, and only the wider context and the Jewish faith tradition prevented the reader from interpreting Isaiah as a figure who was able to perform great miracles without God's help. Ben Sira apparently considered God's covenant with David broken, and did not emphasize the role of the king.[12] The king's normally primary role is reduced. The author was not awaiting a Davidic king. Other figures, like prophets, took the role of David's divinely inspired dynasty.

JEREMIAH

When Jesus asked his followers to tell him who he was thought to be, according to popular opinion, they replied, "Some say John the Baptist; others say Elijah; and still others, Jeremiah or one of the prophets" (Matthew 16:14). This answer is one of the several fragments illuminating the role of Jeremiah in the later tradition. The scripture only tells about his prophecies, but early Judaism knew more. Unfortunately, we only have fragments of this tradition. However, *Second Maccabees* reports that in Judah's vision, Jeremiah gives a sword from heaven to the Jews (2 Macc 15.13–16). The *Lives of the Prophets*, a collection of small biographies of the biblical prophets, refers to Jeremiah's miracles in Egypt where he was exiled. He offered protection against snakes and crocodiles, a role that Egyptians used to give Horus. In the *Life of Jeremiah*, the prophet also takes and hides the ark, which is protected from the enemies, and causes a rock to swallow it. There it waits for the resurrection and the end of the world. This is only one of the several versions of the story of how the ark was rescued when the enemies destroyed Jerusalem.[13] Apparently, Jeremiah became a strong, eschatological figure. Some of his extrabiblical miracles were militant.

DANIEL

The figure of Daniel, the sage at kings' courts, offers a good example of how the tradition of the biblical miracles unfolded in early Judaism. The book of Daniel was not yet written when the Egyptian Jews translated the scripture into Greek as the Septuagint (LXX). The Aramaic and the Greek texts found their final form very slowly. The role of miracles and miracle-workers varies between these two different versions. But the later writings in particular reworked the traditions that had already been written before the book of Daniel, and set new accents. *The Life of Daniel*, for example, pays attention only to the story told in chapter 4, and introduces Behemoth, the demon who tortured the king. Daniel's faithful intercession during seven years led to forgiveness for the king's sins and to his healing. This all shows how flexibly stories could be used in the later tradition.

EZEKIEL

Sometimes the later tradition needed only a few biblical words to produce a miracle story. At other times a long passage was reinterpreted and a miracle was introduced into it. The use of the long biblical book of Ezekiel offers examples of both, and more. Ezekiel 47:10 mentions fishermen ("Fishermen will stand along the shore; from En Gedi to En Eglaim there will be places for spreading nets"). Apparently, these words were enough to produce a tradition, which the *Life of Ezekiel* (v. 11a) summarizes as follows. "Through prayer he furnished them of his own accord with an abundant supply of fish." The *Life* does not tell more, and apparently the author considered it needless. The background story was apparently well known to the ancient audience, but unfortunately not to us.

A completely different history of tradition is revealed when another passage in the *Life of Ezekiel* is examined.[14] The biblical book of Ezekiel includes in chapter 37 a vision of dead bones that are miraculously resuscitated. The historical sense of the vision is unambiguous: The people of Israel will rise again and return from the exile. Now, however, the interpretation is very concrete. The prophet showed the miracle of resuscitation to the enemies of Israel. The *Life* is not the only source in which the concrete interpretation is attested. It appears in fragments at Qumran (4Q385) and surprisingly often in early Christian sources. The prophecy made Ezekiel a prophet who revived dead people, and this tradition could be used in various ways.

CONCLUSION

The modern reader no longer lives in the world of the people who lived in the time of the NT. Historical analysis helps us to understand how ancient people interpreted what they heard and read. When dealing with miracles, the task has been and is very difficult. However, it should be clear that the vivid Jewish miracle tradition has been widely neglected. The biblical stories of the OT miracles were frequently retold, often freely and innovatively. Biblical passages that do not include miracles at all were reinterpreted. This tradition of telling and retelling miracles often included narratives of battles between good and evil spirits. Miracles could be militant, but they could also happen in ordinary daily life and play no political role. Consequently, the traditions could empower political leaders, attempting to legitimate themselves with traditional miracles. It could also encourage people to apply to the Jewish world all the Mediterranean magic and call themselves followers of Solomon the wise. This fascinating setting forms the background of Jesus' miracles in the Gospels.

The history of investigation shows that it has not been easy for scholars to deal with miracles. We have often been tempted to think we are much smarter and understand everything better than ancient people. The scholarly failures that have derived from that supposition should make us cautious.

NOTES

1. See my article "The Religious-Historical Background of the New Testament Miracles" in this volume, chapter 7.

2. The term "Rewritten Bible" was first used by Geza Vermes and soon by several scholars who, unfortunately, used the phrase differently. See Erkki Koskenniemi and Pekka Lindqvist, *Rewritten Bible, Rewritten Stories*, Studies in Rewritten Bible 1, Antti Laato and Jacques van Ruiten, eds., in press.

3. Pekka Lindqvist investigates the story of Moses, who broke the tablets of the Law, and presents how problematic early Jewish writers found the story, in her book, *Sin at Sinai: Early Judaism Encounters Exodus, 32, Studies in Rewritten Bible 2,* Åbo, in press.

4. See especially Artapanus, Fr. 3.1–4, and *Biblical Antiquities* 9, but also Philo, *Moses* 1.1–33 and Josephus, *Antiquities* 2.205–37.

5. See especially the ancient book about Pharaoh's magicians, *Jannes and Jambres*, preserved today in fragments, but referred to by Pliny, Philo, Origen, and the *Decretum Galasii.* A strong ancient tradition on magic preceded this work.

6. See Wendy E. Helleman (1990), Philo of Alexandria on Deification and Assimilation to God, *The Studia Philonica Annual* 2, 51–71.

7. According to Numbers 16:32, Korah and his sons were killed, but they are subsequently mentioned in Numbers 26:11. Consequently, Pseudo-Philo allows the sons to reject their father's call and confess their commitment to the Law (16:5).

8. Kahl has helped scholars to consistently ask who is making, who is mediating, and who is praying for a miracle, or in his terms, who is the BNP ("Bearer of the Numinous Power" actually causing the miracle), who the MNP ("Mediator of the Numinous Power" used as the agent of the BNP), and who the PNP ("Petitioner of the Numinous Power" asking the BNP to make the miracle). See Werner Kahl (1994), *New Testament Miracle Stories in their Religious-Historical Setting. A Religionsgeschichtliche Comparison from a Structural Perspective, Forschungen zur Religion und Literatur des Alten und Neuen Testaments (FRLANT)* 163, 62–65, Göttingen: VandenHoeck und Ruprecht.

9. See Shemaryahu Talmon (1996), Fragments of a Joshua Apocryphon— Masada 1039–211 (Final Photo 5254), *Journal of Jewish Studies (JJS)* 47, 128–39.

10. See chapter 7 of this volume.

11. See the sermon, De Sampsone, translated in German in Folke Siegert's work (1980 and 1992, respectively), *Drei hellenistisch-jüdische Predigten Ps.-Philon, "Über Jona," "Über Jona" (Fragment) und "Über Simson." I. Übersetzung aus dem Armenischen und sprachliche Erläuterungen; and II. Kommentar nebst Beobachtungen zur hellenistischen Vorgeschichte der Bibelhermeneutik, Wissenschaftliche Untersuchungen zum Neuen Testament (WUNT),* Tubingen: Mohr-Siebeck, 60–61.

12. See Helge Stadelmann (1980), *Ben Sira als Schriftgelehrter. Eine Untersuchung zum Berufsbild des vormakkabäischen Sofer unter Berücksichtigung seines Verhältnisses zu Priester-, Propheten, und Weisheitslehrertum, Wissenschaftliche Untersuchungen zum Neuen Testament (WUNT)* 2.6, Tübingen: Mohr-Siebeck, 204–205.

13. See Anna Maria Schwemer, *Studien zu den frühjüdischen Prophetenlegenden Vitae Prophetarum I–II*, 1995–96, *Texte und Studien zum Antiken Judentum (TSAJ)* 49, 203–10, Tübingen: Mohr-Siebeck.

14. See Brook W. R. Pearson, "Dry Bones in the Judean Desert: The Messiah of Ephraim, Ezekiel 37, and the Post-Revolutionary Followers of Bar Kokhba," *Journal for the Study of Judaism (JJS)* 29 (1998): 192–201.

REFERENCES

Helleman, Wendy E. (1990), Philo of Alexandria on Deification and Assimilation to God, *The Studia Philonica Annual* 2, 51–71.

Kahl, Werner (1994), *New Testament Miracle Stories in Their Religious-Historical Setting. A Religionsgeschichtliche Comparison from a Structural Perspective*, Göttingen: VandenHoeck und Ruprecht, *Forschungen zur Religion und Literature des Alten und Neuen Testaments (FRLANT)* 163.

Koskenniemi, Erkki (2005), *The Old Testament Miracle-Workers in Early Judaism, Wissenschaftliche Untersuchungen zum Neuen Testament (WUNT)* II/206, Tübingen: Mohr-Siebeck.

Koskenniemi, Erkki, and Pekka Lindqvist, *Rewritten Bible, Rewritten Stories*, in *Studies in Rewritten Bible* 1, Antti Laato and Jacques van Ruiten, eds., Åbo Akademi, in press.

Lindqvist, Pekka, Sin at Sinai: Early Judaism Encounters Exodus 32, in *Studies in Rewritten Bible* 2, Antti Laato and Jacques van Ruiten, eds., Åbo Akademi, in press.

Pearson, Brook W. R. (1998), Dry Bones in the Judean Desert: The Messiah of Ephraim, Ezekiel 37, and the Post-Revolutionary Followers of Bar Kokhba, *Journal for the Study of Judaism (JSJ)* 29, 192–201.

Schwemer, Anna Maria (1995–96), *Studien zu den frühjüdischen Prophetenlegenden Vitae Prophetarum I–II, Texte und Studien zum Antiken Judentum (TSAJ)* 49, Tübingen: Mohr-Siebeck.

Shemaryahu, Talmon (1996), Fragments of a Joshua Apocryphon—Masada 1039–211, (Final Photo 5254), *Journal for Judaic Studies (JJS)* 47, 128–39.

Siegert, Folke (1980), *Drei hellenistisch-jüdische Predigten Ps.-Philon, "Über Jona," Über Jona" (Fragment) und "Über Simson" I, Übersetzung aus dem Armenischen und sprachliche Erläuterungen.* Tübingen: Mohr-Siebeck; Folke Siegert (1992), *Drei hellenistisch-jüdische Predigten Ps.-Philon, "Über Jona," Über Jona" (Fragment) und "Über Simson" II, Kommentar nebst Beobachtungen zur hellenistischen Vorgeschichte der Bibelhermeneutik. Wissenschaftliche Untersuchungen zur Neuen Testament (WUNT)* 60–61, Tübingen: Mohr-Siebeck.

Stadelmann, Helge (1980), *Ben Sira als Schriftgelehrter. Eine Untersuchung zum Berufsbild des vormakkabäischen Sofer unter Berücksichtigung seines Verhältnisses zu Priester-, Propheten und Weisheitslehrertum, Wissenschaftliche Untersuchengen zum Neuen Testament (WUNT)* 2, 6, Tübingen: Mohr-Siebeck.

CHAPTER 6

Moses' Competition with Pharaoh's Magicians

Andre LaCocque

There is miracle and miracle. Or, more accurately, there is miracle and there is prodigy, two aspects of the "wonderful" that need to be mutually distinguished. The Hebrew vocabulary does not always differentiate the two in the Old Testament (OT) stories. Their domains overlap and there is a reason for this, as we shall see: *interpretation* of the sign is decisive.

This chapter focuses on a somewhat embarrassing text, which is strategically situated at the heart of Israel's self-consciousness, namely, in the book of Exodus. The story has to do with Moses' training before his return to Egypt, where a price has been put on his head (Ex 4:1–9). After repeated objections by Moses to God's mission, he is commissioned to perform a series of three awesome acts that should convince Egyptians and Hebrews alike of God's presence and power. Convincing Pharaoh was designed to get him to let the Israelites out of bondage. Convincing the Hebrews was intended to encourage them effectively to leave.

Let us reflect upon the differentiations to be made between the supernatural and the miracle proper, concentrating on this most intriguingly relevant text. Exodus 4:1–9 presents all the appearances of magic. Scholars have regularly stumbled over these verses that, biblically speaking, are unexpected and paradoxical. The very fact that Egyptian magicians are capable of duplicating most of the wonders displayed by Moses and Aaron at Pharaoh's court seems sufficient to give any reader a spontaneous impression of unease.

Yet, that initial reaction may be premature and bypass the essential message of the text. Moses' signs are *polyvalent*, differing in their psychological bearing according to three elements: the person of the miracle-worker, the nature of the wonder, and the conflicting standpoints of the witnesses. The Egyptians and the Hebrews do not see the same phenomena eye to eye. We can draw substantial conclusions if we sharpen our definition of the miracle and the sign within it.

THE SUPERNATURAL AND THE MIRACLE

Edgar Poe considered that when the supernatural is approached through the "Calculus of Probabilities," it is an anomaly to apply "the most rigidly exact in science . . . to the shadow and spirituality of the most intangible in speculation."[1] Belief in a miracle or in a prodigious event rests upon the conviction that there exists an invisible powerhouse, a *heaven*, that at times breaks through from the invisible to the visible (see Is 64:1).

The miracles that the present world acknowledges are of the medical order, of the electronic sphere, of special exploration, of genetic manipulation, and the like. Today, Moses' burning bush would be a technical creation at Hollywood. Such wonders leave us blasé or desperate. For, in a one-dimensional technological world, the human being is a senseless speck lost in a meaningless horizontal cosmos. Desperation leads to violence, for the feeling of emptiness must be assuaged by something to fill it, even though it be artificial or compulsory. Hitler found fellow Germans that had lost all vision of a goal, and he provided the illusion of a transcending goal, through rage and outrage.

Regarding Exodus 4 and its display of prodigies, the word "technical ethos" comes from the pen of Martin Buber in his book on Moses.[2] In that Exodus narrative, we are facing manifestations of wonders presented as "proofs of truth," an idea otherwise generally foreign to biblical literature. Martin Buber reminds us that, for the prophets, a miracle is a signification of some transcendent truth, and such a sign is the incarnation of that revealed truth. That is different than the miracle being a proof (see Is 20:3; Ez 4:3).

One of the terms used in the Bible for the miraculous is *niphla'oth*, a problematic designation. It properly means marvels and suggests something contradicting the natural and scientific laws; though Buber erroneously says that the miraculous in the Bible is never contrary to nature. On the contrary, the term *sign* (*'oth* in Hebrew; in the New Testament [NT] Greek, *semeion*), signifies a heavenly or divine truth. The miracle does not suppress the natural, but transfigures it; "eternity changes it," says Mallarmé. When the prophet Elisha heals Naaman the Syrian, the latter's leprosy is not denied but, as it were, set within God's intent for creation, which does not include the maladies that plague humanity (cf. 2 Kgs 5).

A biblical miracle is an *historical* act, that is, a history-shaping event, as can be seen, for example, when the fleeing Hebrews crossed the Sea of Reeds. As such, the witness of the sign does not focus on the materiality of the phenomenon, but upon its value as revelation of a transcending reality. This is especially clear in the reports of Jesus' miracles (see the Lukan theology in 2:20; 17:15; 18:43; 19:17; Acts 5:13).

The Hebrew discourse about miracles does not always distinguish clearly between the miraculous and the prodigious. The Gospel of John is more precise on the topic. Jesus' miracles are called signs, *semeia*, while what the populace demands are supernatural-appearing wonders, *terata*. We find both words in the same saying of Jesus in John 4:48. They are not, however, synonymously used. Remarkably, the Nazarean's miracles invariably enjoin the beneficiaries to praise God. That way, the attention is deflected from the miracle-maker and from any self-reference of the phenomenon. The miracle "rends the veil" (cf. Mt 27:51 and para.) and reveals the divine intervention in human time and space. In other words, the miracle is prophetic (cf. Ps 74:9).[3]

As such, the sign demands interpretation, itself interpreting the human reality in a sense that surprises, in that it does not remain at the surface level of meaning but renders audible or visible a more profound message or proclamation begging to be revealed (cf. Mt 8:4; Lk 17:14). On this score, the miracle is less the irruption of the *extraordinary* than of *God's ordinary*. It puts the creation back on track towards its plenitude. It is an "anti-sin." Characteristically, Jesus says, "Go and sin no more" (Jn 5:14; 8:11). That is why miracles are the presence of eternity, that is, eschatological markers at the heart of human development and the unfolding of human history.

This cannot be said of a prodigy or wonder. Of course, miracle and prodigy have something in common: they are both *wonder*ful. They are arresting. A prodigy can even at times become a sign. However, while the miracle has prodigious dimensions, the prodigy does not necessarily have a miraculous value. In Exodus 4, for example, it is conceivable to have an Egyptian magician duplicating, at least to some extent, Moses' wonders (cf. 7:9–12:22; see 8:3), but it is unimaginable that magicians work a miracle proper, in the sense of their action signifying some divine or heavenly meaning. Of this, the biblical texts are unanimous in their denial (see Gn 41:8, 24; Dan 1:20; 2:2, 10, 27; 5:7–8; Acts 13:6–12). This is evident when the Egyptian magicians are defeated in their own game by Moses' wonders, although we are at that point still in the domain of sheer extraordinary manifestations.

Moses, ever since the beginning of his dialogue with God, set himself on the terrain of magical performances as the means for establishing three things: his personal authority, the foundation of his call, and his immunity from the Egyptian death threat against his life. His only excuse is his belief that magic is the sole language capable of persuading both Pharaoh and the Israelites in Egypt. Pure miracles, so to speak, would have isolated Moses and Aaron. For the miracles are valid only within the parameters of the people of Israel. Their effectiveness is intramural because they occur each time as a kind of theophany for Israel; and there is no theophany of Israel's God outside of Israel. Hence, what Exodus 4 displays is not a series of miracles, but a series of wonders; a more neutral term susceptible of designating either a prodigy or a prophetic sign, or perhaps both at the same time, according to whomever is interpreting it.

The prodigious aspect of Moses' demonstration puts the whole scene on a stage familiar to Egyptian soothsayers: magic. In this sense, the performance and counter-performance are elements of a *dialogue*. Moses, like St. Paul later, becomes "all things to all people" (1 Cor 9:22). The psychological lesson is of great importance. Moses in Egypt behaves and acts as an Egyptian. We are at the antipode of arrogance. Moses does not import a worldview so foreign to his audience as to be totally incomprehensible. Yet, if he does at all, it must be veiled (cf. Ex 34:33) and "as in a glass darkly" (cf. 1 Cor. 13:12), lest it be so strong as to blind instead of to illumine the Egyptians. And the Israelites, perhaps? The competition with the Egyptians has an aspect of compassion. Moses' purpose is not to destroy his competitors, but to convince them. From this perspective, there *must* be a margin of freedom left to the magicians in their response to Moses. Pure miracles would paralyze them. Soon this will be demonstrated in full when the miracle of the Sea of Reeds will occur; it will open itself to the Hebrews and close itself upon the drowning Egyptian army. Evidently, at that point the dialogue was over. Meanwhile, at the court of Pharaoh, Moses must defeat the Egyptians at their own game.

A closer look at the vocabulary of Exodus 4, describing the future of Moses' performance in Egypt, will help one focus on the nature of these extraordinary phenomena. Throughout the pericope, the word *'oth* (sign) is used. In verse 8, for instance, we find the term repeated twice; in verses 17, 28, 30, the same word appears in the plural, *'othoth*. We have encountered the same situation above about the Gospel of John (*semeia*). Moses' signs may, however, be called, by some and in some circumstances, marvels. In verse 21 the term *mophthim* is found with this meaning; but, whether in the former case or in the latter, the wonders here are *signs*. They are no gratuitous and random acts; they *signify* something. So it is not surprising that we see the miracles associated with the term *qol* (voice) (verses 1, 8, 9), or with *peh* (mouth) (verses 10, 11, 12, 15 [three times], 16); three times with *peh* and seven times with *qol*.

The expressed purpose of the signs is to earn the trust and faith of the people (see verses 1, 5, 8 [two times], 9, 31), and to convince Pharaoh to let God's people go (verses 21, 23 [two times]; note that the verb "to send" is again used five times in associated contexts: verses 4 [twice], 13 [twice], 28). This duality of purpose corresponds to the duality of interpretation offered by the ambivalence of the signs. The latter may appear to the Egyptians as sheer performance challenging their own know-how. To the Hebrews, in contrast, the signs are fraught with divine message, with proclamation *(ker-ygma)*. Exodus 11:3 makes a clear distinction between "in the sight of Pharaoh's officials and in the sight of the people" (of Israel).

ON EXODUS 4:1–9

Let us take one example from among the three wonders Moses performed in Egypt. It seems clear that for the water of the Nile to be changed into blood (verse 9) is no random transubstantiation. To the Egyptians, this meant death. To the Hebrews, it was something like an unveiling of their suffering under Egyptian taskmasters. Therefore, we should probe all the signs as to what kind of message they may convey.

In fact, there are three elements involved: the signs themselves; the recipients of the signs (Egyptians and Hebrews); and the person of the sign-worker (God/Moses/Aaron). This latter element must be emphasized and singled out as the main one of the three. Moses is the performer, but God is the giver of the wonders. The text's attribution of them to God thwarts, from the outset, all magical interpretation. Only their duplication by the Egyptians is magical and, therefore, the competition at the court of Pharaoh is not magic against magic but *logos* against *magos*.[4]

Moses is the carrier of a message, he is no magician. Of course, he can be mistaken as one, like Daniel later will be considered as the chief of Nebuchadnezzar's magicians (Dan 4:9; 5:11). Yet, this is an optical illusion, as it were, on the part of the gentiles. For in reality the Pharaoh is facing, in the person of Moses, a prophet (cf. Dt 34:10); a servant of the Lord (Dt 34:5; Ps 105:26); God's elect (Ps 106:23); indeed the mouthpiece of God himself (Ex 4:16; 7:1). The pagan confusion is powerfully denounced in Daniel's declaration to King Nebuchadnezzar, "The mystery about which the king inquires, no wise man, astrologer, magician, or diviner can set forth before the king, but there is a God in heaven who reveals mysteries" (Dan 2:27–28). As usual in the Bible, the messengers are hidden behind their message. Joseph, Moses, Daniel, all the prophets in Israel, deflect the attention from themselves to God who sent them. Is, then, a psychological approach to the human heralds made inappropriate or improper? Indeed not, as we shall see below; but some aspects of the signs must first be clarified.

From what precedes, we may conclude that Moses' demonstration is *revelatory*. The Egyptian courtiers' misunderstanding is reported tongue in cheek. Their blindness is incurable. They have eyes but do not see (cf. Ps 135:16). They are fascinated by the spectacle and ignore its meaning. However, when their eyes are opened, the spectacle becomes highly symbolic, as when Jesus changed the water into wine at Cana (Jn 2), unmistakably referring to the sacrament of the Eucharist ushering in Christ's passion (see Jn 2:4).

THE SIGN AS SYMBOL

Are Moses' signs symbols? Moses performs an act of transubstantiation, the change of the Nile waters into blood. Here also the context is clear. It is the truth of the matter that the channel of life to the land of Egypt is a river of blood, metaphorically the blood of the slaves compelled to build mausoleums to dead pharaohs and dignitaries. It is the truth that the "house of slavery" is obsessed with death and pours the blood of the living on the stones of funerary monuments. Thus, the pouring by Moses of the Egyptian water on the ground goes much beyond witchcraft. It broadens the perspective to the whole land of oppression and metaphorically signifies its destruction. What used to be the vital artery of the country is punctured and the blood gushes out until Egypt is bloodless. Some time, in the near future, the tenth plague hitting Egypt will actualize that which the third sign in Exodus 4 signified (see Ex 12:20 ff.).

Another reference to blood spilled on the ground is Cain spilling Abel's blood, of which we read in Genesis 4 (see verses 10–11). Here again, the blood is shed by a wicked agent, Cain. Hence, Exodus 4 may allude to Egypt as a collective Cain the murderer, as both pericopes are from the hand of the same author. There are also other biblical texts denouncing the scandal of human blood polluting the soil. It clamors for justice or vindication (see Is 26:21; Ez 9:9; Jb 16:18). Only blood can redeem the victims' blood (Nm 35:33; Ps 106:38). Moses and the people are living in an impure land, polluted by crime, violence, and inhumanity. It tries to hide its pollution behind a deceptive culture and other architectural artifacts; but the hiding is in vain, for the Egypt unveiled by Moses' sign is like a bloody naked rock (Ez 24:8).

"To the one a fragrance of death to death, to the other a fragrance of life to life" (2 Cor 2:16; cf. Ws 18:8). If the Egyptians do not understand the portentous bearing of the sign, soon the first plague will fulfill the omen in a terrible way: Moses strikes the Nile with his staff "and there was blood in the land of Egypt" (Ex 7:21).

With this last of the three signs given by God to empower Moses, we have gone from metamorphosis to metamorphosis. The other two signs follow suit in terms of their bearing. Even Moses' stick upon which he leans is something of a serpent, that is, something impure to God and a fiend to the humans. Does it look like a staff or does it look like a snake? Is it a serpent or a support? Moses leaning on such a dubious staff is surely no possessor of immortality. He is fundamentally vulnerable, constantly accompanied by tokens of death: serpent, leprosy, spilled blood. The threatening signs that he brings with him to the Egyptians appear not to make him immune to the same fate. A certain analogy with Cain's story holds true if we remember that Cain may have thought that by killing the competition he guaranteed his own survival: you die, I live.

Moses, to be sure, is not Cain, but he also, it seems, is humbled by God with the realization that as messenger, he is not some kind of Nietzchean superman. Not really unexpectedly, he is physically laid hold of by the very God who sent him back to Egypt as God's champion (Ex 4:24–26). Thus, the clash with Pharaoh is between two wounded men, one deeply aware of his injury, like Jacob at Jabbok (Gn 32:22–32), the other unconscious of being stabbed to death by the God he chooses to ignore. The blows they inflict upon each other are enormous, though the sparring in Exodus 4 is only a kind of warm-up before the unremitting match in 10 rounds from which Moses comes out the victor.

So, the first wonder God gave Moses concerns the staff that he leans upon. We soon learn that the various signs given him are as many onslaughts against his person before becoming weapons against Egypt. Is not Pharaoh a "broken reed of a staff, which will pierce the hand of anyone who leans on it" (Is 36:6 [NRSV])? Such concordance between the message-giver and the message-recipient is food for thought. There is here an uncanny consubstantiality of *traditor—traditio—receptor* that very much falls in parallel with the prophetic process. We are at a far cry from the prodigy where, on the contrary, there often is dissociation between the performer, the performed, and the witnesses.[5]

In analogy with the prologue to the book of Job, Moses is first hit in the realm of his belongings: "What is in your hand?" (Ex 4:2). Then, the second sign becomes intimately personal: Moses' bodily integrity is impaired: his hand becomes leprous before it is again healed. As regards the third and last wonder, the water of the Nile changed into blood, it is clear that it puts Moses in a very awkward situation vis-à-vis his Egyptian hosts, who no doubt will take umbrage at such an insult to or violation of the Nile and the whole of Egypt. When the magicians also succeed in transmogrifying the water into blood (Ex 7:22), they prolong the duel with Moses/Aaron as well as their own blindness; while in a way unwittingly rescuing Moses from the lethal wrath of Pharaoh! In short, the three wonders do involve Moses as dramatis persona in the scheme of liberating the Hebrews from thralldom.

Of course, the wonders could have been confined to the realm of artifices contrived by human skill, leaving intact the person of the performer. However, they are precisely not mere artifices in this case. Moses' staff becomes a serpent and he must grab it by the tail. Then his flesh is rotting under his eyes and we can imagine his distress. Eventually, Moses is literally attacked by God who "sought to kill him" (Ex 4:24)—that is, Moses returning to Egypt is under no status of immunity! The signs he is equipped with are too closely personal to constitute an efficient shield of protection. If the wonders do not work as expected, Moses is no better than dead. The point is important. Moses' bargaining dialogue with God has the double purpose of getting a magical protection for his person and providing an inescapable argument for the fulfillment of his mission.

On both counts, Moses does not get what he wants, *as he did not earlier when he asked to be privy to the Name of God* (Ex 3:13–14). What he gets is less and it is more. On both occasions God shifts the realms from *magos* to *logos*. No divine sacred "name of power" is at Moses' disposal. Similarly, no magical shield will immunize him from harm, and no argument he will formulate will appear incontrovertible to his audience. As messenger, he passes from a desired automatic outcome to a feared responsibility. The liberation of the people of Israel from the land of graves (Ex 14:11) demands that Moses first shares the present endangerment of the Hebrews (cf. Nm 20:15; Dt 26:6; Jgs 10:11), as later when Queen Esther must first put herself in harm's way ("If I perish, I perish" Est 4:16). Exodus 4, or more accurately Exodus 3–4, is about the training of Moses for leadership, but also for some sort of martyrdom.[6]

POLYVALENCE OF MOSES' SIGNS

"What is in your hand?—A staff!" We, the rereaders of the old Bible stories know that Moses' staff will have multiple functions. Marvelously as a scepter or a serpent, it will hit the Nile waters and change them into blood; it will also be stretched over the Sea of Reeds and part its waters to let the people ford to the other side; further, it will again hit a rock and water will gush out. A magical wand of sorts, its multilayered function transcends any flat interpretation. In the eyes of the Egyptians, Moses' stick effects lethal signs for the present and in the future: serpent; blood; drowning tide (Ex 14:26). Not so in the Israelites' eyes. Moses' staff is salvific: the "Hebrew" serpent swallows up the Egyptian serpents (Ex 7:12); the sea's waters are split and its bottom turns into dry land for the people (Ex 14:11–22); the rock is hit and gushes drinking water in the desert (Ex 17:6). Therefore, the so-called "Aaron's rod," after it miraculously bloomed, is deposited within the Ark as a token of divine interventions (Nm 17:23–26 [Engl. 17:8–11]). Elsewhere, it is called "the staff of God" (Ex 4:20; cf. Is 10:26).

This polyvalence is verified once more as regards the intermediary sign granted by the Lord to Moses: the leprous hand.[7] This second wonder belongs to the category of "miracle of trial," in the same way that Exodus 15:25 says that the Lord "tested them" by the sweetening of the bitter waters of Marah (cf. also 16:4). Moses' staff was already a sign testing its owner; now the probing becomes more personal.[8] The message is branded in his own flesh. For the physical limitation and transience of Moses' disease must not blind us. From now on, as a matter of fact, one will wonder whether his body is whole and wholesome (and accidentally plagued), or unhealthy (and graciously, incessantly restored to wholesomeness).

"Skin for skin! All that people have they will give to save their lives," says Job 2:4 (NRSV). Between the property and the proprietor, the difference is biblically one of degrees. But now, the divine onslaught reaches its apex, for Moses' leprosy signifies his death (see Nm 12:12; *ExR* 11.23). Moses' mission is to save from death an enslaved people. He must first go himself through death (see Ex 4:24). In no way will Moses be an outsider or a diplomat. His testing in Midian before his daring return to Egypt implies his going down into the crucible, in common with those that Pharaoh submits to a slow genocide (cf. Ex 1:22: the drowning of the Hebrew boys is symbolically a forced disintegration, a return to chaos).

Of significance is the fact that Moses is not hit from above by his vulnerability and humanness, but from the mere contact with his own flesh. When facing himself Moses discovers his impurity (Lv 13:2 ff.). Even the partial spread of the disease contributes to the demonstration, for were he entirely leprous he would retrieve his purity by the laws of cleansing (see Lv 13:13, 45–46). Moses is impure because he is a sinner before God (see Nm 12:9–15, 19: Miriam; 1 Kgs 13:4–6: Jeroboam; 2 Kgs 5:27: Gehazi). The return to health (Ex 4:7) is thus Moses' "resurrection" by the grace of God (cf. King Jeroboam's recovery; and in a different context, see Isaiah's purification before being sent on a mission, Is 6). Moses experiences his "exodus from Egypt" before he leads the people out of the "land of darkness" (Ex 10:22).[9] Earlier, he had shown his commitment to and his capacity for leadership and liberation in Exodus 2:17.

We must stress the idea of substitution as the basis of Exodus 4, including, of course, the rite of circumcision in verses 24–27, "prerequisite for the participation in the Passover."[10] Moses is not merely a messenger; by substitution he incarnates his people. Had he been killed in Egypt, there would be no Israel in history. True, his incarnation is in the form of a servant (cf. Nm 11:11; Dt 34:5; Jos 1:2; Heb 3:5; Rv 15:3), humble to the point of death (cf. Ex 32:32; Nm 12:3; cf. *DeutR* Ki Tavo 7.10). God's testing purported to exalt him as the promise of his people's glorification (cf. Ws 19:22).

SUMMARY AND ELABORATION

Let me highlight a few points and develop further some of their implications. The very ambiguity of the signs granted to Moses and performed in Egypt is revealing. These phenomena are considered magical or prodigious by the Egyptian witchcraft workers, while Israel interprets them as miraculous and thus worthy of being told from generation to generation. It is not surprising that the Exodus history is absent from the Egyptian annals. That is in keeping with the skewed Egyptian interpretation of Moses' wonders as little more than circus performance. Yair Zakovitch is thus right to emphasize the nature of the reception of a sign as decisive to how it is experienced.

He writes, "The decisive factor is a literary one: the expression of excitement and wonder in the face of an incident and the amount of words devoted to its description."[11]

That is somewhat one-sided. First, it is true that the marvelous has the property of stirring a feeling of wonderment, while "most people think they sufficiently understand a thing when they have ceased to wonder at it," as Spinoza says.[12] Yet, we must also insist with Franz Rosenzweig that a miracle is intelligible only when it is experienced as miracle at the time of its occurrence. "When it no longer seems a thing of the present, all there is left to do is explain. . . . In fact nothing is miraculous about a miracle except that it comes when it does."[13] This effect in the moment of the miracle being perceived as a miracle prevents the development of any supernaturalism as the basis of religion.

For it is quite clear that the very notion of the miraculous implies a confrontation between transcendence and nature. This philosophical problem was hotly debated already by Renaissance thinkers. Much earlier, Tertullian famously exclaimed, "credo quia absurdum" (I believe such and such because it is absurd, i.e., there is no way to apprehend or handle this absurd reality but to embrace it by faith). Theology, in such a case would be in opposition to nature; a proposition rejected by Thomas Aquinas for whom the mysteries *transcend* nature.

On this point, Aquinas is closer to the Hebrew worldview, namely, that the universe is *wrapped up in transcendence.* At times, there occurs, as it were, a tear in the heavenly envelope and transcendence becomes visible, like sunshine piercing the clouds—"O that you would tear open the heavens and come down . . . so that the nations might tremble at your presence!" (Is 64:1, 2 [NRSV]). This does not strike out nature; it makes nature meaningful. Moon, wind, earth, are St. Francis's brothers and sisters!

This same conception lies, for instance, at the basis of Jeremiah "seeing" a branch of an almond tree with its signification. "Then Yahweh said . . . 'You have seen well, for I am watching over my word to fulfill it'" (Jer 1:11–13). It has nothing to do with idealism or with pantheism. As the earth cannot live without the sun's light and warmth, so the world draws its substance, sustenance, and meaning from the beyond. Although, to be sure, not everyone in ancient Israel was a saint, everyone was religious because no other kind of existence was conceivable.

Furthermore, I emphasize not only the referential quality of the sign, but also the person of the performer.[14] An Egyptian wizard is able to change a stick into a snake and the act looks the same whether performed by him or by the Hebrew man, but there is a world of difference between the magician and Moses producing the same phenomenon. The problem arises not so much on the cognitive as on the psychological level. Before becoming a literary feature, the miracle is *experienced* as a miracle, not by all to be sure but by some eyewitnesses; and then remotely through tradition by generations of hearers and readers, for whom the miracle is then explained, as Rosenzweig said.[15] The explanation of a miracle does not consist in displaying its hidden controls but in the revelation of its proclamation *(kerugma)*. That is why Jesus spoke of persuasion or belief and said, "If they do not listen to Moses and the prophets, neither will they be convinced (believe) even if someone rises from the dead" (Lk 16:31 [NRSV]).

The witness to a wonder faces the impossible. It takes hard-won will and humility to accept a manifestation of the miracle. Such attitude amounts to commitment. When acknowledged, the miracle, as a matter of fact, does not constitute an end but the starting point of a new life ("Go and sin no more!" Jn 8:11; 5:14). This indeed is a strong criterion for determining the nature of the wonder, whether it is a prodigy or a miracle. The miracle's property is to reorient life in the right direction; the prodigy, at the least, leaves one indifferent and, at the most, gravely disturbed, as it destroys an elementary trust in the stability of nature.[16] Hence, the decisive question regarding a wonder is: what kind of newness of life does it usher in?

Most of Jesus' miracles are in the form of healing the sick. In fact, it is not an exaggeration to view those healings as a marker of the general nature of Jesus' actions: they heal and restore. "Go to tell John [the Baptist] what you hear and see: the blind receive their sight, the lame walk, the lepers are cleansed, the deaf hear, the dead are raised, and the poor have good news brought to them" (Mt 11:5; Lk 7:22). The point is valid also as regards our Exodus text: Moses' signs eventually bring Israel's liberation from the "house of bondage," to their liberation from the dangerous sea waters (Ex 14), from the bitter waters in the desert through their being changed into sweet water (Ex 15); and from the snakes' venom, which is neutralized (Nm 21:4–9).

Remarkable is the frequent cooperation of both God and a human agent in the performance of the miracle, until the supreme agent in the NT arrives.[17] Exodus 14:31 states, "The people feared the Lord, and believed in the Lord and in Moses, his servant." As God's word is only proclaimed through human intermediaries, as mouthpieces or interpreters, so God's work is wrought by human agency.[18] Joshua 10:14 and 1 Kings 17:22 say that "God heeded a human voice" before intervening in history, obeying as it were the human injunction. In the case of Exodus 4, it is rather Moses who heeds the voice of God.

THE YAHWIST'S PSYCHOLOGY

With this remark, we enter the domain of the Yahwist's psychology. The Yahwist was the author or editor of the very early narratives in the Hebrew Bible. One of the characteristics of those early biblical narratives is an

emphasis on the necessity of human agency in the fulfillment of divine direc-
tives. From the beginning of the world, there is according to the Yahwist a
cooperation of the divine and the human. Adam works in a Garden planted
by God. The humans are under a divine command that respects their freedom ("You shall / you shall not"). This kind of partnership with the divine
finds an uncanny echo in the familial partnership between man and woman,
and the societal relationship between the one and the many.

On this, the Yahwist is in full agreement with all other biblical sources and
traditions: God and the human race are in an ongoing dialogue, a phenomenon that is highly arresting as God puts himself in a situation of need. God
needs the human labor to cultivate the Garden; God needs the human agency
to actualize his lordship over the whole of creation; God needs prophets and
legislators to spell out his will, and poets to laud his glory. A daring rabbinic
midrash on Isaiah 43:12 amplifies the biblical text as saying, "'So you are my
witnesses, declares the Lord, and I am God.' That is, if you are my witnesses
I am God, and if you are not my witnesses, I am, as it were, not God."[19]

It is within this perspective that the Yahwist's adoption of popular traditions is to be understood. His enthusiasm for his people's unique consciousness of the covenant that binds them with God prompts him to repeat for
them the legends about God's miraculous intervention in the Exodus history. For, as we take into consideration the multiplicity of marvels in the
Yahwist's narratives, especially in the desert between Egypt and Canaan,
their very accumulation creates a certain feeling of uneasiness. Clearly, the
Yahwist has inherited a folkloric trend of interspersing stories with the marvelous. What this suggests is that the biblical author grounds our trust less
upon the actuality of the reported events *than on their signification.*

On the other hand, we need also to be reminded of the irrefutable historicity of miracles attributed to modern personalities such as the *Curé d'Ars*
or Don Bosco[20]; within Judaism, the Hasidic tradition in particular, reports
of miraculous rabbis.[21] Thus, the miracle exists, and its exploitation by the
populace also exists. This fact puts in relief the limit of the psychological in
our interpretation of miracles. Psychologically speaking, there is a similarity
of attitude and expectation on the part of people motivated either by faith or
by superstition. Theologically, however, the difference between them is an
unbridgeable divide. A rationalistic approach to miracles presses the psychological beyond its proper limits and reduces the transcendent to the trivial.
As in everything that pertains to human existence, interpretation is the decisive factor. I have tried to put in relief some features of the marvelous that
can serve as criteria of authentication. To repeat the main point, it is less a
matter of historicity than of signification. Moses' signs signify.

While the prodigy can be said to be "monologic," the miracle is fundamentally dialogic. The prodigy demands, it is true, an audience like the miracle,
but the witnesses remain passive. All that is required is awe and amazement.

Not so with the miracle: when there is only a watching, there is no miracle. Miracle demands the witnesses' *participation*, that is, *faith*. As long as the Nile waters, changed into blood, remain a spectacle, as for the Egyptians, the event is prodigious, merely a wonder. When the Nile is revealed for what it actually represents, as for the Hebrew slaves in Egypt, namely, divine intervention for their salvation, the prodigy itself is also changed into miracle. Interpretation is what gives breath to the lump, so to speak.

However, interpretation is a two-edged sword. On this score, the Egyptians in Exodus 4 are confounded by an act that negates the apparently immutable laws of nature. After that, they cannot trust anything in the world. They have become subjected to the arbitrary. The sun can be obscured; the rivers can be streams of blood; the fields' crops can swarm with frogs or insects. Nothing makes sense anymore; existence has become as meaningless as the prodigy itself was. The Egyptian interpretation results in a nihilistic view of the world. The prodigy is destructive and produces only despair.

For the Hebrews, by contrast, the marvel, after some hesitation on their part as to its message, has opened up an entirely new perspective on life. What their experience in thralldom meant to them is now broken open for all to see. The Nile, the life artery of the land of Egypt, is in truth flowing with their blood. The Egyptian civilization is in fact a broken reed that pierces the hand of anyone leaning on that unreliable staff (see Is 36:6). It can be revealed anytime as a lethal poisonous serpent. The Egyptian toleration of the Israelites, as long as they were useful as laborers, is a transparent veil thrown over what all now can see as impurity, indeed leprosy.

We remember Manetho's contemptuous depiction of the Hebrews as being themselves leprous. Manetho certainly expresses the persistent Egyptian sentiment regarding the non-Egyptians and especially their northern neighbors.[22] Moses' move with his hand becoming leprous in contact with his own flesh would thus fill the role assigned to him as a Hebrew. For it goes without saying that, in the eyes of the Egyptians, the leprous Moses did confirm an ingrained Egyptian opinion of the Hebrews. But in a second phase of this story, Moses demonstrates his purity and, consequently, the purity of his people. By contrast, among the plagues that eventually afflict the Egyptians, there are a deadly pestilence and boils (Ex 9), but none for the despised but exalted Israelites.

While the prodigy leaves all people voiceless with awe, the miracle is always dialogical in that it invites conversation about and response to the signification: divine interventions of healing and deliverance. No healing performed by Jesus left his audiences indifferent. Besides stirring a reaction of praise to God, there was always the possibility of the signification of the miracle being contested. In other words, the conviction, the persuasiveness of the miracle and its signification, is never coerced. The Egyptian side in the audience is safeguarded and respected.

There is no reasonable reply to the prodigy, but with the miracle there is the ongoing invitation to *believe*, that is, to agree with being reoriented toward a different way of life. For the Hebrews, the process starts with the miraculous Exodus from Egypt, the metaphoric value of which has defined the life and destiny of the people of the Bible ever since. Not an easy life, but a life of freedom and purposefulness. That signification is the core of Judaism and Christianity. Happy are those who have eyes to see and ears to hear; they will leave the land of oppression, while the mere rationalists will stay there forever.

NOTES

1. Edgar Allen Poe (2002), The Mystery of Marie Roguet, in *Edgar Allan Poe: Complete Tales and Poems*, Edison, NJ: Castle Books, 141.

2. Martin Buber (1947), *Moses, the Revelation and the Covenant*, London: East and West Library.

3. As Yair Zakovitch states, "A clear and frequent purpose of the miracle is to inspire faith in God" (see Ex 4:30–31; 1 Kgs 18:37–39; Nm 14:11; Jo 4:23–4; etc.). "A strengthened faith in God is frequently combined with a strengthened trust in God's messenger" (see Ex 14:31; 1 Kgs 18:36; 2 Kgs 2:15). See his article, Miracle (OT), *Anchor Bible Dictionary (ABD)* 4, 855.

4. The book of Deuteronomy also recognizes that "signs and wonders" can be worked by false prophets (see Dt 13:3).

5. This does not apply to the shaman who, nevertheless, remains a magician.

6. A strong Jewish tradition states that Moses was a martyr and died as such; see for instance *Sifre Deut*, Ha'azinu, 306, fol. 131 b.

7. On the ambivalence of the *'oth*, see, for example, Exodus 12:13.

8. The Deuteronomy insists on God testing his people; see 4:34; 7:19; 29:2–3.

9. A bitterly ironic expression to designate a country worshipping the sun.

10. Johannes Pedersen (1940), *Israel, Its Life and Culture*, volumes iii–iv, London: Geoffrey Cumberlege, 736.

11. Miracle (OT), *ABD* 4, 848a.

12. Baruch Spinoza (1951), *A Theologico-Political Treatise*, R. H. Elwes, trans., Mineola, New York: Dover, 84. Abraham Heschel (1959) speaks of a "radical amazement" in his *God in Search of Man*, Philadelphia: Jewish Publication Society (JPSA), 43.

13. Franz Rosenzweig (2000), A Note on a Poem by Judah ha-Levi, in Nahum N. Glazer, *Franz Rosenzweig, His Life and Thought*, Indianapolis: Hackett, 290.

14. See a negative example in the person of Gehazi, for example (2 Kgs 4:31).

15. See above note 13. Refer especially to Psalm 78:2–8.

16. Baruch Spinoza warns against nature's disruption, which, he says, "not only can give us no knowledge of God, but, contrariwise, takes away that which we naturally have, and makes us doubt God and everything else." See (1951), *A Theologico-Political Treatise*, R. H. Elwes, trans., Mineola, New York: Dover, 85. He refers here to Deuteronomy 13:2–4. This Spinoza stance is countered by Samuel Hirsch (1808–1888), who says that the miracle demonstrates that nature is not omnipotent in (1841, republished in 1986) *Die Religionsphilosophie der Juden oder das Prinzip der Jüdischen Religionsanschauung*, Hildesheim: Georg Olms. See Wisdom 19:6, "the whole creation in

its nature was fashioned anew, complying with your commands, so that your children might be kept unharmed."

17. No text, however, went so far in the same direction as Exodus 7:1 (see also 4:16): "Yahweh said to Moses, 'Behold, I have made you God to Pharaoh, and your brother Aaron shall be your prophet.'"

18. A. Lefèvre (1957), "Miracle" (*Dictionnaire de la Bible Supplément* [*DBS*] col. 1307), Paris: Letouzey et Ane, says re the miracle, "le critère dernier est la conformité avec la Parole (Dt 13:2–6; Matt 24:24 and //; Rev 13:12–18; 16:13–14; 19:20)."

19. *SifreDeut* 346, Babylonian Talmud, Finkelstein ed., 1956, New York: Jewish Publication Society.

20. A. Lefèvre, "Miracle," in *DBS* col. 1303.

21. In the Talmud already, we find, for instance, rabbis like Honi ha-Me'aggel (= the Circle Maker) in the first century BCE and Hanna ben Dosa in the first century CE (see Taanit 23–25, Babylonian Talmud, Finkelstein ed., 1956, New York: Jewish Publication Society).

22. See Manetho's *History of Egypt*, This is a lost work of the third century BCE, but according to Josephus's, *Contra Apionem* 1,232–51, it is alleged that Manetho had an anti-Judaic description of the Hebrews as unclean lepers. The Hebrews, he says, were in fact an Egyptian rubble "deported from Egypt for leprosy and other diseases" (1,229), thus "cleansing the whole country of lepers and other 'unclean' people" (1,233), "with deformed bodies" (1,234), with "some learned priests afflicted with leprosy among them" [Moses and Aaron, Miriam?]. (See also 1,241, 248, and 251.) Their leader was a priest from Heliopolis, an Egyptian who "changed his name and was called Moses" (1,250).

REFERENCES

Babylonian Talmud, Finkelstein ed. (1956), New York: Jewish Publication Society of America (JPSA).

Buber, Martin (1947), *Moses, the Revelation and the Covenant*, London: East and West Library.

Glazer, Nahum N., see under Rosenzweig.

Heschel, Abraham (1959), *God in Search of Man*, Philadelphia: Jewish Publication Society of America (JPSA).

Hirsch, Samuel (1841), *Die Religionsphilosophie der Juden oder das Prinzip der Jüdischen Religionsanschauung*, Hildesheim: Georg Olms. Republished in 1986.

Josephus, *Contra Apionem*, in William Whiston, ed. (1987), *The Works of Josephus Complete and Unabridged*, Peabody, MA: Hendrickson.

Keller, Carl A. (1946), *Das Wort OTH als "Offenbarungszeichen Gotte,"* Basel: E. Hoenen.

Lefèvre, A. (1957), Miracle, in *Dictionnaire de la Bible Supplément (DBS)*, col. 1299–1308, Paris: Letouzey et Ane.

Manetho, *History of Egypt*, see: Josephus, *Contra Apionem* 1, 232–51.

McCasland, S. V. (1957), Signs and Wonders, *Journal of Biblical Literature (JBL)*, 76, 149–52.

McKenzie, John L. (1952), God and Nature in the Old Testament, *Catholic Biblical Quarterly (CBQ)* 14, 18–19, 124–45.

Pedersen, Johannes (1940), *Israel, Its Life and Culture*, volumes iii–iv, London: Geoffrey Cumberlege.

Poe, Edgar A. (2002), The Mystery of Marie Roguet, in *Edgar Allan Poe: Complete Tales and Poems*, Edison, NJ: Castle Books.

Polhill, J. B. (1977), Perspectives in the Miracle Stories, *Review and Expositor* 74, 389–400.

Rosenzweig, Franz (2000), A Note on a Poem by Judah ha-Levi, in *Franz Rosenzweig, His Life and Thought*, Nahum N. Glazer, ed., Indianapolis: Hackett.

SifreDeuteronomy, Ha'azinu, 306, fol. 131 b.

Spinoza, Baruch (1951), *A Theologico-Political Treatise*, R. H. Elwes, trans., Mineola, New York: Dover.

Stolz, F. (1972), Zeichen und Wunder, *Zeitschrift für Theologie und Kirche (ZTK)* 69, 25–44.

Zakovitch, Yair (1992), Miracle (OT), David N. Freedman, ed., *Anchor Bible Dictionary (ABD)* Vol. 4, Nashville, TN: Abingdon, 845–56.

CHAPTER 7

THE RELIGIOUS-HISTORICAL BACKGROUND OF THE NEW TESTAMENT MIRACLES

Erkki Koskenniemi

The biblical miracles have never been easy to understand and have not always been easy for theologians to explain.[1] Long before the beginnings of scientific interpretations of scripture and critical exegesis, Spinoza formulated the relation between the Jewish-Christian belief and the critical mind (1670): God has created the universe and the laws of the Nature. If something like a miracle accidentally broke these laws, it would contradict God's wisdom and the good harmony in his world. So miracles, in his view, do not support religion but contradict it.[2] This concept is a good example of how miracles may lose their religious relevance completely.

The laws of nature, a concept unknown to the people of the Old and New Testament, have come to be perceived as independent from God, and the immanent reality of God present in his creation is what matters, even to many religious persons. God is not understood so much as a fascinating or awesome mystery, but as something which is compatible with our reason. He is the source of all rationality, as in large parts of medieval scholastic theology. Consequently, much biblical material, such as miracles, was marginalized. Many attempts have been made to marginalize it further with rational or scientific explanations.

Albert Schweitzer skillfully served some of these attempts in his history of *Leben Jesu-Forschung (Research on the Life of Jesus)*.[3] H.E.G. Paulus, for example, avoided no means to show that Jesus' miracles were simply based upon misunderstandings of his disciples. Today we may find these interpretations humorous, but the challenge was once considered serious. Otto Weinreich, a prominent scholar of Classical antiquity, who contributed to the early religious-historical investigation with his work *Antike Heilungswunder*,[4] quotes in his preface the words of Björnstjerne Björnsson: "*Ich bin der Ansicht, dass die Mirakel einer ebenso grossen Gesetzmässigkeit unterliegen wie alle andern Dinge, ob wir gleich das Gesetz nicht schauen*" ("I believe that miracles follow a similar order as all other matters, although we do not see it").[5] These words illumine the atmosphere in which religious-historical work was done in the beginning of the last century.

GREEK NARRATIVE AND LITERARY MODELS

A decisive innovation in the New Testament interpretation of the early twentieth century was the introduction and adaptation of the form-critical method, which had formerly been used in the investigation of the Old Testament (OT). Form-criticism, as Laato pointed out in chapter 2, is an analysis of texts on the basis of the type of literature an author uses: poetry, stories, historical report, mythic imagination, miracle story, and the like. The German masters, K. L. Schmidt, Martin Dibelius, and Rudolf Bultmann, developed a toolbox that is still used today, although perhaps with reservations. Scholars tried to define the genres of the New Testament (NT) material. In this concept, the evangelists were considered collectors and bearers of tradition rather than independent authors and theologians: it meant that scholars thought that they were able to go over their works that belonged to "Kleinliteratur," to the oral tradition, and to listen to anonymous mediators of the Jesus tradition. This concept also drastically influenced the investigation of the miracle stories.

According to Dibelius, some early Christian teachers only briefly stated what had happened, and the genre was then "paradigm."[6] There were, however, others, who were able to expand the tradition, and the narrative skills caused the brief "paradigms" to grow to "novels." All this meant that the scarce Christian material was expanded according to models of the Graeco-Roman folklore. Miracle stories attested how early Christians increasingly adapted themselves to literary models and forms of their world.

Dibelius's work, completed and introduced with Bultmann's *Geschichte der synoptischen Tradition*, often led scholars to consider miracle stories alien to real, original Christianity.[7] It is easy to understand that several scholars later tried to rescue every NT writer who could be rescued. Luke could not, and that is why he was sometimes vehemently criticized for adaptation to his world.[8] But Paul allegedly fought a battle against his opponents, who were all too fond of miracles.[9] Few scholars, if any, observed what he proudly wrote on his own "signs that mark an apostle" (2 Cor 12:12), and how proudly he wrote about what he had done "by the power of signs and miracles, through the power of the Spirit" (Rom 15:19). Mark allegedly criticized the theology of his sources or even all the disciples of Jesus.[10] It took time before scholars[11] noted that Mark does not speak critically or skeptically of miracles. According to Fortna, for example, John was critical of miracles, and it is partly true (cf. Jn 4:48).[12] However, John pays attention to several miracles and emphasizes them, as for example, in John 9 and 11.

The classical form-critical research took the genre of miracle story for granted. However, miracle stories strongly differ from each other and it might be problematic to treat them as a single category. Klaus Berger denied the existence of the literary model or genre called miracle story, claiming that this category includes several different genres containing miraculous elements.[13] Theissen tried to improve the form-critical method with his work.[14] Accurate works on how every NT writer dealt with miracles were already published during the 1980s, but the task is huge. It is clear that miracle stories should not be investigated superficially. As Laato presents in chapter 2 of this volume, even the concept of miracle is problematic and by no means identical in the usage of early Judaism and of the modern world.

GREEK "DIVINE MEN"

The most important contribution of the religious-historical investigation of the biblical miracles was the theory of divine men, which influenced scholarship almost the entire twentieth century. The rise and fall of the theory illumines the dangers of comparative investigation of religions. Simultaneously with and partly influenced by the form-critical research, scholars were impressed by the Greek parallels of Jesus' miracles. The first to use the words *divine men* was Reitzenstein (1906, 1910), but very soon Wetter (1916) contributed to the study of comparative religion and adapted his results to the study of the NT, especially of the Gospel of John. According to Wetter, classical antiquity knew several men who were considered divine, sons of god or gods. They originated from different nations or of different religions, but the classical world considered them belonging to a certain category of divine men.

To verify his claim he referred to numerous classical texts. However, he neither gave exact definitions of divine men nor dated his sources, which understandably led to problems later. Moreover, it is crucial to recognize Wetter's background. Like several of his fellow scholars, he believed that religion was originally alike in all primitive societies and developed later towards higher religions. Wetter apparently considered it irrelevant to date his ancient sources, because he still could recognize the same primitive traits of early religion on the streets of the Orient in his own days.[15] This concept should be problematic to a modern scholar, who does not believe in the evolution of religions.[16] However, although it is easy to understand that the view was held in Wetter's time and that most prominent scholars referred to concepts like *mana* or *taboo*, adapting them to the NT miracle stories, it is curious that the view could survive in the derivatives of the divine men hypothesis.

Moreover, Bieler, the famous Austrian classicist, added philosophical color to the debate with his influential book in 1935–36. This expert of the classical Greek and Roman literature offered an immense collection of material, not only from classical antiquity, mostly from the Christian era, but even of tales from Africa, Lithuania, and early North America. He explicitly says that the concept of divine man is a Platonic model, with great universal appeal.[17] No wonder that he did not pay attention to the date or provenance of his sources, because in his view every holy man was predestined to go the way of Socrates, Apollonius of Tyana, or Jesus. It is curious that it took more than 40 years before Bieler's views were thoroughly criticized,[18] and even then scholars overlooked the circular reasoning of the later research.

Christian texts, both the Gospels and later writings, formed a crucial element in Bieler's pattern. It was not a problem for Bieler, because he openly assumed a Platonic model, but it should have been a problem for scholars using Bieler's pattern to investigate the Gospels. However, they compared, for example, the theology of the Gospel of Mark with Bieler's pattern and found them widely similar. This would not have surprised anyone who had analyzed how the Christian texts helped Bieler to construct his pattern. The reason for the error was, of course, that only a few NT scholars were able to deal with classical texts and did not realize that Bieler had used texts that were mainly substantially later than the NT.

The pattern of *divine men* was already used in NT scholarship before World War II. However, the redaction critical method at first meant an explosion of books and articles using the concept. Since Hans Conzelmann and Willi Marxsen, scholars asked questions that had been neglected for a long time. They no more considered the Gospels mere collections of individual pearls but as pearl necklaces, and asked for the role of the writers who had decided to select precisely these pearls and put them exactly in this order. Mark, Matthew, Luke, and John were considered authors and theologians again. It was now current to ask again for the role of the miracles in the Gospels or in their sources. The work of the previous generations was now carefully observed. It is hard to overestimate the role of Rudolf Bultmann, who had early[19] accepted the pattern of *divine men* and used it to interpret the Gospels. Talented students went to study at Marburg, and after some decades, his pupils sat on chairs overall in the learned world.

Once activated, the concept of *divine man* was widely used in the New Testament exegesis. Scholars used it to interpret the miracles in Mark, Matthew, Luke, John, and their sources. It was used to define the theology of the opponents of Paul in 1 Thessalonians, Philippians, and especially in 2 Corinthians. However, the use of this hypothesis peaked and began to decline in the 1980s. Scholars investigating Mark were increasingly critical,[20] as well the ones investigating John.[21] Only a few, however, rejected the entire concept, which had and still has prominent supporters.[22] Critical voices have been louder, and today I consider it difficult to defend the traditional hypothesis. Actually, it would be difficult to define what is meant with the "traditional hypothesis." The views of Reitzenstein, Wetter, and Bieler differed so much that it is impossible to speak of *the* hypothesis.

After a century of religious historical work some points seem clear.

1. The classical world called some men divine (*theios*), but did not construct a fixed pattern of *divine men* (*theios aner*) although the words sometimes occur.[23] This is not an ancient category, but a modern concept, which may be useful if defined and used critically.

2. We do not know Greek or Roman historical miracle workers or works about them that could have served as models for Jesus or the Gospels. Actually, we know virtually no Greek miracle workers from 300 BCE to about the year 150 CE.[24] When constructing the pattern of *divine men*, scholars used sources that date later than the Gospels, and did it uncritically.

3. Ancient people believed in miracles and magic. The most important parallels for Jesus' mighty deeds are the miracles of rulers and gods, and the miracles performed by anonymous magicians.[25]

4. Scholars have badly neglected the rich Jewish tradition. In this volume, it is treated in the articles written by Antti Laato and me.

THE JEWISH TRADITION

I have briefly presented the rich tradition of the Old Testament miracle workers and their role in the later Jewish writings.[26] The mighty deeds of Abraham, Moses, Elijah, Elisha, and several other figures played an important role in early Judaism. This tradition was part of the past that defined the identity of the nation. Several historical figures attempted to use this tradition to legitimate themselves as leaders. They were not, however, the only Jewish miracle workers in the times of Jesus.

Political Jewish Miracle Workers

Our sources tell of several Jewish men whose miracles played a political role. The New Testament briefly mentions Theudas in a speech by Gamaliel: "Some time ago Theudas appeared, claiming to be somebody, and about four hundred men rallied to him. He was killed, all his followers were dispersed, and it all came to nothing" (Acts 5:36).[27]

Josephus too mentions Theudas (*Ant.* 20.97–98):

[He] . . . persuaded the majority of the masses to take up their possessions and to follow him to the Jordan River. He stated that he was a prophet and that at his command the river would be parted and would provide them an easy passage. With this talk he deceived many.

Cuspius Fadus, the procurator (ca. 44–46 CE), sent cavalry against the crowd. Theudas was captured in the massacre and his head was cut off and sent to Jerusalem. If Josephus' version is correct, the events happened between 44 and 46 CE, namely, years after Gamaliel's speech described in Acts. At any rate both writers mention Theudas and say that he was one of several of his kind. Luke does not report precisely Theudas' claims, which were clearly political, saying only "claiming to be somebody." Josephus calls him a sorcerer, and says that the man claimed to able to repeat the miracles of Moses at Red Sea and of Joshua at the Jordan. The changed function of the miracle illumines the role of mighty deeds. People who followed Moses were rescued by the miracle, and the parting of the Jordan made the invasion into the Promised Land possible in Joshua's time. Now, the people did not need to be rescued and there were several ways to the Land of Canaan without a miracle. However, the miracle was needed to legitimate Theudas as a leader like Moses and Joshua once were. The Roman army did not need more hints to know what the intention of the crowd was. A right to collect people and to freely talk to them may belong to the modern human rights, but it was not allowed in Rome and still less in the provinces. It mattered not whether the people were armed. The Romans first sent in the constabulary and only afterwards asked for the reason for the people assembling.

Luke informs us that the Romans identified Paul mistakenly with a famous man when they detained him in Jerusalem:

> "Do you speak Greek?" he replied. "Are you not the Egyptian who started a revolt and led four thousand terrorists out into the desert some time ago?" (*Acts* 21:38)

This Egyptian,[28] who had appeared between 56 and 60 CE, was a famous man and Josephus mentions him twice in two not fully compatible passages (*War* 2.261–63; *Antiquities* 20.169–72). The Egyptian called 30,000 men (*War*), at first in the desert (*War*) and then to the Mount of Olives (*War* and *Antiquities*), and wanted to show how his words could cause the walls of the city to fall down (*Antiquities*). Claudius Felix let the soldiers kill 400 and take 200 men (the numbers only in *Ant.*), but the Egyptian escaped his enemies, as even Luke takes for granted. The words (in *Ant.* 20.172), "the Egyptian became invisible," are easily interpreted as referring to a miracle, causing people to wait for his return.[29] The Egyptian was not the only one with this art. Josephus himself links him tightly with some other troublemakers: The Egyptian serves in *Antiquities* as an example of impostors and deceivers; in *War* Josephus tells immediately after him that the miracle workers and the robbers joined their powers (*War* 2.264).[30] Although they often were conventional robbers and the miracles are not mentioned (*War* 2.271), Josephus often uses with regard to them words he also uses describing the Egyptian (*War* 2.565).

It is interesting that no one of the three sources gives the name of the man: He is always "the Egyptian." The strange detail that the Egyptian Jew is not supposed to speak Greek, although Greek was their most important language, may reveal that anonymity is not the issue. Maybe it did not refer to his provenance but to his claims. The man did not came from Egypt but from the countryside of Palestine, and was called "Egyptian" because he wanted to repeat the miracles made in Egypt by Moses, and during the conquest by Joshua, both of whom had come up out of Egypt. As Joshua came from Egypt and conquered the land from the Canaanites, the man claimed to be able to repeat the miracle of Jericho and expel the Romans. We cannot be certain of all this, but his models were certainly taken from the sacralized past. Miracles were politically important. Religion and revolt were intimately interwoven.[31] It is important to observe that, according to Josephus, the Jerusalemites fought side by side with Romans against the man. This certainly shows the tension between the rich, Hellenized aristocrats in Jerusalem, and the religious poor people in the countryside.

The last events of the Jewish war dramatically attested the power of the militant miracles. When the fall of Jerusalem was imminent, a prophet led people to the temple to see God's saving miracles; or rather, to be burned alive with the temple (Josephus, *War* 6.281–287). But even after the end of the last rebels in Masada, a man named Jonathan still gathered poor people to the desert to show them God's miracles. Catullus, the Roman governor, cruelly used the option to fight his own Jewish war and killed the unarmed people (*War* 7.437–442 and *Life* 423–425).

Nonmilitant Jewish Miracle Workers

Sources also inform us of less militant Jewish miracle workers, who helped people in their daily life. The best known of them is Honi the Circle-Drawer, or Onias, as Josephus calls him. He lived about 65 BCE and his successful prayer that ended a long drought made him famous.[32] Josephus mentions the miracle only briefly and tells how he was stoned to death when he refused to curse his fellow Jews during their civil wars. His death by stones apparently refers to his miraculous skills: Deuteronomy 13:1–6 orders this punishment to false prophets. The fragmentary and often suppressed evidence of Honi in the Rabbinic sources attests to how difficult it was for the mainstream rabbis to accept people with miraculous skills. Miracles were present, and they divided the opinions of the teachers; and the danger of magic made the majority of them cautious. However, Honi was slowly and carefully "rabbinized," though this process was present initially only in the later texts. A similar process was apparently required before Hanina ben Dosa, who lived about 70 CE and was allegedly the last of the "men of deed," was accepted by the rabbinic authorities.[33]

Two figures in particular inform us of Jewish people who healed by throwing out demons. The Gospel of Mark informs us of a man who started to use Jesus' name in his exorcisms. Jesus' disciples tried to hinder him because the man was not identified with Jesus' band (Mark 9:38–41; cf. Luke 9:49–50). We only can regret that the interest of the gospel writers is not focused on the anonymous exorcist but on the attitude of the disciples. Even the Old Testament contains a similar story (Num 11:26–29), which might have been a model for Mark, or even his source. At any rate, we here meet a Jew who healed by exorcism. Another Jew who threw out demons had, according to Josephus, famous spectators and made a great success. Vespasian, his sons, tribunes and other soldiers were watching when Eleazar performed the exorcism:

> He put to the nose of the possessed man a ring, which had under its seal one of the roots prescribed by Solomon, and then, as the man smelled it, drew out the demon through his nostrils, and, when the man at once fell down, adjured the demon never to come back into him, speaking Solomon's name and reciting the incantations which he had composed. Then, wishing to convince the bystanders and prove to them that he had this power, Eleazar placed a cup or foot basin full of water a little way off and commanded the demon, as it went out of the man, to overturn it and make known to the spectators that he had left the man. (*Antiquities* 8.42–49)

Eleazar was only one of the Jewish wise men deeply informed of "Solomon's wisdom."[34] Apparently, this wisdom was a door that made it possible to adapt and apply all kinds of Hellenistic knowledge, occult as well as nonoccult, among Jewish people.

We also know of several Jewish miracle workers who acted as professionals. In general, Roman mighty men seem to have appreciated the help of oriental wise men. Tiberius had many astrologers and especially Thrasyllus filling his needs; and Otho took a man named Ptolemy with him when traveling to Spain. Both of them are mentioned by the skeptical Tacitus (*Annals.* 6.20–21, and *Histories* 1.22). Apparently, oriental sages were a kind of status symbol, and Jews were appreciated among them. The New Testament tells how Barjesus Elymas served Sergius Paulus (Acts 13), and according to Josephus a man called Atomus helped Antonius Felix, the procurator of Judea about 53–58 CE, who had fallen in love with a Jewish married lady named Drusilla:

> He sent to her one of his friends, a Cyprian Jew named Atomus, who pretended to be a magician, in an effort to persuade her to leave her husband and to marry Felix. Felix promised to make her supremely happy if she did not disdain him. She, being unhappy and wishing to escape the malice of her sister Berenice, for Drusilla was exceedingly abused by her because her beauty, was persuaded to transgress the ancestral laws and

to marry Felix. By him she gave birth to a son whom she named Agrippa (*Ant.* 20.141–143).

We do not know what the methods were that Atomus used to persuade the lady, but the text shows the power of the Jewish magician. Apparently, the "Seven Sons of the High Priest Sceva" in Acts 19, hardly sons of a high priest and hardly brothers, were a band of professionals, who sought their clients among the lower layers of the people in Ephesus.

CONCLUSION

It is curious that this material has been so rarely observed during the decades of the *divine man* hypothesis, and I cannot explain it. Perhaps early Judaism was not a popular subject in Germany before World War II. At any rate, the scholars seem to have had an inadequate grasp of the ancient Jewish tradition. They considered the most important parallels to be found in the Greco-Roman world, the reason being the huge influence of the German History of Religions School *(Religionsgeschichtliche Schule)*. According to the basic view of this school, the research of the New Testament starts with the idea that early Christianity was a syncretistic religion. Greek and Roman influence were sought and found in it, but sometimes, as in the investigation of miracles, influential patterns were uncritically developed, without adequate foundation in fact. Such modern constructions do not help, but hinder, the critical understanding of biblical miracle stories. It is time to return to the religio-historical work without distorting our lenses. The first task is to observe the rich Jewish tradition properly.

NOTES

1. See, for example, Gerhard Maier (1986), Zur neutestamentlichen Wunderexegese im 19. und 20. Jahrhundert, in David Wenham and Craig Blomberg, eds., *Gospel Perspectives* 6, Sheffield, Scotland: Sheffield Academic Press, 49–87.

2. See Gerhard Maier (1986), 50–51.

3. See Albert Schweitzer (1951), *Geschichte der Leben Jesu-Forschung*, 6th edition, Tübingen: Mohr, 51–6.

4. Otto Weinreich (1909), *Antike Heilungswunder: Untersuchungen zum Wunderglauben der Griechen und Römer*, in his *Ancient Salvation-miracles, Research into the Greek and Roman Faith in the Miraculous*, Giessen: Toepelmann.

5. Ibid.

6. Martin Dibelius (1933), *Die Formgeschichte des Evangeliums*, 2nd edition, Tübingen: Mohr. First published (1919), Tübingen: Mohr.

7. Rudolph Bultmann (1934), *Geschichte der synoptischen Tradition*, Göttingen: VandenHoeck und Ruprecht.

8. See, for example, Karl Ludwig Schmidt (1923), Die Stellung der Evangelien in der allgemeinen Literaturgeschichte, in *Eucharisterion Hermann Gunkel zum 60ste*

Geburtstag, H. Schmidt, ed., Göttingen: VandenHoeck und Ruprecht. Republished by Ferdinand Hahn, ed. (1985), as *Formgeschichte des Evangeliums*, in the series, *Wege der Forschung*, No. 81, 225, Darmstadt: WB.

9. See Dieter Georgi (1986), *The Opponents of Paul in Second Corinthians*, Edinburgh: T&T Clark.

10. Theodore J. Weeden (1968), The Heresy that Necessitated Mark's Gospel, *Zeitschrift fuer Neutestamentliche Wissenschaft (ZNW)* 59, 145–58.

11. See Jack Dean Kingsbury (1981), The "Divine Man" as Key to Mark's Christology: The End of an Era?, *Interpretation* 35, 243–57, and Eduard Schweizer (1982), Zur Christologie des Markus, *Neues Testament und Christologie im Werden, Aufsätze*, Göttingen: VandenHoeck und Ruprecht, 86–103.

12. Robert Tomson Fortna (1970), *The Gospel of Signs. A Reconstruction of the Normative Source Underlying the Fourth Gospel*, Monograph Series of the Society for New Testament Studies *(MSSNTS)* 11, Cambridge: Cambridge University Press.

13. Klaus Berger (1984), *Formgeschichte des Neuen Testaments*, Heidelberg: Quelle und Meyer, 305–6.

14. Gerd Theissen (1974), *Urchristliche Wundergeschichten, Ein Beitrag zur formgeschichtlichen Erforschung der synoptischen Evangelien, Studien zum Neuen Testaments (StNT)* 8. Gütersloh: Gutersloher Verlag.

15. Gillis P. Wetter (1916), Der Sohn Gottes, in his *Eine Untersuchung über den Charakter und die Tendenz des Johannes-Evangeliums. Zugleich ein Beitrag zur Kenntnis der Heilandsgestalten der Antike*, Göttingen: VandenHoeck und Ruprect, 187–88.

16. See, for example, James Waller and Mary Edwardson (1987), Evolutionism, *The Encyclopedia of Religion*, vol. 5, 214–18.

17. Ludvig Bieler (1935–36), *Theios Aner: Das Bild des "Göttlichen Menschen" in Spätantike und Frühchristentum*, Vienna: Hofels, vol. 1, 4.

18. Carl R. Holladay (1977), *Theios Aner in Hellenistic Judaism. A Critique of the Use of this Category in New Testament Christology, Society for Biblical Literature Dissertation Series (SBLDS)* 40, Missoula, MT: Scholars Press; Eugene V. Gallagher (1982), *Divine Man or Magician? Celsus and Origen on Jesus, Society for Biblical Literature Dissertation Series (SBLDS)* 64, Chico, CA: Scholars Press.

19. Bultmann had previously been rather critical of the concept. See his (1925), Die Bedeutung der neuerschlossenen mandäischen und manichäischen Quellen für das Veständnis des Johannesevangeliums, *Zeitschrift für Neutestamentliche Wissenschaft (ZNW)* 24, 100–146. He later changed his mind. See his commentary on John: Bultmann (1941), *Das Evangelium des Johannes, Kritisch-exegetischer Kommentar ueber das Neue Testament (KEK)*, Göttingen: VandenHoeck und Ruprecht.

20. Thomas Söding (1985), *Glaube bei Markus, Glaube an das Evangelium, Gebetsglaube und Wunderglaube im Kontext der markinischen Basileiatheologie und Christologie, Stuttgarter Biblische Beitraege (SBB)* 12, 72, Stuttgart: Katholisches Bibelwerk. See also Dieter Lührmann (1987), *Das Markusevangelium, Handbuch zum Neuen Testament (HNT)* 31, 94–5, Tübingen: Mohr-Siebeck; and Barry B. Blackburn (1991), *Theios Aner and the Markan Miracle Traditions, Wissenschaftliche Untersuchungen zum Neuen Testament (WUNT)* 2, 40, Tübingen: Mohr-Siebeck.

21. Wolfgang J. Bittner (1987), *Jesu Zeichen im Johannesevangelium. Die Messias-Erkenntnis im Johannesevangelium vor ihrem jüdischen Hintergrund, Wissenschaftliche Untersuchungen zum Neuen Testament (WUNT)* 26, Tübingen: Mohr-Siebeck.

22. The most important supporter of the concept is Hans Dieter Betz (1983), Gottmensch (II), *Reallexikon fuer Antike und Christentum (RAC)* 12, 234–312, Stuttgart: Hiersemann. For the current status of the debate, see Hans Josef Klauck (2000), *The Religious Context of Early Christianity: A Guide to Graeco-Roman Religions, Studies of the New Testament and its World*, Edinburgh: T&T Clark, 174–77.

23. See David S. du Toit (1997), *Theios anthropos: zur Verwendung von theios anthropos und sinnverwandten Ausdrücken in der Literatur der Kaiserzeit, Wissenschaftliche Untersuchungen fuer Neuen Testament (WUNT)* 2, 91, Tübingen: Mohr-Siebeck

24. The Greek and Roman miracle-workers are listed by Blackburn (*Theios Aner*, 185–87), and by me (*Apollonios von Tyana*, 207–27).

25. See my book *Apollonius von Tyana*, 219–29.

26. See my book *The Old Testament Miracle-Workers in Early Judaism* (Tübingen: Mohr-Siebeck, 2005), *Wissenschaftliche Untersuchungen fuer Neuen Testament (WUNT)* II/206, and my second article in this work.

27. On Theudas, see Rebecca Gray (1993), *Prophetic Figures in Late Second Temple Jewish Palestine: The Evidence from Josephus*, New York and Oxford: Oxford University Press, 114–16; and Stefan Schreiber (2000), *Gesalbter und König. Titel und Konzeptionen der königlichen Gesalbtenerwartung in frühjüdischen und urchristlichen Schriften; Beihefte zur Zeitschrift für die neutestamentliche Wissenschaft und die Kunde der Älteren Kirche*, Berlin and New York: De Gruyter, 293–94.

28. On the Egyptian, see Gray (1993), *Prophetic Figures*, 116–18; Schreiber (2000), *Gesalbter und König*, 291–92.

29. Morton Smith (1999), The Troublemakers, *Cambridge History of Judaism*, vol. 3, *The Early Judaism*, William Horbury, W. D. Davies, and John Sturdy, eds., Cambridge: Cambridge University Press, 501–68. Even Luke presupposes that the man was not taken by the Romans. Josephus uses the words *afanes egeneto*, describing the end of Moses and Elijah (*Antiquities* 9, 28).

30. Otto Betz (1974) considers them no miracle-workers: Das Problem des Wunders bei Flavius Josephus im Vergleich zum Wunderproblem bei den Rabbinen und im Johannesevangelium, in his *Jesus der Messias Israels: Aufsaetze zur biblischen Theologie*, Tübingen: Mohr-Siebeck, 398–419. The reference is specifically to page 407. In contrast see Emil Schürer (1973), *The History of the Jewish People in the Age of Jesus Christ [175 B.C.–A.D. 135]*, 1–3, Geza Vermes and Fergus Millar, eds., Edinburgh: T&T Clark, 464. Morton Smith (1999), in his article "The Troublemakers", emphasizes that Josephus connects the elements from the outset (p. 517).

31. Prominent scholars disagree whether rebellion and revolt were closely connected. Martin Hengel (1989), with his famous book *The Zealots: Investigations into the Jewish Freedom Movement in the Period from Herod I until 70 A.D.*, Edinburgh: T&T Clark, linked rebels and militant religion very closely, and many scholars agree with him. Morton Smith was critical until the end; see The Troublemakers, 542–44, 566.

32. On Honi, see Michael Becker (2002), *Wunder und Wundertäter im frührabbinischen Judentum. Studien zum Phänomen und seiner Überlieferung im Horizont von Magie und Dämonismus, Wissenschaftliche Untersuchungen zum Neuen Testament (WUNT)* 2, 144, 290–346, Tübingen: Mohr-Siebeck.

33. On Hanina ben Dosa, see Becker (2002), *Wunder und Wundertäter*, 347–77.

34. On Eleazar, see Bernd Kollmann (1996), *Jesus und die Christen als Wundertäter. Studien zu Magie, Medizin, und Schamanismus in Antike und Christentum, Forschungen*

zur Religion und Literatur des Alten und Neuen Testaments (FRLANT) 170, 147–51, Göttingen: VandenHoeck und Ruprecht.

REFERENCES

Becker, Michael (2002), *Wunder und Wundertäter im frührabbinischen Judentum. Studien zum Phänomen und seiner Überlieferung im Horizont von Magie und Dämonismus, Wissenschaftliche Untersuchungen zum Neuen Testament (WUNT)* 2, 144, Tübingen: Mohr-Siebeck.

Berger, Klaus (1984), *Formgeschichte des Neuen Testaments*, Heidelberg: Quelle und Meyer, 305–6.

Betz, Hans Dieter (1983), Gottmensch (II), *Reallexikon fuer Antike und Christentum (RAC)* 12, 234–312, Stuttgart: Hiersemann.

Bieler, Ludvig (1935–36), *THEIOS ANER. Das Bild des "Göttlichen Menschen" in Spätantike und Frühchristentum*, Vienna: Höfels.

Bittner, Wolfgang J. (1987), *Jesu Zeichen im Johannesevangelium. Die Messias-Erkenntnis im Johannesevangelium vor ihrem jüdischen Hintergrund, Wissenschaftliche Untersuchungen zum Neuen Testament (WUNT)* 26, Tübingen: Mohr-Siebeck.

Blackburn, Barry B. (1991), *Theios Aner and the Markan Miracle Traditions, Wissenschaftliche Untersuchungen zum Neuen Testament (WUNT)* 2, 40, Tübingen: Mohr-Siebeck.

Bultmann, Rudolph (1921), *Geschichte der synoptischen Tradition, Forschungen zur Religion und Literatur des Alten und Neuen Testaments (FRLANT)* 12, Göttingen: Vandenhoeck und Ruprecht.

Bultmann, Rudolph (1925), Die Bedeutung der neuerschlossenen mandäischen und manichäischen Quellen für das Verständnis des Johannesevangeliums, *Zeitschrift zur Neutestamentliche Wissenschaft (ZNW)* 24, 100–146.

Bultmann, Rudolph (1941), *Das Evangelium des Johannes, Kritisch-exegetischer Kommentar über das Neue Testament (KEK)*, Göttingen: Vandenhoeck und Ruprecht.

Dibelius, Martin (1919), *Die Formgeschichte des Evangeliums*, Tubingen: Mohr. 2nd edition, 1933, Tübingen: Mohr.

du Toit, David S. (1997), *Theios anthropos: zur Verwendung von theios anthropos und sinnverwandten Ausdrücken in der Literatur der Kaiserzeit, Wissenschaftliche Untersuchungen zum Neuen Testament (WUNT)* 2, 91, Tübingen: Mohr-Siebeck.

Fortna, Robert Tomson (1970), *The Gospel of Signs. A Reconstruction of the Normative Source Underlying the Fourth Gospel, Monograph Series of the Society for New Testament Studies (MSSNTS)* 11, Cambridge: Cambridge University Press.

Gallagher, Eugene V. (1982), *Divine Man or Magician? Celsus and Origen on Jesus, Society of Biblical Literature Dissertation Series (SBLDS)* 64, Chico, CA: Scholars Press.

Georgi, Dieter (1986), *The Opponents of Paul in Second Corinthians*, Edinburgh: T&T Clark.

Gray, Rebecca (1993), *Prophetic Figures in Late Second Temple Jewish Palestine: The Evidence from Josephus*, New York and Oxford: Oxford University Press.

Hengel, Martin (1989), *The Zealots: Investigations into the Jewish Freedom Movement in the Period from Herod I until 70 A.D.*, Edinburgh: T&T Clark.

Holladay, Carl R. (1977), *Theios Aner in Hellenistic Judaism: A Critique of the Use of this Category in New Testament Christology, Society of Biblical Literature Dissertation Series (SBLDS)* 40, Missoula, MT: Scholars Press.

Kingsbury, Jack Dean (1981), The "Divine Man" as Key to Mark's Christology: The End of an Era? *Interpretation 35*, 243–57.

Klauck, Hans Josef (2000), *The Religious Context of Early Christianity: A Guide to Graeco-Roman Religions, Studies of the New Testament and its World*, Edinburgh: T&T Clark.

Kollmann, Bernd (1996), *Jesus und die Christen als Wundertäter: Studien zu Magie, Medizin und Schamanismus in Antike und Christentum, Forschungen zur Religion und Literatur des Alten und Neuen Testaments (FRLANT)* 170, Göttingen: Vanden-Hoeck und Ruprecht.

Koskenniemi, Erkki (1994), *Apollonios von Tyana in der neutestamentlichen Exegese. Forschungsbericht und Weiterführung der Diskussion, Wissenschaftliche Untersuchungen zum Neuen Testament (WUNT)* 2, 61, Tübingen: Mohr-Siebeck.

Koskenniemi, Erkki (2005), *The Old Testament Miracle-Workers in Early Judaism, Wissenschaftliche Untersuchungen zum Neuen Testament (WUNT)* II/206, Tübingen: Mohr-Siebeck

Lührmann, Dieter (1987), *Das Markusevangelium, Handbuch zum Neuen Testament (HNT)* 31, 94–95, Tübingen: Mohr-Siebeck.

Maier, Gerhard (1986), Zur neutestamentlichen Wunderexegese im 19. und 20. Jahrhundert, in *Gospel Perspectives* 6, *Journal for Studies in the Old Testament (JSOT)*, 49–87, David Wenham and Craig Blomberg, eds., Sheffield, Scotland: Sheffield Academic Press.

Reitzenstein, Richard (1906), *Hellenistische Wundererzählungen*, Leipzig: Teubner.

Reitzenstein, Richard (1910), *Die hellenistischen Mysterienreligionen nach ihren Grundgedanken und Wirkungen*, Leipzig: Teubner.

Schmidt, Karl Ludwig (1923), Die Stellung der Evangelien in der allgemeinen Literaturgeschichte, in *Eucharisterion Hermann Gunkel zum 60ste Geburtstag*, H. Schmidt, ed., Gottingen: VandenHoeck und Ruprecht. Republished by Ferdinand Hahn, ed. (1985), as *Formgeschichte des Evangeliums*, in the series, *Wege der Forschung*, No. 81, Darmstadt: WB.

Schreiber, Stefan (2002), *Gesalbter und König: Titel und Konzeptionen der königlichen Gesaltenerwartung in frühjüdischen und urchristlichen Schriften, Beihefte zur Zeitschrift für die neutestamentliche Wissenschaft und die Kunde der Älteren Kirche (BZNWKAK)*, 293–94, Berlin and New York: de Gruyter.

Schürer, Emil (1973), *The History of the Jewish People in the Age of Jesus Christ (175 BC–AD 135)*, Volumes 1–3, Geza Vermes and Fergus Millar, eds., Edinburgh: T&T Clark.

Schweitzer, Albert (1951), *Geschichte der Leben Jesu-Forschung*, 6th edition, Tübingen: Mohr.

Schweizer, Eduard (1982), Zur Christologie des Markus, in *Neues Testament und Christologie im Werde, Aufsätze*, 86–103, Göttingen: VandenHoeck und Ruprecht.

Smith, Morton (1999), The Troublemakers, in *Cambridge History of Judaism*, vol. 3, *The Early Judaism*, William Horbury, W. D. Davies, and John Sturdy, eds., Cambridge: Cambridge University Press.

Söding, Thomas (1985), *Glaube bei Markus: Glaube an das Evangelium, Gebetsglaube und Wunderglaube im Kontext der markinischen Basileiatheologie und Christologie*, Stuttgarter Biblische Beitraege *(SBB)* 12, 72, Stuttgart: Katholisches Bibelwerk.

Theissen, Gerd (1974), *Urchristliche Wundergeschichten, Ein Beitrag zur formgeschichtlichen Erforschung der synoptischen Evangelien, Studien zum Neuen Testament (StNT)* 8, Gütersloh: Gütersloher Verlag.

Waller, James, and Mary Edwardson (1987), Evolutionism, *The Encyclopedia of Religion* 5, 214–18.

Weeden, Theodore J. (1968), The Heresy That Necessitated Mark's Gospel, *Zeitschrift fuer Neutestamentliche Wissenschaft (ZNW)* 59, 145–48.

Weinreich, Otto (1909), *Antike Heilungswunder, Untersuchungen zum Wunderglauben der Griechen und Römer*, Giessen: Töpelmann.

Wetter, Gillis P. (1916), *"Der Sohn Gottes": Eine Untersuchung über den Charakter und die Tendenz des Johannes-Evangeliums, Zugleich ein Beitrag zur Kenntnis der Heilandsgestalten der Antike*, Göttingen: VandenHoeck und Ruprecht.

CHAPTER 8

THE MIRACLE OF CHRIST'S BIRTH

John W. Miller

It is not generally recognized that there are two views of the miracle of Christ's birth in the Bible. The purpose of this essay is to point out that this is in fact the case and to indicate when and how these two views originated and came to be included in the same Bible. The better known of these views is set forth in vividly told stories in the Gospels of Matthew (1:18–25) and Luke (1:26–35). Here we learn—in the Greek text of Matthew 1:18—that Jesus was conceived *ek pneumatos hagiou* ("of the Holy Spirit") in the womb of a virgin without a human father. Luke describes this event similarly in Luke 1:35. Being conceived in this manner is so extraordinary that we expect it to be referred to again and again in the scriptures that follow, but this is not the case. The miraculous conception of Jesus *ek pneumatos hagiou* ("of the Holy Spirit") is never mentioned again in the entire New Testament.

Silence about a miracle of such import is perplexing until it is realized another perspective on the conception of Christ was pervasive in the first Christian communities. This is the view alluded to by the Apostle Paul at the beginning of his letter to the Romans where he writes (Romans 1:1–4) about the gospel he was called to proclaim to the world. It is a gospel, he states, about "God's Son," Jesus Christ, "promised beforehand . . . in the Holy Scriptures who according to the flesh was conceived of the sperm of David" (*ek spermatos David*). Referring to Christ's conception in this way reflects the thinking of the time regarding how life begins. A human life began, it was thought, when male sperm was deposited in a woman's womb where it co-agulated like milk (Job 10:10–12) and grew into a child. There was no aware-ness as yet of the part played by the female ovum.[1] The origins of children were thought to be totally in the sperm of their fathers. This is why the genealogies of children were traced through the sperm-line of their fathers—as in genealogies of Jesus in Matthew 1:1–17 and Luke 3:23–38—and why Paul in Romans 1:3 can write of Jesus being conceived "of the sperm of David" (*ek spermatos David*).[2] Paul was signaling to his readers that Jesus truly is, "according to the flesh," the "son" or descendent of David.

EXPLORATION OF THE ISSUE

So what is miraculous about that? The very question indicates one of the reasons why this view is not as well known as the other. The miraculous nature of Jesus being conceived in the womb of a virgin "of the Holy Spirit" (*ek pneumatos hagiou*) is at once recognizable, but what is unusual about his being conceived "of the sperm of David" (*ek spermatos David*)? An explanation is required. We must be reminded that Jesus was a Jew—and first-century Jews were hoping and praying as never before for the coming of God's kingdom through a divinely anointed descendent of David.[3] We need to know as well that David was Israel's most illustrious king and had been promised a dynasty that would last forever. When therefore Paul states in Romans that Jesus Christ was conceived *ek spermatos David* he was announcing this promise had been fulfilled and the much hoped for kingdom of God was already dawning and about to appear in its fullness. Hence, this view of Christ's conception was as miraculous for those who espoused it as was the view of his virgin birth for those who espoused it, but in a different way. The view that he was conceived "of the Holy Spirit" (*ek pneumatos hagiou*) was a miracle of divine origins, the view that he was conceived "of the sperm of David" (*ek spermatos David*) was a miracle of providence related to God's rule on earth.

TWO VIEWS SIDE BY SIDE

How did two such different views of Christ's miraculous conception originate? The already mentioned fact that only two texts in the entire New Testament tell of or allude to Christ's miraculous conception "of the Holy Spirit" (Matthew 1:18–25 and Luke 1:26–38) hints at a possible answer. On closer inspection we observe that these two texts are located side by side with two genealogies—Matthew 1:1–17 and Luke 3:23–38—that trace the paternal sperm-line of Jesus to David and Abraham. This is hardly accidental. It suggests that these two texts which tell of Christ's miraculous conception "of the Holy Spirit" might have been secondarily inserted where they are in each Gospel to supplement or modify the view of Christ's conception "of the sperm of David" in the genealogies.

Textual oddities in the genealogies confirm this impression. At the beginning of Luke's genealogy (Luke 3:23–38) unexpected words occur between "son" and "of Joseph" (3:23): "Now Jesus himself . . . was about thirty years old

being the son—as was supposed—of Joseph, of Heli, of Matthat, of Levi. . . ."
Given their location, the words "as was supposed" cast doubt on the validity of
the opinion of those who prepared this genealogy—implied is that they were
sincere but mistaken. They "supposed" Jesus to be the son of Joseph but were
mistaken about that. It is hard to imagine that those who wrote the genealogy
would question the accuracy of their own account in this way. By contrast it is
easily imaginable that these words were expressive of the sentiments of those
who might have inserted the prior story of Christ's virgin birth (Luke 1:26–
38). When they did this, they were mindful of the discrepancy between their
view of Christ's conception and the view of the genealogy.[4] They could have
deleted the genealogy—but for reasons to be discussed they decided to retain
it. Instead, they modified it with a few words questioning its assumptions.

Matthew's Gospel posed a similar dilemma to the person or persons who
inserted the virgin birth stories in this Gospel. In this instance the original text
likely said that Joseph "begot" Jesus, as Joseph was "begotten" by a line of fathers
before him beginning with David and Abraham (Mt 1:1–16). So in their case
too they faced a choice of deleting the genealogy or changing it at the point
where it stated, "Joseph begot Jesus who is called Christ." They too chose
to retain the genealogy but changed it in the following way: After the word
"Joseph" they deleted the word "begot" and between "Joseph" and "Jesus who
is called Christ" substituted for the deleted "begot" the words, "husband of
Mary who gave birth to" (Mt 1:16). By doing so, they erased the fact that Jesus
was Joseph's son and emphasized instead that Joseph was nevertheless Mary's
husband—a fact referred to in the story they placed right after the genealogy,
relating how Joseph and Mary were engaged, but before coming together,
Jesus was conceived "of the Holy Spirit" (Mt 1:18). With these changes Matthew's genealogy is made to dovetail with the following virgin birth story.

ORIGINS OF THE OLDER VIEW

As to the origins of these two views, it seems evident that the view reflected in the genealogies is the older of the two. Where did that view come
from? From various sources it can be concluded that this was the view of
Jesus' family and first disciples. Since Jesus did not object to being called
David's son (Mt 20:29–34; Mk 10:46–52; Lu 18:35–43), it may be that the
Davidic descent of his family was common knowledge. Paul's letters, which
were written in the middle of the first century and circulated widely among
the churches of that period, indicate as much. They were among the earliest
extant writings of the Christian movement—hence, that Paul could write
as he does in his letter to the Romans that Christ's conception was "of the
sperm of David" (Rom 1:3), and take for granted that he would be understood, indicates this was the accepted view of the time.[5]

But from where did Paul obtain his views in this regard? He was not personally acquainted with Jesus or his family before his conversion. He likely

would not have known of Christ's descent from David unless someone had told him. Who might have told him? In one of his letters Paul writes of going to Jerusalem to spend time with the "pillars" there, to consult about the message he was preaching (Gal 1:18–2:10). Among the "pillars" he mentions was Jesus' brother James, who was their leading elder (Acts 15:13–20). How James would have felt about his brother's sperm-line is indicated in an incident recorded by the church historian Eusebius. In his *Ecclesiastical History* he mentions an attempt by the Roman emperor Domitian (81–96 CE) to execute "all who were of David's line" among the Jews of Jerusalem. Quoting from an older historian, he describes Domitian's action as follows: "And there still survived of the Lord's family the grandsons of Jude, who was said to be His brother, humanly speaking. These were informed against as being of David's line, and brought . . . before Domitian Caesar who was as afraid of the advent of Christ as Herod had been. Domitian asked them whether they were descended from David, and they admitted it." After interrogating them further—and discovering the "kingdom" they were hoping for was no threat to his own—"Domitian found no fault with them . . . and issued orders terminating the persecution of the Church" (*Ecclesiastical History* 3.20). Eusebius concludes his report with these words: "On their release they became leaders of the churches, both because they had borne testimony and because they were of the Lord's family; and thanks to the establishment of peace they lived on into Trajan's time" (98 CE).[6]

From this report it seems apparent that the brothers of Jesus and their children and grandchildren were utterly convinced of their descent from David. In all likelihood, this was the reason that Jesus' conception "of the sperm of David" (*ek spermatos David*) was the taken-for-granted view of the Christian movement from its inception—and also why, later on, this Judean sector of the church stubbornly rejected the notion of Christ's virgin birth when it arose. It was not their "vanity" that made them do so, as Irenaeus would assert in *Against Heresies* in 185 CE when it was published—but their integrity.[7] Being convinced of their family's descent from David, his brothers and their offspring had no other option—they knew for a fact that Jesus was of "David's line" too.[8]

ORIGINS OF THE LATER VIEW

When and how then did the alternative view of Christ's conception arise—that he was conceived "of the Holy Spirit" (*ek pneumatos hagiou*) without a human father? And when and why was this view included in two Gospels of the Bible? We have come to a point of considerable uncertainty among researchers of these issues. A respected Catholic biblical scholar has recently concluded that all proposals to date regarding the origins of the "virgin birth" stories are "meager and disappointing"—and that he too, does not know where these traditions originated (Meier 222).[9]

My own view is that more can be known about this matter than is generally acknowledged. The two blocks of virgin birth stories in Matthew and Luke are themselves suggestive in this regard. It can be readily observed how different they are. While they agree on certain core details (name of Jesus' parents, miraculous conception, birth in Bethlehem) their accounts of what occurred before and after his birth are astonishingly different. Matthew's version begins with Jesus' parents living in Bethlehem—and there is where his miraculous conception occurs; then, when Jesus is born, fearing he might be killed by soldiers of Herod, they flee to Egypt and from there go to Nazareth where Jesus grew up. In Luke's version Jesus' parents were living in Nazareth before Jesus was born—and Nazareth is where his miraculous conception occurs; then the parents go on a brief trip to Bethlehem where the birth takes place; shortly afterwards they return to Nazareth with a stopover in Jerusalem to visit the temple. What shall we make of these differences? At the very least they testify to a lack of fixed traditions.

Do we have any clues as to who might have composed these accounts? I have begun to think that we do. Several decades ago in a meticulously researched essay, a respected church historian, Hans von Campenhausen (1964), traced the origins of the theology of virgin birth in the ancient church to a church leader named Ignatius, who was bishop of the church at Syrian Antioch from about 69 to 107 CE. This church was one of the oldest and largest of the time. It was made up of Jews and Gentiles (Acts 11:19–21). Here Christ's "disciples were first called Christians" (Acts 11:26) and it was from here that Paul and Barnabas started on their first missionary journey (Acts 13:1–3). This too was the church where a controversy erupted over whether Gentiles should be circumcised (Acts 15:1–2). This led to the first consultation of church leaders in Jerusalem in 49 CE (Acts 15:4–29). Another controversy at Antioch was over food laws and this time there were sharp differences between Paul and Peter that could not be resolved (Gal. 2:11–14). It was over this large conflict ridden church that the man presided—Bishop Ignatius—who was the sole source of the virgin birth theology of the early church according to Campenhausen.

When reading Campenhausen's monograph I sensed its insights might be relevant for discovering the source of the virgin birth stories as well. To understand why, it will be necessary to understand why he came to believe Ignatius is the sole source of the virgin birth theology in the early church. His reasoning is as follows. "It seems to me," he writes, "that too little account is taken of the fact that all the so-called 'apostolic fathers'—with one important exception—do not seem to know of the virgin birth. . . . The exception is Bishop Ignatius of Antioch, the Bishop of Syria as he calls himself. . . . No other fragments of Christian writings up to the middle of the second century that have been handed down to us, other than his writings, speak of the virgin birth" (Campenhausen 1964, 19).

To get the full weight of Campenhausen's argument we must ask what "fragments of Christian writings" he is referring. They are not mere "fragments," as he calls them, but substantial documents like the long letter Clement, the bishop of Rome, wrote (in 96 CE) to "the Church of God" at Corinth; the letter Polycarp, the bishop of Smyrna, wrote to the Philippians; the *Epistle to Diognetus*, a treatise on the beliefs and customs of Christians; the strident *Epistle of Barnabas*; the imaginative *Shepherd of Hermes*. These copious writings were written by contemporaries of Ignatius, yet in none of them is there a single reference to Christ's virgin birth. The only writer in the first century to even mention this miraculous birth is Ignatius, bishop of Antioch.

Even more remarkable, Campenhausen goes on to point out, is the fact that Christ's "virgin birth" is not just mentioned in the writings of Ignatius, but is at "the centre of his conviction." For him, Campenhausen continues, "The virgin birth is the very special sign of salvation in the Christian faith. Indeed, the whole of Ignatius' theology revolves around the great contrast between the human and the divine, the realm of death and the realm of life. . . . The primary miracle of redemption depends on the incarnation, on the paradoxical fact that Christ was both the Son of God and, in a new sense that expressly emphasizes the earthly aspect of his being, the Son of man, or, what comes to the same thing, that he is descended on the one side from the seed of David, but on the other from the Holy Spirit" (29). In summary, before Ignatius, there was not a whisper of Christ's virgin birth in the extant writings of his contemporaries; by contrast, in the writings of Ignatius, Christ's virgin birth is at the center of an innovative theology.

The conclusion Campenhausen draws from this remarkable fact is paradoxical. He believes Ignatius to be "the starting point" of the ancient church's theology of virgin birth but not of the accounts of Christ's virgin birth in the Gospels (Campenhausen 1964, 25). He is persuaded that the Gospel accounts of Christ's virgin birth predate Ignatius and were already part of the version of Matthew's Gospel which he and others of this region were reading. As such, he speculates, these Gospel accounts were the starting-point of all later expositions of virgin birth theology in the early church. This is the point at which I find his research flawed but relevant for an understanding of the origins of the virgin birth accounts in the Gospels as well—for I want now to indicate why I believe it was the other way around. The starting point of Ignatius' theology was not the Gospel accounts of Christ's virgin birth but Ignatius' theology was the starting point for the Gospel accounts. The total silence about Christ's virgin birth in the extant writings of his contemporaries would alone suggest this. If the virgin birth stories were already part of Matthew's Gospel, why would Ignatius be the only one in his time to comment on them? Moreover, we know of Jewish-Christians living in this region and time who were devoted to Matthew's Gospel but opposed to the idea of Christ's virgin birth when it arose—so obviously, in their version of Matthew's Gospel these stories were missing.[10]

However, the most compelling reason for thinking Ignatius did not derive his virgin birth theology from the stories in Matthew's Gospel is that he never even hints at doing so, but on the contrary, gives every indication that the source of his thoughts in this regard was himself. Virtually all that we know about Ignatius is found in seven letters written while he was on his way to a martyr's death in Rome (in 107 CE). Most of them were drafted on the spur of the moment in response to delegations from the churches who visited him during this momentous journey. Like Paul, whom he admired and sought to emulate, he wrote candidly about his fears, thoughts, and concerns. Also like Paul, he was a man of exceptional talent who felt called by God to foster the unity of the churches of his region in a time of strident conflicts due in large part to the fact that they did not yet have a set of agreed upon scriptures—and those they did have only acerbated their disagreements. Among these were scriptures Christians inherited from Judaism, the letters of Paul, and the Gospel of Matthew.

All Christians, more or less, respected the scriptures of Judaism but they interpreted them in increasingly different ways. One faction embraced the perspective on these scriptures in the writings of Paul, the other faction embraced the views in Matthew's Gospel.[11] The faction devoted to the letters of Paul inclined more and more to an interpretation that viewed Christ as a God of grace that had come to earth from a totally different realm to liberate human beings from the material world and its laws for a spirit-home in heaven where Christ now lived. The faction that embraced the Gospel of Matthew viewed Christ as the divinely anointed Son of David who had come as a messianic teacher to fulfill the law and prophets and bring about God's kingdom on earth as it was in heaven. These two groups were increasingly in conflict with each other. Those who espoused Matthew's Gospel regarded Paul and his letters as subversive of the Law of Moses and the promises of the prophets; those who espoused Paul's letters thought the adherents of Matthew's Gospel were fostering a kind of legalism and materialism that was the exact opposite of the spiritually liberating Gospel of Paul.

We know from his letters that Ignatius was searching for a way to unite these divided factions.[12] An aspect of his strategy was to exalt the role of the bishop in each and every church—but in what would the bishops be united? From his letters, we sense this was the question preoccupying him and he was excited by the answers welling up within him. It would be a shared new perspective on the centrality and importance of Jesus Christ as both God and man. It was of this that he began to write at the end of his letter to "the deservedly happy church at Ephesus in Asia," as he calls it.[13] He characterizes his thoughts in this regard as a "preliminary account for you of God's design for the New Man, Jesus Christ. It is a design for faith in Him and love for Him, and comprehends His Passion and Resurrection" (*Letter to Ephesians* 20). He adds, "I hope to write you a further letter—if in answer to your prayers, Jesus Christ allows it, and God so wills—in which I will continue this preliminary account. . . ." He had previously written in this same letter about the "mysteries" of Christ's Death and Resurrection as set forth in the letters of Paul (*Letter to Ephesians* 12), but Paul did not have much to say about Christ's birth. His own thoughts about this, is what Ignatius now wants to share. And so, perhaps for the first time (in the middle of paragraph 18 of his letter), abruptly and without forewarning, he begins to put down on paper a "preliminary account" of his thinking in this regard. He writes as follows:

> [18.] Under the Divine dispensation Jesus Christ our God was conceived by Mary of the seed of David and of the Spirit of God; He was born, and He submitted to baptism, so that by His Passion He might sanctify water.
> [19.] Mary's virginity [he continues in a new paragraph] was hidden from the prince of this world, so was her child-bearing, and so was the death of the Lord. All three trumpet-tongued secrets [literally, "these mysteries of a loud shout"][14] were brought to pass in the deep silence of God. How then were they made known to the world? Up in the heavens a star gleamed out, more brilliant than all the rest; no words could describe its luster, and the strangeness of it left men bewildered. The other stars and the sun and moon gathered round it in chorus, but this star outshone them all; the spells of sorcery were all broken, and superstition received its deathblow. The age-old empire of evil was overthrown, for God was now appearing in human form to bring in a new order, even life without end. Now that which had been perfected in the Divine counsels began its work; and all creation was thrown into a ferment over this plan for the utter destruction of death.

The theological premise with which Ignatius began this "preliminary account"—namely, that "Jesus Christ our God was conceived by Mary of the seed of David and of the Spirit of God"—is exactly what is conveyed through the genealogy of Matthew's Gospel, showing Jesus to be "of the seed of David," and its follow-up account of Christ's virgin birth, showing him to have been conceived "of the Spirit of God." Either Ignatius found this theological premise when reading Matthew's Gospel, or he created it. In the light of the fact that none of Ignatius's contemporaries testifies to finding it in Matthew, nor does Ignatius, the probability is that he created it and the follow-up stories in Matthew's Gospel (2:1–23) about Jesus' birth at Bethlehem and the "star" that led the magi to worship the newly born "Emmanuel" ("God with us"; Mt 1:23). All are themes touched on by Ignatius in his "preliminary account of God's design for the New Man, Jesus Christ."

There can be little doubt as to Ignatius's motives for wanting to divulge his novel thinking in this regard, for after doing so he spells them out. At the very end of his letter he writes of his desire to write further about these matters "if the Lord reveals to me that you are all, man by man and name by name attending your meetings in a state of grace, united in faith in Jesus Christ, who is the seed of David according to the flesh and is the Son of Man and Son of God, and are ready now to obey your bishop and clergy with undivided minds" (*Letter to Ephesians* 20). To unite the churches of his time in his newly coined vision of Jesus Christ as both Son of David and Son of God was right then, as his martyrdom in Rome approached ever nearer and nearer, his passion and calling.

THE CREATION OF THE BIBLE

When and why was a block of virgin birth stories inserted in Luke's Gospel; and when and why were Matthew and Luke assembled along with other writings and published in a one-volume Bible such as we have today? There is evidence that both actions, the insertion of virgin birth stories in Luke's Gospel and the creation of the first one-volume Bibles, were made in response to the same controversies in the churches of the first half of the second century. These controversies were similar to those Bishop Ignatius had to contend with at the end of the first century. As a first step toward understanding them it is important to note what the results might have been of his efforts to address them.

There is evidence that soon after his death a new edition of Matthew's Gospel, with the virgin birth stories added, was accepted by a growing number of churches. The chief witness to this development is to be found in the writings of Justin Martyr (110–165), born shortly after Ignatius' martyrdom in Rome. Justin is the first to mention these stories as they appear in the Gospels (Campenhausen 1964, 30–33). He accepts them at face value, and makes ample use of them as proof of Christ's divinity, even while acknowledging that there are Christians who reject them (*Dialogue with Trypho* 48). So in this sense the endeavors of Ignatius appear to have been successful.

At the same time the theological proposals he had made did not reconcile the contending Christian factions of his time: namely, the adherents of Matthew's Gospel and the devotees of Paul's letters. Above all, Ignatius's endeavors did nothing to deter those devoted to Paul's letters from developing their theology in new, more radical directions that would turn out to be more divisive than ever.

The writings of Justin Martyr also bear witness to this development. They are not only the first to mention the virgin birth stories in the Gospels but the first to warn of a new, more virulent threat to the unity of the churches in the teachings of Marcion, "a man of Pontus," as Justin refers to him. He describes this threat as follows: "And there is Marcion," he wrote, ". . . who is even at this day alive, and teaching his disciples to believe in some other god greater than the Creator. And he, by the aid of devils, has caused many of every nation to speak blasphemies, and to deny that God is the maker of the universe, and to assert that some other being, greater than He, has done greater works" (*First Apology* 26). What Justin is referring to is a theological movement that was arising from within the church and threatening to take it over. The "god greater than the Creator" that Marcion was proclaiming was Jesus Christ. Marcion had come to believe in him as such through studying the letters of Paul. In other words, the churches of Asia Minor, and the world, were now, with Marcion on the scene, more bitterly divided than ever and facing an unprecedented crisis. How had this happened?

From all that we can know about Marcion, the "man from Pontus" must have been an extraordinary individual.[15] He was a pastor's son who had become a wealthy shipbuilder. He was also an innovative and assiduous student of the church's older and newer scriptures, the letters of Paul in particular. When studying the latter, Marcion was struck by what Paul wrote in Galatians about the revelation of Jesus Christ from which he derived his Gospel, a Gospel of grace and forgiveness that stood in sharp contrast with the Law of Moses in the scriptures of Judaism.[16] This is what likely led Marcion to the radical conviction that there were two Gods: the just, law-obsessed God of Judaism, who created this miserable world; and Jesus Christ the God of grace who came to rescue those who believed in him for a totally different spirit-world in heaven where he now lives.

Utterly convinced of his insights, Marcion felt compelled to act. First, he wrote a book called *Antitheses* in which he tabulated the differences he observed between Jesus Christ, as revealed to Paul, and the law-obsessed God of Judaism as he perceived to be portrayed in the scriptures of Judaism. Next, as a replacement for the scriptures of Judaism, which he called upon Christians everywhere to stop reading, he created a first Christian "Bible" consisting of a version of the Gospel of Luke, a companion of Paul, and ten letters of Paul (nine to seven churches: Galatians, Corinthians, Romans, Thessalonians, Ephesians, Colossians, Philippians; plus Philemon). Then Marcion went to the church at Rome, the leading church of the time now that Jerusalem was destroyed. After giving its elders a large sum of money, he presented his ideas in a bid for their support. His ideas were rejected and his money returned, whereupon he began propagating his teachings on his own.

His teachings and Bible, a single codex, spread like wildfire to all parts of the church. Scholars estimate that Marcion's followers outnumbered non-Marcionites in the decades of the 160s and 170s (Miller 2004, 49). His success stunned and energized those who opposed him. They rightly sensed a definitive moment had come. Marcion had called upon the churches to get rid of their Jewish scriptures and embrace as their scriptures his own newly created Bible. Instead, those who opposed him did an amazing thing. They quickly produced an alternative Bible by having the entire body of Jewish scriptures, still on scrolls, copied onto the pages of a single codex (as Marcion had done) and then added, in the same codex, many additional

Christian writings, including those that Marcion had in his Bible. By this act alone those who did this were saying in effect: Jesus Christ is not a new God; Christianity is not a new religion. Christians believe in God the Creator, Maker of heaven and earth. Christianity is part of the same story, guided by the selfsame God that is witnessed to in the scriptures of Judaism (Miller 2004, 60–75).

This alternative Bible, a prototype of Bibles today, was huge! Nevertheless, it too was disseminated and embraced by more and more churches worldwide (Trobisch 106). It was at this time, for example, with this alternative Bible in hand, that Irenaeus (130–200 CE), bishop of the church in Lyons, France, wrote *Against Heresies* in which he subjected the teachings of Marcion, and other like-minded teachers, for the first time, to a thorough theological critique. Fifteen years later Tertullian of Carthage (160–230) did the same in a treatise entitled *Against Marcion*. Three manuscript copies of these first alternative Bibles have survived. They are known as Codex Alexandrinus, Codex Sinaiticus, and Codex Vaticanus.

Usually dated to the fourth or fifth centuries, they are examples of what the "first edition" Bibles of the second century looked like (Trobisch 24; Miller 2004, 52–54). A treatise of Tertullian (160–230 CE), *Prescription against Heresies*, published at the end of the second century indicates not only when but where these first one-volume Bibles were first published (Miller 2004, 130). In it he praises the church at Rome for having at some point earlier in that century "united the law and prophets" (scriptures of Judaism) with "the writings of evangelists and apostles" (Christian scriptures) in a volume from which the church "drinks in her faith" (*Prescription* 36).

Vibrant testimony to the creation of a compendium of this kind in mid second-century Rome is also to be found in an ancient text called the *Muratorian Fragment*. It reports on a conclave to draw up a list of books that would be read "publicly to the people in the church" (line 78).[17] It refers to disputes over scriptures that were being discussed and settled. The "heresy of Marcion" is mentioned. The name used for the scriptures under discussion is "Prophets" ("Old Testament") and "Apostles" ("New Testament"). The list of "Apostles" to be read publicly is one that resembles the list of books in the New Testament of Bibles today. The document's first lines were destroyed. So it begins as follows: "The third book of the Gospel is that according to Luke"—and then we read the following: "The fourth of the Gospels is that of John." So we can surmise that the four Gospels in the order we have them in Bibles today were being singled out for a collection of books that would be read publicly in those churches that agreed with this conclave.

TWO VIEWS IN ONE BIBLE

We have confirmation of the work of this conclave in the three codices referred to above: Codex Alexandrinus, Vaticanus, and Sinaiticus.[18] In all three the four Gospels are grouped together at the forefront of what would become known as the "New Testament" of this Bible. The Gospel of Matthew is first, undoubtedly because some version of this Gospel had played a vital role from the beginning of the Christian movement—but also because of its opening genealogy. That genealogy, linking Jesus to a line of fathers going back to Abraham, now serves a dual purpose within this newly formed one-volume Bible: showing the ancestry of Jesus—but also now connecting his story (and the story of the world-mission of his disciples) to the story recounted in the prior scriptures of Judaism beginning with creation (Genesis 1). So with Matthew's Gospel now an integral part of this one-volume Bible, the story of Christ's virgin birth, which follows, is now also an integral part of this larger story extending from creation to the world-mission of Christ's disciples. Hence, as it turns out, the lofty goals that Ignatius had in mind for its theological perspectives were being realized—to unify and strengthen the churches of the whole world (and the world itself) with a "preliminary account of God's design for the New Man, Jesus Christ . . . a design which provides for faith in Him and love for Him and comprehends His Passion and His Resurrection" (*Letter to Ephesians* 20).

What then are we to make of the quite different stories of Christ's virgin birth a few chapters later in this same Bible, in Luke's Gospel? When were these stories added to Luke's Gospel—and why were they also included in the first one-volume Bibles? As previously indicated, this may have occurred at the time this one-volume Bible was created and for similar reasons—to combat Marcion's teachings and Bible. A similar thesis is proposed by veteran biblical scholar Joseph B. Tyson in a recently published study (Tyson 2006). Marcion taught that since Jesus is God, it was absurd to think that he was born as a baby or really died. He was eternal, but manifest on earth as a fully grown man. So in all likelihood, Tyson suggests, the version of Luke's Gospel Marcion had in his Bible did not begin with infancy stories. Marcion's version may have been the original version of Luke's Gospel, Tyson argues. "Quite apart from the Marcionite issues," he writes, "there are good reasons to think that the infancy narratives of Luke's Gospel were late additions to an earlier version of Luke's Gospel" (Tyson 90). The earlier version began with the third chapter where Jesus is introduced, as he is in Mark's Gospel, as an adult. So the infancy stories in Luke 1:5–2:52 were inserted into Luke's Gospel, Tyson suggests, after Marcion's Bible was published and in circulation, with the intent of combating his mistaken ideas about Jesus only appearing to be human.

How, in Tyson's opinion, do the infancy narratives of Luke's Gospel do this? Tyson points to three ways. First, "Above all, the narratives maintain that Jesus was born of a woman; he did not suddenly descend from heaven to Capernaum. . . . For the author of canonical Luke [Tyson observes], although Jesus was born without the agency of Joseph . . . his is nevertheless a human birth. The language that the angel Gabriel uses in addressing Mary in Luke 1:31 seems to have been selected specifically to offend the Marcionites: Mary is to conceive in her womb and produce a son. . . . Anatomical references are also stressed in the meeting between Elizabeth and Mary (Luke 1:39–45), when the child of Elizabeth leaps in her womb (Luke 1:41–44). . . . The language throughout Luke 1:5–2:52 emphasizes the humanity of Jesus" (Tyson 98–99).

Secondly, "The Lukan infancy narratives also stress the relationship of Jesus to Israel," Tyson writes. "Jesus' relationship to the Jewish people is made clear in the references to Joseph and Jesus as of the house of David (Luke 1:27; 1:69; 2:4) and to David as Jesus' father (Luke 1:32). . . . The fidelity of the family to Jewish practices is shown in Luke 2:22–24, the stories of the presentation of Jesus and of Mary's purification. . . . The author also implies that Jesus himself incorporated these practices, noting that as a child he was obedient to his parents (Luke 2:51). But Jesus' Jewishness is nowhere more emphatically signified than in the story of his circumcision (Luke 2:21). . . . Together with others, this passage indicates that the legitimacy and right of Jesus to speak and act in the name of the God of Israel for salvation on behalf of the people and nations is beyond doubt. For our purposes," Tyson summarizes, "it is important to observe that the vital link with Judaism signified by Jesus' circumcision would have been highly offensive to Marcion and his followers" (Tyson 99).

A third feature of these stories that would have been offensive to Marcion, Tyson points out, is "the pervasive influence of the Hebrew Scriptures . . . notable in Luke 1:5–2:52. Allusions to a number of books may be found throughout the narratives, but the author makes prominent use of Daniel and Malachi. . . . These considerations make it highly probable," Tyson concludes, "that the Lukan birth narratives were added in reaction to the challenges of Marcionite Christianity. It would be very difficult to explain why Marcion would choose a gospel with these, to him, highly offensive chapters at the beginning only to eliminate them. Further, it would be difficult to imagine a more directly anti-Marcionite narrative than what we have in Luke 1:5–2:52. . . . The author of Luke 1:5–2:52 wants his readers to know that Marcion is wrong in denying the human birth of Jesus, his Jewish connections, his fulfillment of Jewish expectations, and the role of the prophets in predicting his coming. In a relatively short span our author has succeeded in challenging and rejecting major Marcionite claims" (Tyson 100).

Tyson's thesis includes more than the infancy narratives in Luke's Gospel. He believes other inserts were made to this Gospel at this time and an additional volume was created, the New Testament book of Acts, to produce a work "that would clearly and forcefully respond to the claims of the Marcionites" (Tyson 120). He visualizes this as a stand-alone project. He does not consider what, in my opinion, is the more likely possibility, namely, that the infancy narratives were added to Luke's Gospel in the process of adding this Gospel to a one-volume Bible that the church was preparing to combat Marcion's teachings and Bible. Viewed in this light, the infancy narratives in Luke's Gospel can be seen as a corrective response not only to the mistaken ideas of Marcion but as a corrective supplement as well to the infancy narratives in Matthew's Gospel, which are located just a few pages earlier.

In any case, in their present setting, as part of a one-volume Bible, these two blocks of virgin birth stories will inevitably be compared and it will be noticed how the infancy narratives in Luke's Gospel do in fact supplement and correct certain possibly wrong impressions that might be taken from the infancy narratives of Matthew's Gospel. For all their differences, Luke's virgin birth stories are sufficiently like the stories in Matthew's Gospel that it can be assumed that Matthew's account served as a model for the stories in Luke, but the stories in Luke are more human, more realistic, more credible, conveying a picture of Jesus' family as it really might have been in the times in which Jesus grew up. In this way the stories in Luke serve to humanize and historicize Jesus not only vis-à-vis Marcion's Bible but vis-à-vis Matthew's infancy narratives.

Do we have any clues as to who might have written the stories in Luke's Gospel? There is one possible candidate—it turns out to be someone Ignatius of Antioch knew and admired. On his way to his martyrdom in Rome Bishop Ignatius arranged for a prolonged stopover at the port-city of Smyrna, where a much younger man was bishop. Over the next fifty years, until his own martyr's death, this young man, Bishop Polycarp of Smyrna, would become the pre-eminent leader in the whole of Asia Minor and Rome, in the struggle against Marcion.[19] That stopover in Smyrna was the setting in which Ignatius received his first church delegations, and where he drafted his letter to the Ephesians (cited above). In that letter he went public for the first time with a "preliminary account" of his new thinking about Christ's virgin birth (*Letter to Ephesians* 20). During that stopover a bond was formed between Ignatius and Polycarp that is evident in their subsequent letters (Staniforth 126).

Polycarp not only went on to lead the fight against Marcion in Asia Minor and Rome but there is evidence that he may have had a hand as well in helping design the first one-volume Bible to combat Marcion.[20] History is an inexact science, but sources at hand all point to Ignatius as having shaped, if not written, the virgin birth stories in Matthew's Gospel, and to Polycarp as having influenced, if not written, the virgin birth stories in Luke's Gospel. The older view of the miracle of Christ's birth, that he was conceived *ek spermatos David*, is also still present in this one-volume Bible, but in modified form. Even so, this older view continues to serve as a reminder that the story of Christ's virgin birth is not to be interpreted too literally, but, to repeat, in the way Ignatius hoped it would be read, namely, as "a preliminary account of the New Man, Jesus Christ . . . which provides for faith in Him and love for Him" (*Letter to Ephesians* 20).

NOTES

1. In his essay "On the Generation of Animals," the fourth-century Athenian philosopher, Aristotle, spelled out the reproductive science of the time as follows: "Male is that which is able to concoct, to cause to take shape, and to discharge semen possessing the 'principle' of the 'form'." Whereas "female is that which receives semen, but is unable to cause semen to take shape or discharge it" (Lefkowitz and Fant 84). The persistence of such reproductive concepts in Middle Eastern culture is indicated by a reference in the eighth-century Qur'an to a child being fashioned by Allah from a "sperm drop" (Sura XVIII:37). For details on these views and their relevance for interpreting the Bible, see Miller (1999), Chapter 3, "Male-Centered Reproductive Biology and the Dynamics of Biblical Patriarchy."

2. David Mace (1953) has noted how consistent this reproductive view is with the biblical principle of succession from father to son, for if children originate in the sperm of the father, then "the continuity of the 'line' can logically exist only through the males of the family," he writes, and "the particular woman who happens to bear sons to a man is from the point of view of succession a matter of indifference; hence the complete absence in Hebrew thought of our modern conceptions of 'legitimacy.' The woman supplies nothing of her essential self. She merely provides in her womb the human incubator in which the man's seed becomes his child, the reproduction of his image" (206).

3. On the intensification of these hopes right at this time, see Collins (1995) who summarizes the situation as follows: "the expectation of a king from the Davidic line, which is dormant for much of the postexilic era, resurfaces after the restoration of native, nonDavidic, Jewish kingship in the Hasmonean period (late second to early first centuries BCE). It then reappears in more than one setting. By the first century CE it can fairly be said to be part of the common heritage of Judaism" (49).

4. The opinion of Vermes (1973), a respected Jewish scholar, is similar. He writes that "the logic of the genealogies demands that Joseph was the father of Jesus"—but "To make place for the dogma of the virgin birth, this logic had to be tampered with by the compilers of Matthew and Luke" (215). However, as will be seen, I differ with Vermes about who did this and their reasons for doing so.

5. The failure of Paul to refer to Christ's virgin birth counts especially heavily against its being known to him, since his theological legacy is so large and rich in Christological formulae. In several places he would surely have referred to it, or expressed himself differently, if he or his churches were aware of it. One such place is Galatians 4:4 where, to stress his abasement, Paul writes of Jesus being born, not of a virgin, but of a "woman." This is consistent with his view that Christ's conception was *ek spermatos David* (Rom 1:3; 2 Tim 2:8).

6. These citations are from the translation of Eusebius' *Ecclesiastical History* (3.19–20) by Williamson (1965).

7. This is the charge Irenaeus (in 185 CE) levels against Jewish Christians he calls "Ebionites" in the fifth volume of *Against Heresies* (5.1.3). "Ebionite" means "the poor"—which may refer to "the poor among the saints at Jerusalem" (Rom 15:26). Irenaeus had earlier written (in volume one of *Against Heresies*) of the Ebionite belief that Jesus was "the son of Joseph and Mary according to the ordinary course of human generation" (*Against Heresies* 1.26.1). Now here, in volume five, he takes them

to task for not accepting "by faith" the story of Christ's virgin birth. For information regarding the "Ebionites" and other Jewish Christians of this period, see Wilson
(143–59).

    8. Meier (1991), after an exhaustive investigation of the Catholic view that the
"brothers" of Jesus were not Jesus' biological brothers, concludes that they were. The
Greek word, *adelphous*, he writes, except when used metaphorically, always means
"blood brother," not cousin or step-brother (328). But then he goes on to hypothesize
that they might have been "half-brothers"—and cites as proof of this novel notion,
Mark 6:17, where Philip is called the "brother" of Herod Antipas, when in fact he
had a different mother. Meier is therefore of the opinion that the word "brother" in
this text "has to mean half-brother, since Herod Antipas was the son of Herod the
Great by still another wife. Hence, the blood bond [Meier writes] was only through
the common biological father, and so Philip (whoever he was) was the *adelphos* of
Antipas in the sense of being a half brother" (328). Meier's conjecture in this instance
is flawed. As noted earlier in this essay, in the culture of the time sperm, not blood,
defined genealogical relationships. "Brothers" were brothers by virtue of being begotten by the same father, regardless of their mothers. When therefore it is written
that Jude was brother of James (Jude 1), as James was brother of the Lord (Gal 1:19),
this is tantamount to saying all three had the same father.

    9. He writes that, "Taken by itself, historical-critical research simply does not
have the sources and tools available to reach a final decision on the historicity of
the virginal conception as narrated by Matthew and Luke. . . . Once again, we are
reminded of the built-in limitations of historical criticism. It is a useful tool, provided
we do not expect too much of it" (Meier 222).

    10. Once again, we are referring to the Ebionites. For them and their views about
Christ's virgin birth, see footnote 7. According to Irenaeus they "use the Gospel according to Matthew only" (*Against Heresies* 1.26.2). Campenhausen is aware of this
group and their beliefs but believes they deleted the stories of Christ's virgin birth
from their version of Matthew's Gospel (Campenhausen 1964, 20). This is improbable. Why would they be devoted to a Gospel from which they first had to delete
an important account like that? On the other hand it is completely consistent with
everything else we know about them that they would cherish a Gospel that began (as
Matthew's Gospel does) with a genealogy showing that Jesus was "begotten" by a
line of fathers beginning with Abraham and David (Mt 1:1).

    11. It is notoriously difficult to give a credible account of the controversies among
Christians in this region and period. This and the following summary description are
based partly on what we are told in the New Testament about the controversies that
plagued the church at Antioch (see Acts 15:1–35; Galatians 2:11–14), partly on what
Ignatius writes in his letters, and partly on what I learned from my research on controversies of this region when the churches opposing Marcion created the first one-
volume Bibles such as we have today. For the latter development, see Miller (2004)
and the discussion that follows.

    12. The letters of Ignatius address now this faction, now that. Two address the
perils of Docetism (or "spiritualism" as I prefer to call it)—his letters to the Ephesians
and Tralles; three address the "old leaven" of Jewish thinking and observances—his
letters to the Magnesians, Philadelphians, and Smyrnians. Staniforth (1968), who
has prepared an excellent translation of these letters, describes the "disunity" in the

church to which they are addressed as follows: "He [Ignatius] found it split into three divergent parties, which we might describe in modern terms as left, right and centre. On the left were Docetists [spiritualists], whom he saw as the most serious of the dangers threatening the Catholic faith, and against whom he launches his sharpest shafts. On the right were those whose Christianity was still deeply impregnated with the 'old leaven' of Judaism. Midway between the two stood the congregation of faithful believers, with Ignatius as their leader. The paramount need, therefore, as he [Ignatius] saw it, was to find some means of creating an undivided church by inducing the dissidents on either side to unite themselves with this central body" (67). My impression is that "central body" may not have been as united as Stanisforth implies, at that time at least—but a "central body" of this kind is certainly what Ignatius was trying to foster.

13. I am quoting from the translation of these letters in Staniforth.

14. Staniforth offers the following explanation of the peculiar wording used here. This is "a deliberately paradoxical expression," he writes. "They [the secrets] were prepared in the silence of God, in order to be proclaimed abroad to the world."

15. Virtually all that we know about Marcion is through the writings of those who wrote against him, since none of his own writings have survived, except possibly the so-called "Marcionite Prologues" to Paul's letters, present in all branches of the Latin Vulgate and thought by some to be a surviving remnant from Marcion's Bible. Of those who wrote against him, the most informative are Irenaeus in his magnum opus, *Against Heresies* (185 CE), and Tertullian in his five volume work, *Against Marcion* (200 CE). The latter volumes are completely devoted to critiquing Marcion, both his teachings and his Bible. All students of Marcion are indebted to the painstaking research of Harnack (1924), corrected and supplemented by Hoffman (1984), summarized and updated by Wilson (1995), synopsized and related to the formation of the first Bibles by Miller (2004).

16. This is likely why Galatians was at the forefront of Marcion's letter collection in his Bible, right after his version of the Gospel of Luke. Galatians was important to Marcion not only for his interpretation of the teachings of Paul, but for his belief that Paul was the only faithful apostle of Jesus Christ—for in Galatians Paul writes of how he had to rebuke the leading Apostle Peter for his failure to stand up for the Gospel of God's grace revealed in Jesus Christ (Gal 2:11–14).

17. For date and description of this intriguing manuscript, see Miller (2004, 127–30).

18. For a chart showing the books in each of the three codices, listed side by side for purposes of comparison, see Miller (2004, 57).

19. Irenaeus (130–220), a younger contemporary of Polycarp (70–156), who as a boy saw him in action and greatly admired him, says this about him (among other things): "But Polycarp . . . was not only instructed by apostles and conversed with many who had seen Christ, but was also, by apostles in Asia, appointed bishop of the Church in Smyrna. . . . He it was, coming to Rome in the time of Anicetus [155–66] caused many to turn away from the aforesaid heretics [Valentinus and Marcion] to the Church of God" (*Against Heresies* 3.3.4).

20. Based on a comparison with Polycarp's letter to the Philippians, Campenhausen (1977) believes Polycarp (or his associates) may have been responsible for some of the letters in the end-section of the Bible, namely, 1 and 2 Timothy, and Titus. These letters, he writes, are charged with "the same strength of feeling and with almost the

same phrases" as Polycarp uses in his Philippians letter (181). It is also apparent from their content that they, like Polycarp's letter to the Philippians, are aimed at Marcionites. There is a possible allusion to Marcion himself in the first of these letters. It was widely known that Marcion was a "shipbuilder"—in 1 Timothy those "who have put conscience aside" are said to have "shipwrecked" their faith (1:19). At the end of this same letter (1 Tim) there is also a likely allusion to a book Marcion wrote called *Antitheses*—the final verse of 1 Timothy reads as follows: "O Timothy, guard the deposit, turning away from profane empty utterances and the contradictions [Greek: *antitheseis*] of the falsely called knowledge" (1 Tim 6:20).

REFERENCES

Campenhausen, H. von (1964, original German edition 1962), *The Virgin Birth in the Theology of the Ancient Church*, London: SCM.

Campenhausen, H. von (1977, original German edition 1968), *The Formation of the Christian Bible*, Philadelphia: Fortress.

Collins, John J. (1995), *The Scepter and the Star, The Messiahs of the Dead Sea Scrolls and Other Ancient Literature*, New York: Doubleday.

Harnack, Adolph von (990, original German edition, 1924), *Marcion: The Gospel of the Alien God*, Durham: Labyrinth.

Hoffmann, R. J. (1984), *Marcion: On the Restitution of Christianity, an Essay on the Development of Radical Paulinist Theology in the Second Century*, Chico, CA: Scholars Press.

Lefkowitz, M. R., and Fant, M. B. (1982), *Woman's Life in Greece & Rome*, Baltimore: Johns Hopkins University.

Mace, D. (1953), *Hebrew Marriage: A Sociological Study*, London: Epworth.

Meier, J. P. (1991), *A Marginal Jew*, Volume One: *Rethinking the Historical Jesus*, New York: Doubleday.

Miller, John W. (1999), *Calling God "Father"—Essays on the Bible, Fatherhood & Culture*, New York/Mahwah: Paulist.

Miller, John W. (2004), *How the Bible Came to Be: Exploring the Narrative and Message*, New York/Mahwah: Paulist.

Staniforth, M., trans. (1968), *Early Christian Writings: The Apostolic Fathers*, Hammondsworth: Penguin Books.

Trobisch, D. (2000), *The First Edition of the New Testament*, New York: Oxford.

Tyson, J. B. (2006), *Marcion and Luke-Acts: A Defining Struggle*, Columbia: University of South Carolina.

Vermes, Geza (1973), *Jesus the Jew: A Historian's Reading of the Gospels*, New York: Macmillan.

Williamson, G. A., trans. (1965), *Eusebius: The History of the Church from Christ to Constantine*, Harmondsworth: Penguin Books.

Wilson, S. G. (1995), *Related Strangers: Jews and Christians 70–170 C.E.*, Minneapolis: Fortress.

CHAPTER 9

"That They May Believe": Distinguishing the Miraculous from the Providential

Stephen J. Pullum

In October 2005, the unthinkable happened to Shana West. In what must be every skydiver's worst nightmare, after she leaped from the plane, Shana's tangled parachute only partially deployed, leaving her to fall toward the earth at an astounding fifty miles per hour. The resulting collision broke multiple bones in her face and body but did not kill her. To complicate matters, unknown to her, Shana was two weeks pregnant. Amazingly, she not only survived what was almost a total free fall, but in time gave birth to a healthy baby boy. In reporting the story in March 2007, Robin Roberts, coanchor for *Good Morning America*, called Shana's survival miraculous.[1] It is doubtful that many people, especially people of faith, would have disagreed with Roberts's assessment.

A few days later, *ABC News* reported that Christa Lilly of Colorado Springs had slipped into a coma in October 2001. After six years, though, she suddenly and unexplainably woke up. Calling her ordeal mystical, Christa's neurologist could not explain why. Family members, however, had a different take. They called it a miracle from God.[2] It is doubtful that many people would have disagreed with their assessment either.

A few weeks afterwards, *Good Morning America* reported yet another story, in which a teenager by the name of Levi Draher survived after passing out for five minutes, during which time his brain was deprived of oxygen. Draher was participating in a fad known as the choking game, in which teenagers intentionally choke themselves in an attempt to get high. Fortunately, Draher was resuscitated in time to save his life. Despite the fact that he suffered a dramatic loss of speech and motor skills and would have to spend the next two years in rehabilitation in order to fully recover, reporter Chris Cuomo hailed Draher's survival as "nothing short of a miracle."[3] In a speech to a group of high school students Draher himself recounted, "Do I consider myself a miracle? Yes, I do."[4] As in the above cases, few would probably disagree with Cuomo's and Draher's assessments either.

In early May 2007 a tornado that was about a mile and a half wide, with winds greater than two hundred miles per hour, ripped through the small town of Greensburg, Kansas. It destroyed about 85 percent of the town and caused the deaths of what was reported at the time to be eight people. *ABC News* titled their story "Miracle in Kansas." Even though the town had been warned a few minutes earlier by the National Weather Service, the alleged miracle was the fact that more people were not killed from such a large and powerful storm.[5]

These examples illustrate the fact that we are quick to label as miraculous things that we cannot explain. Is this correct procedure? Whenever an individual narrowly avoids what could have been a major automobile accident while traveling at a high rate of speed, or trapped coal miners are extracted alive from deep within the earth after several days without food and water, or individuals with terminal diseases who are given weeks to live suddenly go into remission, individuals of faith are quick to call these incidents miraculous. However, do any of the above examples actually qualify as miracles?

My purpose in this chapter is to address this issue from a biblical perspective. Specifically I want to examine how miracles are depicted in both the Old and New Testament narratives. Additionally, and equally important, I want to analyze what differences, if any, there may be between the miraculous and the providential. What role, if any, does God play in these two areas according to the Bible?

Before going further, a few preliminary issues may be addressed. Why should we analyze miracles as depicted in the Old and New Testaments? The answer is relatively simple. Many people, who are quick to call miraculous those seemingly unexplainable events that defy the odds, are usually people of faith, primarily Christians, who have read at least portions of the Bible. In many cases it is *because* they have read stories about the miraculous in the Bible that they believe in the possibilities of miracles today in the first place. But should they?

Because people are quick to label unexplainable, positive outcomes as miraculous with little thought to what they are saying, this topic is important. Furthermore, there are a number of televangelists and faith healers today, such as Benny Hinn, Gloria Copeland, and Pat Robertson, who make the claim to an unsuspecting public that they can and should receive some type of miracle in their life, be it financial, physical, social, or emotional, provided they have enough faith. However, if miracles do not exist today, what televangelists are teaching is problematic. For example, unsuspecting individuals may decide that they have indeed received a miraculous healing. This in turn may lead them to stop taking badly needed medicine or throw away essential medical apparatuses and die. Even if these individuals do not die but never improve when they think they should, simply because some preacher is telling them to believe in miracles, this is torturous. Boggs rightly points out that, "It is a very serious thing to raise the hopes of multitudes of sick people with assurances that God will always reward true faith by healing diseases, and then to lead the great majority of these people through disillusionment to despair."[6]

In analyzing the Old and New Testament narratives, my intention here is not to argue one way or the other regarding their veracity. I understand that there are a number of people who dismiss the biblical narratives as mere myth. By doing so, one does not have to grapple with the issue of miracles in the first place, at least as the Bible portrays them. They can be simply dismissed as impossible. However, there are thousands of people who accept the claims regarding the miraculous as revealed in the Bible. Moreover, as was suggested, in most cases it is because individuals read stories about the miraculous in the Bible that they believe they occur nowadays. My intention is to provide a better understanding of miracles as they are depicted in the Bible for people of faith today. I want to offer these individuals a clearer understanding of what constitutes the miraculous and what constitutes the providential from a biblical perspective without throwing God out of the picture.

Differentiating the miraculous from the providential is not merely a matter of semantics. Knowing what a miracle is, what providence is, and the differences in the two is very important in helping individuals to have realistic expectations. I will argue that, in spite of whether a person believes in God, miracles do not occur today because their original purpose has ceased. I will also suggest that what some claim to be miracles today, especially those related to physical healings, in no way resemble what one reads about in the biblical literature. However, despite the fact that it cannot be verified today, one may continue to believe in the providential, which is different from the miraculous. Let us turn our attention first to the miraculous.

MIRACLES

Miracles Violated Natural Law

One of the first things that we should understand about miracles, as they are revealed to us in the Bible, is that they always violated the laws of nature. McCarron argues that it is one thing to pray on the way toward the ground that one's tangled parachute open, and it does so, and another to stop in midair and untangle it before proceeding further.[7] Stopping in midair would constitute a violation of the laws of gravity, making it miraculous.

In the Old Testament when God called Moses to lead the Israelites out of Egypt some fifteen hundred years before Christ, Moses was not confident he could do the job. Part of his problem was that he was not convinced that the Jewish elders would believe him when he would go to them with the message that God had called him to lead.

Exodus 4 records that God gave Moses three "signs," that is, miracles, to demonstrate to the Jews that he had chosen him as their leader. God first told Moses to cast his rod on the ground. When he did, it turned into a snake. When Moses picked the snake up by the tail, it turned back into a rod. The second sign involved Moses putting his hand into his bosom and taking it out. At that point it turned leprous. God then instructed Moses to return his leprous hand to his bosom and to remove it a second time, at which point it was restored. The third sign God gave Moses was to pour water from the river onto the ground. When Moses did so, it turned into blood. All of these involved a violation of nature. Rods left alone do not morph into snakes. Hands do not naturally change instantaneously from healthy to leprous and back to healthy again. In nature, whenever skin diseases heal, they take time—weeks, months, or even years—but they certainly do not heal immediately. Water does not change into blood in nature if left on its own.

Another popular story from the Old Testament that illustrates that miracles were a violation of the laws of nature involved Elijah the prophet and his contest with the prophets of Baal on Mount Carmel. 1 Kings 18 records how Elijah, in an attempt to persuade the Israelites to believe in God, suggested that they build two altars on which to offer a sacrifice, one for Baal and one for Elijah's God. Elijah proposed that the God who "answereth by fire"[8] would thereby demonstrate that he was the true God. He allowed the prophets of Baal to go first. After these prophets invoked their god from morning until noon, nothing happened. Then came Elijah's turn. He commanded the people to douse his altar three times with water before he invoked his God to consume it. The narrative tells us that "the fire of Jehovah fell, and consumed the burnt-offering, and the wood, and the stones, and the dust, and licked up the water that was in the trench."[9] What makes this miraculous is the fact that in nature fire does not rain down from heaven or burn up stones.

One of the best examples of nature being violated is the conception of Christ to the Virgin Mary as recorded in the New Testament.[10] Christ's conception is considered miraculous because the laws of nature tell us that women, especially virgins, do not conceive children without being inseminated by a man. Before we go further, let us be clear that conception and birth are two different things. Births in any species are in no way miraculous, even though they are often speciously referred to as miracles.[11] The fact is, births occur every day in nature and have been occurring for millennia. As I argue elsewhere, they are as common in nature as thunderstorms.[12] So, while babies being born are glorious events, they hardly qualify as miraculous. However, among some Christians, Mary's conception of Christ is a different matter. It is miraculous.

At least once in the Bible a miraculous conception occurred even with normal sexual intercourse as in the case of Sarah, wife of Abraham. What makes this conception miraculous is that the laws of nature do not allow women who have gone through menopause to conceive babies even though they may engage in sexual intercourse. Sarah was 90 years old when she conceived Isaac. When she overheard messengers from God tell her husband that she would have a son, the Bible records how Sarah "laughed within herself, saying, 'After I am waxed old shall I have pleasure, my lord being old also?' "[13] Sarah was fully aware of the laws of nature regarding conception for women of her age. She knew that left on their own, she and Abraham were not going to have any children at that stage in their life together.[14]

As stated earlier, while the conceptions of Christ and Isaac were miraculous, the physical births themselves were not. We assume that both Mary and Sarah, once they had conceived, carried their babies to full term and delivered them in the natural way that women give birth. The only way these births would have been miraculous is if Mary and Sarah had delivered them in some mode that would have violated the laws of human gestation and delivery. C. S. Lewis suggests, "If God creates a miraculous spermatozoon in the body of a virgin, it does not proceed to break any laws. The laws at once take it over. Nature is ready. Pregnancy follows, according to all the normal laws, and nine months later a child is born."[15]

Other examples of the laws of nature being violated or suspended can be found in the New Testament (NT). According to the narratives, Jesus, for example, walked on water[16] and turned water into wine.[17] On other occasions he stilled the storm on the Sea of Galilee,[18] restored the right ear of Malchus, which had been cut off by Peter in the Garden of Gethsemane,[19] and even raised a dead person.[20] The above-mentioned miracles are just a few of the many types recorded for us in the Old and New Testaments that demonstrate a violation of natural law.

Miracles Were Unlimited in Scope

Throughout the Bible miracles dealt with a wide variety of phenomenon. Perhaps this is most easily seen, though not exclusively, in the ministry of Jesus in the NT. Cogdill points out that Jesus demonstrated authority over nature when he calmed the storm on the Sea of Galilee. He also demonstrated authority over material things when he multiplied the loaves and fishes and fed five thousand people. In healing lepers as well as "all manner of disease and . . . sickness," Jesus demonstrated power over physical ailments. He also demonstrated power over demons by casting them out. Ultimately he showed his authority over death when, for example, he raised Lazarus from the dead.

In short, nothing was impossible for Jesus. After arguing that contemporary faith healers would not attempt to do what Jesus did but, nonetheless, would have people to believe that nothing is impossible with God and that Jesus heals today through them, Cogdill persuasively asks, "If Jesus is doing the healing now why doesn't He heal now like He did then?"[21]

Miracles Caused Astonishment

Vine suggests that the word *miracle* in the New Testament comes from two Greek words: *dunamis* and *semeion*. *Dunamis* carries the idea of power or inherent ability and "is used of works of a supernatural origin and character, such as could not be produced by natural agents and means." *Semeion* "is used of miracles and wonders as signs of Divine authority." Another word that is frequently found in the same context with signs and/or mighty works is the word *wonder*. Vine points out that wonder, from the Greek *teras*, causes the beholder to marvel. He suggests that while "A sign is intended to appeal to the understanding," and "power (dunamis) indicates its source as supernatural . . . a wonder appeals to the imagination."[22] Miracles, in other words, caused astonishment on the part of those who witnessed them.

There was a "wow" factor involved in beholding miracles as they are revealed to us in the Bible. For instance, when Jesus healed the man with palsy in Mark 2, the narrative tells us that those who looked on "were all amazed and glorified God."[23] When he healed Jairus' daughter, witnesses "were amazed . . . with a great amazement."[24] When many saw a man possessed with a demon be healed, the narrative says that "amazement came upon all."[25] When Peter healed the lame man who was laid daily at the gate of the temple in Acts 3, Luke records how the people who witnessed it "were filled with wonder and amazement at that which had happened unto him."[26]

This particular incident caused many problems for Peter and John. When the authorities heard of the healing, they arrested them. In deciding what to do with Peter and John, the authorities huddled together. Their conversation is telltale: "What shall we do to these men? for that indeed a notable miracle hath been wrought through them, is manifest to all that dwell in Jerusalem; and we cannot deny it."[27] The point to be understood here is that even the very enemies of Peter and John could not, nor did they try to, deny that a miracle had occurred. The New Testament also suggests that when Jesus raised Lazarus from the dead that the religious leaders asked, "What do we do? For this man doeth many signs."[28] They could not, nor did they try to, deny the miraculous event. A similar situation occurred in Matthew 12 where Jesus reportedly cast a demon out of a man. The narrative says, "the multitudes were amazed."[29] Rather than try to deny the miracle, which they honestly could not, the enemies of Christ put the worst possible slant on it by saying that Jesus was able to do what he did only because he was in allegiance with the devil himself.

What I am trying to illustrate in this section is that whenever a miracle occurred, people did not question it. Biblical miracles did not cause skepticism like many so-called "miracles" today do. Miracles in the biblical narratives caused astonishment, even to the point that hardened critics could not deny what had occurred. While they may have been inconvenient for various religious leaders, miracles were nonetheless astounding. Moreover, these miracles never occurred in an emotionally charged atmosphere where people had been whipped into a frenzy to believe.

Miracles Were Immediate

A fourth characteristic of miracles, particularly as they related to healings, is that, with one exception, which I will discuss momentarily, they were always immediate. In other words, there was no waiting period. A person who was healed miraculously, for example, did not have to go home, lie around the house for a few days or weeks, and experience ups and downs before gradually being cured. The healing occurred instantaneously. In the story of a man cured of leprosy, for instance, the New Testament records how he was healed "straightway."[30] In fact, "straightway" is often used to describe individuals' healings. The scriptures say that when Jesus healed a paralytic man who had been let down through the ceiling "he arose, and straightway took up the bed."[31] The woman with "an issue of blood" was healed "straightway."[32] The narrative records how Peter's mother-in-law was healed of a fever and "immediately . . . rose up." This implies that there was no waiting period for her healing.[33] Returning to the lame man of Acts 3 who had been laid daily at the gate of the temple, the scriptures suggest that when Peter healed him, "immediately his feet and ankle bones received strength" and he leaped up and ran around.[34]

In his book *Healing: A Doctor in Search of a Miracle*, medical doctor William Nolen analyzed over 80 cases of individuals who had supposedly received a miraculous healing during one of the crusades in Minneapolis of the world-renowned faith healer Kathryn Kuhlman. After following up these cases, Nolan concluded that not only had many of these people never received a healing, let alone an instantaneous cure, but many had died from their life-threatening ailments. One case specifically that Nolen cites of an individual who claimed to have received a miraculous healing but did not truly receive one was 23-year-old Rita Swanson. Rita "had blemishes all over her face . . . that is a common consequence of severe adolescent acne," reports Nolen. He reveals how Kuhlman said, "In three days that skin problem will be cured." Even Nolen himself, upon future examination, agreed that

Swanson's face "was very much improved." However, Nolen points out that "skin is highly subjective. You look in the mirror, and unless things are too shockingly obvious, you will see, at least in part, what you want."[35] Even though Rita's skin may have been improved, one can hardly call this miraculous. Nolen concludes that "none of the patients who had returned to Minneapolis to reaffirm the cures they had claimed at the miracle service had, in fact, been miraculously cured of anything."[36]

Popular contemporary faith healer Ernest Angley, like other faith healers, occasionally tells individuals who come through his healing lines to "Go and get well."[37] This is ironic due to the fact that, ostensibly, a person is in the healing line in the first place to immediately get well, not to have to wait a period of time afterward. Where is the miracle in having to wait? What contemporary faith healers claim does not square with the biblical narratives, wherein miraculous cures were always instantaneous.

The story of Jesus healing a blind man in Mark 8 is sometimes offered as evidence that not all miraculous healings had to occur instantaneously. The narrative suggests that, after Jesus "spit on his eyes, and laid his hands upon him," he asked the man if he could see. The man responded that he could see men but he saw them "as trees, walking," which suggests that he was not fully healed. Seconds later, Jesus again laid his hands upon the man's eyes, at which point the man "saw all things clearly."[38] For reasons which we can only surmise, the blind man was not able to see clearly the first time.

Foster argues, "We cannot tell why the miracle was gradual: whether by the purpose of Jesus or because of the slow-moving faith of the man." Christians would probably not concede that it was because Jesus did not have the ability to "get it right" the first time. Regardless of whatever reason the man was not able to see clearly the first time, the point that should be understood is that Jesus did not tell him to go home and gradually improve over time. The man was healed before he left the presence of Jesus, therefore, nonetheless, immediately. In no way should this example be used to justify the fact that miracles were not instantaneous. Foster argues, "it is absurd" to take this example "as the necessary model for all [miraculous healings] when the peculiarities are" an exception to the other examples "in the life of Christ."[39]

Miracles Were Always Complete

Closely related to the idea of immediacy is the notion that miraculous healings in the Bible were always complete. In other words, individuals' ailments were always made whole, the above example from Mark 8 notwithstanding. Never was an individual just a little healed and then sent on his way to get better, perhaps never to fully recover. The man in the gospel of Matthew who had a withered hand, for example, was "restored whole."[40] The lame man in

Acts 3 did not need crutches or a cane after he was healed. There were no recurring side effects to anyone who received a healing in the biblical narratives. Moreover, individuals never lost their miracle once they received it.

Perhaps one of the best examples of individuals in our time who claimed to have received miraculous cures but clearly was not wholly healed is that of a young woman in one of Kathryn Kuhlman's crusades. This woman, who had no knee cap, came to the stage claiming that, until she was just healed, she could not walk without her brace. In what was a noble attempt to demonstrate her "miracle" to the thousands of people in attendance, she had taken the brace off of her leg and hobbled badly, yet courageously, across the stage to thunderous applause. Moreover, she hobbled off the stage as badly as she had hobbled onto the stage, without any obvious improvement because she was still missing her knee cap.[41] This could hardly be called a miracle.

In one of contemporary faith healer Benny Hinn's crusades, a young woman came to the stage, claiming she had been healed of deafness. However, she could not speak. One of Hinn's assistants reminded Hinn and the entire auditorium that because the young lady had not been able to hear since birth, she would have to learn how to speak.[42] Ironically, in other words, the young lady was not whole. Why is it that she could receive a miracle involving hearing but not speaking? This makes no sense.

Miracles Were Empirically Verifiable

One very important characteristic of biblical miracles, especially those involving physical healings, was the fact that they could be seen by everyone present. This principle seems to be lost on many people today. In the biblical narratives one could see, for example, Malchus's ear put back on the side of his head, withered hands restored whole,[43] totally blind men receive their sight, lame individuals leap for joy, lepers' skins completely made whole, or even dead people brought back to life after having been dead for days. There were other types of miracles that were visually verifiable as well, such as water instantaneously turning to wine, a man walking on water, or a storm suddenly being calmed, to name a few.

So-called "miracles" today, especially "miraculous healings" cannot always be verified with one's eyes. We are forced to take people's word for the fact that they were once infirm but now are healed. For example, the types of miracles that one witnesses in faith healing services today involve poor blood circulation, weak eyes, backaches, deteriorated disks, internal cancers, depression, and other emotional problems, heart conditions, bursitis, arthritis, rheumatism, inability to smell, and even cigarette and drug addiction.[44] Body parts are never regenerated like those cases in the Bible, which is one reason an individual will never see glass eyes or other prostheses in the trophy cases of faith healers.

In short, none of the types of "miracles" one supposedly sees are visually verifiable on the spot like those recorded in the Bible. Therefore, they are non-falsifiable. In other words, witnesses cannot say, "No, you were not really healed." Audiences are simply asked to take the word of the person being healed. They cannot see for themselves like audiences in the Bible could. Biblical audiences were never merely asked to take the word of anyone. They could see the healing with their own eyes. Even when people occasionally stand up from wheelchairs today during some healing service as proof of the miraculous, audiences still do not know to what extent the individual could or could not walk prior to coming there.

Miracles Preceded Faith

We are told today that faith is necessary to experience a miracle, especially a miraculous healing. The fact is, in the Bible, miracles almost always occurred *prior* to belief. In other words, most of the time, faith was not a prerequisite to receive a miracle. In fact, quite often, it was because of the miracle that audiences developed faith. This is not to say that in every case where a miracle occurred faith always followed. Rather, what I am suggesting is that miracles were designed to produce faith, not vice versa. For instance, in the case of God giving Moses three signs, these miracles were given "that they may believe."[45] After Moses performed these miracles to the Israelites "the people believed: and . . . bowed their heads and worshipped."[46]

In Elijah's contest with the prophets of Baal in 1 Kings 18, he invoked his God to rain fire from heaven to consume the altar that he had built "that this people may know that thou, Yahweh, art God." The narrative suggests that "when all the people" witnessed the altar consumed with fire from heaven, "they fell on their faces: and they said, Yahweh, he is God; Yahweh, he is God."[47] Shortly before Elijah's confrontation with the prophets of Baal, the Old Testament tells us that he raised the dead son of the widow of Zarephath. Afterward, the woman said to Elijah, "[N]ow I know that thou art a man of God, and that the word of Yahweh in thy mouth is truth."[48] Faith followed both of these miracles in the biblical narratives. It did not precede them.

Jesus performed miracles to produce belief in those around him as well. When he told a palsied man that his sins were forgiven, after realizing that there were some who were skeptical of who he claimed to be, Jesus told his onlookers, "But that ye many know that the Son of man hath authority on earth to forgive sins (then saith he to the sick of the palsy), Arise, and take up thy bed, and go unto thy house." When "the multitudes" witnessed the healing, "they were afraid, and glorified God."[49] When John the baptizer was put into prison, he sent his disciples to inquire about Jesus. "Ask him," John instructed, "art thou he that cometh, or look we for another?" Jesus responded to John's disciples, "Go and tell John the things which you hear and see: the blind receive their sight, and the lame walk, the lepers are cleansed, and the deaf hear, and the dead are raised up."[50] Jesus was saying, in other words, "Go offer John the evidence. Tell him what you see for yourselves. Then he'll know who I am."

Nicodemus understood this idea when he said to Jesus, "We know that thou art a teacher come from God; for no one can do these signs that thou doest, except God be with him."[51] The apostle Peter articulated a similar notion when in his inaugural address of Christianity on the day of Pentecost he described Jesus as "a man approved of God unto you by mighty works and wonders and signs which God did by him in the midst of you, even as ye yourselves know."[52]

The apostles of Christ also performed miracles to produce faith. For instance, when the Apostle Paul smote Elymus blind, Sergius Paulus "believed, being astonished at the teaching of the Lord."[53] Acts records that the people became believers after having seen the "signs and wonders" performed by Peter and other apostles.[54] Hebrews explains how the apostles were validated as messengers of God "by signs and wonders, and by manifold powers, and by gifts of the Holy Spirit."[55] In fact the Apostle Paul himself reminded the Corinthian church that the "signs of an apostle" were performed among them "by signs and wonders and mighty works."[56]

Roberts argues that a miracle was not "just *any* divine intervention. . . . It was a very special type of divine intervention that could serve as a *sign* that the person performing the miracle had the power of God behind him." Roberts contends that miracles "were a very special class of supernatural interventions of particularly astounding nature that were especially designed by God to serve as signs in the hands of certain men that he selected to be his messengers."[57]

To reiterate, miracles were designed to produce faith. Faith was not designed to produce miracles. It is true that on one occasion Jesus demanded faith on the part of two blind men before he healed them.[58] This was the exception to the rule, though. In the majority of cases, faith was not a prerequisite. This *was* the rule. In his text, *Modern Divine Healing*, Miller points out that there were 31 cases of miraculous healings performed by Christ in the synoptic Gospels. Of these cases, only once did Jesus require faith on the part of recipients before he healed them.[59] Miller points out that there were other cases where faith was present but not required.[60] It seems, then, that while Jesus may have rewarded faith, it was not necessarily a condition for one to receive a miraculous cure. Most cases of healing involved no faith whatsoever.[61]

In the biblical narratives, sometimes those who were healed knew absolutely nothing about the healer.[62] Hence, there could be no faith. Sometimes those healed were not even present with the healer when they were healed.[63] Sometimes those healed were not even alive. How could they have faith?

Sometimes people were healed because of the faith of other people.[64] If a miraculous healing failed, it was due to the faithlessness of the healer, not the person being healed.[65] What faith healer today would admit to being the cause of someone not receiving a miraculous cure?

Before closing this section, permit me to deal with a narrative that is sometimes cited to prove that faith is necessary for miracles to occur. Mark 6:5–6 suggests of Jesus, "And he could there do no mighty work, save that he laid his hands upon a few sick folk, and healed them. And he marveled because of their unbelief." The argument is that because the people did not believe (i.e., had no faith), Jesus could not perform miracles at that location. Two observations are in order here: (1) the phrase "mighty work" is much broader than just performing miracles. It probably has reference to Jesus' general teachings and attempts to persuade people to accept him; (2) the phrase "mighty work" obviously does not include miraculous healings because the very next phrase says that he laid hands on a few sick people and healed them. He apparently did this regardless of the lack of faith on the part of the people. So, the phrase "could there do no mighty work . . . because of their unbelief" does not suggest that faith is necessary for miraculous healings to occur. However, this passage does seem to suggest that one cannot be successful in a ministry if that person is rejected by the faithless. Jesus' point about a prophet not being without honor except in his own country emphasizes that the folks in his hometown rejected him. They knew him. They grew up with him. Apparently, for whatever reason, they were not impressed with him. Hence, he could do no "mighty work" there.

THE PROVIDENTIAL

Having discussed the miraculous as depicted in the Old and New Testament narratives, let us now turn our attention to the providential to see what differences there are between the two. If miracles do not occur today, does this mean that we should not believe in God or that we should not believe in his providential care? The answer to these questions, I believe, is no.

The word *providence*, per se, is used only one time in the entire Bible, in Acts 24:2. Here the orator Tertullus explains to Felix, the governor of Palestine, that it was by Felix's providence that "evils are corrected for this nation." The term *providence*, comes from the Greek *pronoia*, which means forethought. It is derived from *pro*, meaning before, and *noeo*, to think.[66] Corroborating Vine, Strong suggests that *pro* and *noeo* carry with them the idea "to consider in advance, i.e., look out for beforehand," to "provide (for)."[67] Citing McClintock and Strong, Jackson (1988) points out that providence comes from the Latin *providentia*, which suggests foresight. Jackson argues, "The word is used to denote the biblical idea of the wisdom and power which

God continually exercises in the preservation and government of the world, for the ends which he proposes to accomplish."

Citing the biblical scholar Merrill Tenny, Jackson (1988) also reports, "Providence concerns God's support care and supervision of all creation, from the moment of the first creation to all the future into eternity." According to Jackson, providence is the opposite of chance or fate, which suggests that events are "uncontrollable and without any element of benevolent purpose."[68] Bowman argues that the concept of providence, "whether in Greek, Latin, or English has to do with getting something ready, preparing something ahead of time, with equipping or furnishing what is needed."[69]

Although the word *providence* appears only once in the Bible, the concept of God looking out for or providing for his people can be found throughout the Bible. In Genesis chapters 37 through 46, for instance, we read about how Joseph's brothers sold him into Egyptian bondage but how Joseph eventually rose to second in command of Egypt and saved his family from a famine, including the very brothers who sold him. Ostensibly, at least, it appears that God was operating behind the scenes providentially to care for both Joseph and the Israelites. In Exodus 2: 1–10 we read about the Egyptian Pharoah's daughter finding baby Moses floating in a basket in the crocodile-teeming Nile river and giving the baby back to his Hebrew mother to nurse him.

This may have been the irony of ironies. The mother who had to give up her son in order to save him was now nursing him. Was this by coincidence or by the providence of God? People of faith would suggest that God was probably behind this action, too. In the book of Esther, we read about the Persian King Ahasuerus (i.e., Xerxes) granting permission to his servant Haman to issue a decree to kill all of the Jews in his kingdom. When Mordecai, Queen Esther's cousin, found out about Haman's plot, he asked Esther (a Jewish woman herself) to risk her life and appear before her husband's throne to intercede for the Jewish people, which she reluctantly did. Haman was ultimately hanged on the very gallows that he had built for Mordecai, and the Jews were allowed to resist their attackers, thus saving them from annihilation.

In Esther 4:14, Mordecai persuaded Esther with these words, which suggest, on their face, possible providential intervention by God for His people: "For if thou altogether holdest thy peace at this time, then will relief and deliverance arise to the Jews from another place, but thou and thy father's house will perish; and who knoweth whether thou art not come to the kingdom for such a time as this." Mordecai is saying, in other words, "Esther, God will take care of us Jews. But how do you know that it was not God's providence that made you queen and put you here for a reason?" The idea behind the above examples is that God dwelt in the affairs of humans. In the New Testament we are reminded that God continues to be active in the lives of people.[70] But how, miraculously or providentially?

PRAYER AND PROVIDENCE ARE BOUND TOGETHER

People of faith pray today because they believe that God will respond in some way to their prayers. Bowman suggests, "If I didn't believe in providence, I would not take the trouble to pray."[71] The apostle John taught that "if we ask anything according to his will, he heareth us."[72] The apostle Peter suggests that "the eyes of the Lord are upon the righteous, and his ears unto their supplication."[73] James suggests that "The supplication [i.e., prayer] of a righteous man availeth much."[74] Jesus himself taught, "Ask, and it shall be given you."[75] He also reminded his disciples, "If you abide in me, and my words abide in you, ask whatsoever ye will, and it shall be done unto you."[76] The whole idea behind prayer is that there is a supernatural being behind the universe who hears the requests and groanings of his people. However, when God grants the requests of an individual, does this mean that he has to do so miraculously? In other words, is everything that God brings about in the lives of individuals who pray a violation of natural law? Stated differently, should we call these events miraculous? I think not, for reasons that follow.

The Providential Involves God Working through Nature

Jackson (1988) rightly points out that whereas "A miracle is God's working on a plain [sic] that is above that of natural law; providence is his utilization of natural law." In the miraculous, God operates directly." "[I]n providence, He operates indirectly, employing means to accomplish the end."[77] Let us be careful here to understand that both the miraculous and the providential involve supernatural intervention. However, supernatural intervention can come through nature, not necessarily through a violation of nature. Let us look at some examples from the biblical narratives to illustrate these points.

Jackson (1988) argues that while Mary's conception of Christ was miraculous, Hannah's conception of her son Samuel was providential. First Samuel 1:6 narrates that "Jehovah had shut up her [Hannah] womb." However, she prayed to God to give her a son. The scriptures say that her husband "Elkanah knew Hannah, his wife; and Yahweh remembered her." The idea behind "knew" is that they had sexual relations. Later, "Hannah conceived, and bore a son; and she called his name Samuel, saying, 'Because I have asked him of Jehovah.'" Hannah's prayer had been answered. Jackson suggests, "Here by means of the law of procreation, God intervened and sent a child into the world."[78] One child (i.e., Jesus) came into the world through a miracle. Another child (i.e., Samuel) came into the world providentially. Nonetheless, God was behind both events.

One might ask, "How is it that Hannah's conception was providential, but Mary's (and Sarah's) were miraculous?" Mary's and Sarah's conceptions were miraculous because both clearly violated natural law in their own way, as stated earlier. However, there is no indication that any natural law was violated with Hannah. Occasionally in nature, even when God is not involved, women can go for years thinking that they cannot have any children, when suddenly, seemingly out of nowhere, they become pregnant with the help of their male mate. This is certainly not miraculous. We do not really know why Hannah could not conceive other than the fact that the narrative tells us that God had closed her womb. What God had closed, God could open through natural means. The point to be understood here is that providence still involves supernatural intervention. However, supernatural intervention does not necessarily come miraculously.

When the Jewish King Hezekiah prayed to God to deliver him from the Assyrian King Sennacherib, who had besieged Jerusalem, the narrative tells us that "an angel of Jehovah" smote 185,000 Assyrian troops. Sennacherib was then forced to withdraw to his capital Nineveh. This was miraculous because an angel—a supernatural being—was responsible for single-handedly slaying thousands of enemy soldiers—something impossible to do naturally. Earlier, God had told Hezekiah that He "will cause him [Sennacherib] to fall by the sword in his own land." But how would God accomplish this? When Sennacherib returned from Jerusalem, two of his sons slew him in the temple as he was praying at the altar.[79] Sennacherib's death came about through natural means. God was behind his death, though, making it providential.

In the New Testament, when King Herod jailed Peter, the narrative tells us that Peter had been "bound with two chains" and was asleep between two guards. Two other soldiers were guarding the doors of the prison. However, "an angel of the Lord stood by him [Peter] and a light shined in the cell: and he smote Peter . . . and awoke him . . . and his chains fell off from his hands." The angel proceeded to miraculously lead Peter out of the prison, past all of the guards and the locked door. Eventually he came to "the iron gate that leadeth into the city." This gate "opened . . . of its own accord" allowing Peter to flee from his captors. This all occurred miraculously.[80] In the natural realm, chains and locked doors do not automatically fall off or unlock themselves.

There was another escape that one could argue occurred providentially. In Acts 19, the Apostle Paul had gone to Ephesus to preach. Demetrius, a silversmith who made shrines of the goddess Diana, took offense at Paul's preaching and stirred up an insurrection against him and his traveling companions Gaius and Aristarchus, who had been "seized." Eventually a man named Alexander quieted the mob and persuaded them to take up their cause peacefully in the courts, thus allowing Paul, Gaius, and Aristarchus to leave.[81] One could make an argument that it was God who allowed Paul and his companions to escape. However, no laws of nature were violated as in the above case with Peter.

In the biblical narratives we read where God destroyed two cities, one miraculously and one providentially. The scriptures say that "Jehovah rained upon Sodom and . . . Gomorrah brimstone and fire from out of heaven."[82] This occurred miraculously for roughly the same reason that Elijah's altar caught fire, because fire and brimstone do not fall from heaven according to any laws of nature. On the other hand, Matthew 24 reveals how God would come in judgment against the city of Jerusalem. This was accomplished in 70 CE by the Romans. One can argue that God was behind this act. However, the destruction of Jerusalem was not miraculous. God operated through the realm of nature, in this case, using a foreign army to destroy the city, making the event providential.

One last example of the providential and the miraculous should suffice. It is one thing to miraculously rebuke "the winds and the sea" and bring about "a great calm,"[83] thus showing power over nature, but another thing to pray to God to send rain. This is exactly what Elijah did after Israel had endured a three-and-one-half-year drought. The scriptures say that "the heavens grew black with clouds and wind, and there was a great rain."[84] There was nothing miraculous about rain clouds even though God had answered Elijah's prayer and brought about the change. God had operated providentially through nature.

This discussion about the miraculous versus the providential means, practically speaking, that God has not performed a miracle even though he may have supernaturally intervened in the lives of people. This is a point that many people today fail to understand, especially when it comes to praying for the sick and afflicted. If a sick or ailing individual recovers, it might be because God effected a change through natural law. In other words, God may have operated providentially. However, we should not make the mistake of calling it a miracle. Nevertheless, we have not thrown God out of the picture simply because we deny that a miracle occurred.

But what role, if any, does faith play in all of this? It is true that God could, at any time, make something happen providentially without anyone invoking him. In other words, no prayer or faith on the part of anyone whatsoever need be involved. Oftentimes, though, individuals beseech God through prayer. It is during these times that faith is required. In fact it would not make sense for a person to pray unless he or she had faith in the first place. The author of Hebrews suggests that "without faith it is impossible to be well-pleasing unto him; for he that cometh to God must believe that he is, and that he is a rewarder of them that seek after him."[85]

Even though faith may be necessary to bring about change under the providential, one must understand that realistically there are limitations here. Individuals who have lost a limb or some other bodily member, for example, may pray with all the faith they can muster that their body parts will grow back, but they will never regenerate themselves because this never occurs in nature. Furthermore, some individuals have gone through multiple surgeries and have such ailing bodies that nothing will ever change organically no matter how full of faith their prayers are. Like the Apostle Paul's "thorn in the flesh,"[86] whatever that might have been, the best that they can hope for is what Paul could hope for—strength to endure it. At the beginning of this chapter, I pointed out that the difference between the miraculous and the providential is not merely a matter of semantics but has everything to do with expectations. Knowing the differences between the two allows us to understand that some things we may be inclined to pray for will never occur. Therefore, we should not expect them to. The fact is, we can pray until we're blue in the face with all the faith in the world but still not see any organic change in our defective bodies. Instead, what individuals ought to be praying for is strength to overcome. This is realistic.

Providence Cannot Be Proven Factually

Often events happen in our day and age that appear on the surface to be the workings of God. The fact is, though, we cannot be so sure. Bowman (1992) argues, "We strongly suspect that in certain instances, God has altered circumstances, changed situations so that our best interests were served, perhaps even in what seems to be the answer to our prayers. But we cannot know for sure; we can be certain only if God has revealed [them]."[87] Similarly Hagewood (1990) warns against being "dogmatic about our interpretation" of God's providence. "Accept the fact that God has simply not made us privy to His providence," he concludes.[88] Likewise, Jackson (1988) contends that "no person can point to particular circumstances of his or her life and confidently assert, 'I know that this was the providential intervention of God at work!'" Jackson concedes that an event may very well be the result of the providence of God at work but our "subjective assertions" can "prove nothing." He goes on to point out that, "while it is true that God does work in the lives of men, they are frequently unaware of it. We may suspect it, believe it, hope it to be the case, and even act in such a way as to accommodate it; but, in the final analysis, we walk by faith and not by sight (2 Cor 5:7)."[89]

Turner (n.d.), too, warns about "thinking a certain event or set of circumstances *definitely* means that God has done this or that or wants this or that to happen." He rightly points out that "an event can happen because God wants it to happen and causes it to happen or it may happen for various other reasons," neither of which we can really know for sure. Citing Morde-cai's words to Queen Esther (i.e., "Yet who knows whether you have come to the kingdom for such as this?") Turner argues that Mordecai was not demonstrating a lack of faith. Instead, he was merely being careful not to assume something he should not be assuming.[90] The fact is, people of faith should be careful about what events, whether good or bad, they attribute to God. It just might be that God had absolutely nothing to do with them.

CONCLUSION

In this chapter, I have tried to demonstrate that there are significant differences between the miraculous and the providential as they are por-trayed in the biblical narratives. Miracles involved a suspension of the laws of nature, were unlimited in scope, caused astonishment on the part of onlookers, were always immediate, were always complete, were always empirically verifiable, and almost always occurred without faith on the part of onlookers or recipients. Providence, on the other hand, is linked to faith and prayer, involves God working through nature, but cannot be proven factually. While both involve supernatural intervention into the lives of people, they are not the same things and, therefore, should not be confused.

Having a proper understanding of each has everything to do with what a person can realistically expect to receive when he or she prays to God, or even what he or she should be praying for in the first place. While God is "able to do exceedingly abundantly above all that we ask or think"[91] there is a limitation to what we can and should expect him to do. This is not a lack of faith, however. This is the reality that is presented for us in the biblical narratives. Specifically with regard to miraculous healings, Miller points out that "the issue" is not "whether we believe God capable of healing the sick today. He most certainly is able to heal the sick today, and possesses abundant power to do so miraculously now, if this were his will. . . . The issue is not what God is able to do, but what he wills to do today."[92]

In the infant Christian church miracles were designed to produce faith and guide it in the will of the Lord during a particular period in history, not to serve as God's way of leading people to him forever and certainly not to benefit society as a whole.[93] In other words, miracles were not intended for all people of all ages for all purposes, Hebrews 13:8 notwithstanding. In 1 Corinthians 13, the Apostle Paul argues that we would no longer need the miraculous after "that which is perfect is come."[94] Perfect, in this verse, does not mean sinless. Nor is it referring to Christ's second coming. Instead, perfect means complete, fully grown, or mature (from the Greek *teleios*).[95] The perfect refers to the completed revelation of God's will (i.e., the canon of scripture). The apostle James argues that "he that looks into the perfect (*teleios*) law, the law of liberty, and so continueth . . . shall be blessed in his doing."[96]

In the context of 1 Corinthians 13, "that which is in part" (i.e., miraculous gifts) is contrasted to that which is "perfect" (i.e., something to be completed). "Childish things" are juxtaposed to the mature. The dim is contrasted to the clear. There would come a time when spiritual gifts and other miracles (i.e., things done "in part," "childish things," or dim things) would give way to the "perfect" (i.e., the complete or mature). Moorhead (2004) argues that the "gist of 1 Corinthians 13:10 is that gifts [miracles] would cease in relation to the universal attainment, or coming of the canon." This has been accomplished today. "The community of faith gathered for edification via the scripture is God's plan for the edification of the church today,"[97] not through signs, miracles, or spiritual gifts.

Moorhead (2004) also argues that the miracles mentioned in 1 Corinthians 13 "enabled the Christian to minister beyond human capacity during transition from [the] old covenant to the new covenant program." Their purposes "were to glorify God by equipping and edifying the body of saints in sound doctrine toward maturation and to serve as a sign to unbelievers." Moorhead freely admits that the "exact time of the cessation of spiritual gifts is up for debate" but that there are at least four "prevailing views" of when this occurred: (1) after the book of Revelation was complete; (2) "after the last Apostle died; (3) after the last gifted person died following the close of the canon; and (4) upon the dissemination of the canon throughout the region."[98] All of these probably occurred at or near the end of the first century.

While the miraculous has ceased, this should in no way alarm people of faith because the providential continues. Nothing in the biblical narratives suggests that God has stopped providing for his people. So, while we should be careful about what we label a miracle, even be so bold as to say that miracles no longer exist, this is not to suggest that God does not exist nor that he does not intervene in the lives of humans. But supernatural intervention does not necessarily equate with the miraculous.

Although Shana West's story, like that of Christa Lilly's and Levi Draher's, may be amazing, they hardly qualify as miracles. Certainly they do not violate any laws of nature. The truth is, many people before them have had similar experiences. And just because we may not fully understand them from a scientific point of view, this does not give us the liberty of labeling them miraculous. Whenever an individual escapes a tornado, a car wreck, a mine cave-in, or a life-threatening illness, although they may be wonderful outcomes, they do not qualify as miracles in the biblical sense of the word. Was God looking out for all of these people? Perhaps he was. Perhaps he was not. It could be that sometimes God simply allows nature to run its course without intervening whatsoever, in other words, to allow "time and chance" to occur "to them all."[99] This is quite possible even though some may not want to admit it. We can never know about every situation with absolute certainty. Even though we may not always know when God is at work, we can still believe in a God that dwells in the lives of people today. We do not have to throw the baby out with the bath water.

NOTES

1. Robin Roberts, *Good Morning America*, ABC, WWAY, Wilmington, NC, March 3, 2007.

2. *ABC News*, WWAY, Wilmington, N.C., March 7, 2007.

3. Chris Cuomo, *Good Morning America*, ABC, WWAY, Wilmington, NC, March 29, 2007.

4. Kirk Johnson, "Back from the Dead, Teenager Casts Light on Shadowy Game," *New York Times*, March 28, 2007, http://web.lexis-nexis.com/universe/document (accessed May 22, 2007).

5. *ABC News*, WWAY, Wilmington, N.C., May 7, 2007.

6. Wade H. Boggs, Jr. (1956), *Faith Healing and the Christian Faith*, Richmond: John Knox Press, 30.

7. Gary McCarron (1987), Lost Dogs and Financial Healings: Deconstructing Televangelist Miracles, in *The God Pumpers*, Marshall Fishwick and Ray B. Browne, eds., Bowling Green: Bowling Green State University Popular Press, 19–31. For a similar definition of miracle, see Richard Swinburne (1970), *The Concept of Miracle*, New York: Macmillan, 14, 70.

8. 1 Kings 18:24 (American Standard Version). All biblical references hereafter come from the American Standard Version unless otherwise noted.

9. 1 Kings 18:38.

10. See Matthew 1.

11. See, for example, Kathryn Kuhlman (1970), *I Believe in Miracles*, Old Tappan, NJ: Fleming H. Revell, 20.

12. Stephen J. Pullum (1999), *"Foul Demons, Come Out!": The Rhetoric of Twentieth-Century American Faith Healing*, Westport, CT: Praeger, 158.

13. Genesis 18:12.

14. For a similar story, see the conception of John the Baptist to Elisabeth and Zacharias in Luke 1. Verse 18 describes Zacharias as "an old man," and Elisabeth as "well stricken in years."

15. Clive Staples Lewis (1947), *Miracles*, New York: Macmillan, 59.

16. Matthew 14:25.

17. John 2.

18. Matthew 8:26.

19. John 18: 2–12; Luke 22:51.

20. John 11.

21. Roy E. Cogdill, *Miraculous Divine Healing* unpublished sermon delivered in Bowling Green, KY, October 5, 1952, 14.

22. W. E. Vine (1939), *An Expository Dictionary of New Testament Words*, Nashville, TN: Royal, 746, 1240.

23. Mark 2:12.

24. Mark 5:42.

25. Luke 4:36.

26. Acts 3:8–10.

27. Acts 4:16.

28. John 11:47.

29. Matthew 12:23.

30. Matthew 8:3.

31. Mark 2:12.

32. Mark 5:29.

33. Luke 4:39.

34. Acts 3:7.

35. William A. Nolen (1974), *Healing: A Doctor in Search of a Miracle*, New York: Random House, 76–77.

36. Nolen, *Healing*, 81.

37. Personal observation of the author who attended a Friday night miracle service at Ernest Angley's Grace Cathedral in Akron, February 19, 1988.

38. Mark 8:24–25.

39. R. C. Foster (1971), *Gospel Studies*, vol. 2, *The Life of Christ: A Chronological Study of the Four Gospels*, Cincinnati: Cincinnati Bible Seminary, 54–55.

40. Matthew 12:13.

41. Kathryn Kuhlman (1975), *Dry Land, Living Waters: Las Vegas Miracle Service*, VHS, directed by Dick Ross, Pittsburgh: Kathryn Kuhlman Foundation.

42. Personal observation of the author who attended a Benny Hinn revival in Nashville, October 23–24, 1997.

43. Matthew 12:9.

44. Personal observation of the author, who attended a Benny Hinn revival in Nashville, October 23–24, 1997; a Gloria Copeland healing school in Nashville, October 17, 1992; and an Ernest Angley miracle service in Akron, February 19, 1988.

45. Exodus 4:5.

46. Exodus 4:31.

47. 1 Kings 18:37–39.

48. 1 Kings 17:24.

49. Matthew 8:1–8.

50. Matthew 11:2–6.

51. John 3:1–3. For other narratives that support the idea that miracles of Jesus were used to produce faith in his audiences, see John 2:11 and 23; John 11:42; and John 20:30.

52. Acts 2:22.

53. Acts 13:12.

54. Acts 8:12–16.

55. Hebrews 2:3–4. Compare to Mark 16:20.

56. 2 Corinthians 12:12.

57. Phil Roberts, "What Is a Miracle?" in *The Plano Provoker*, April 17, 1975, 2–4.

58. Matthew 9:27–31.

59. See the story of two blind men in Matthew 9:27–31.

60. Waymon D. Miller (1956), *Modern Divine Healing*, Fort Worth: Miller, 110–13.

61. Miller, *Healing*, 110–13.

62. John 5:13.

63. Matthew 8:5–13.

64. Matthew 8:5–13; 17:14–21; John 4:46–49.

65. Matthew 17:14–21.

66. Vines, *New Testament Words*, 899.

67. James Strong (1984), A Concise Dictionary of the Words in The Greek Testament, in *The New Strong's Exhaustive Concordance of the Bible*, New York: Nelson, 61.

68. Wayne Jackson (1988), A Study of the Providence of God, *Reason and Revelation* 3, no. 1, 1–2.

69. Dee Bowman, Providence, *Christianity Magazine*, November 2, 1992.

70. See, for example, Matthew 5:45; Matthew 6:33; and Romans 13:1 (compare to Daniel 2:21).

71. Bowman, 2.

72. 1 John 5:14.

73. 1 Peter 3:12.

74. James 5:16.

75. Matthew 7:7.

76. John 15:7.

77. Jackson, A Study of the Providence of God, 2.

78. Ibid., 3.

79. Isaiah 37:5–7, 36–37.

80. Acts 12:1–10.

81. Acts 19:23–41.

82. Genesis 19:24.

83. Matthew 8:26.

84. 1 Kings 18:44–45; Jas. 5:16–18.

85. Hebrews 11:6.

86. 2 Corinthians 12:7.

87. Bowman, Providence, 2.

88. Tommy Hagewood, Is God Showing Me Something through My Circumstances? *Locust Light* 22, no. 10, 1990, 2.

89. Jackson, A Study of the Providence of God, 3.

90. Allan Turner, Is It Possible to Interpret Providence? unpublished manuscript, 4–5. Manuscript is in author's personal files.

91. Ephesians 3:20.

92. Miller, *Healing*, 20.

93. There were at least two examples in the New Testament where the Apostle Paul could have performed a miracle to benefit two people had that been the purpose of miracles. However, he chose not to. In 2 Timothy 4:20 we read where he left Trophimus at Miletus, "sick." In 1 Timothy 5:23 he told Timothy to "use a little wine for thy stomach's sake and thine often infirmities." If miracles were intended as social benefits, why did Paul not heal these two people?

94. 1 Corinthians 13:10.

95. Vine, *New Testament Words*, 845– 46.

96. James 1:25.

97. Jonathan David Moorhead, 1 Corinthians 13:8–13 and Ephesians 4:11–16: A Canonical Parallel, unpublished manuscript presented to Dr. Robert Pyne, Dallas Theological Seminary, in partial fulfillment of RS1001, Research Seminar, August, 2004, 70–73. Manuscript in author's possession.

98. Moorhead, 70–71.

99. Ecclesiastes 9:11.

REFERENCES

ABC News (2007), WWAY, Wilmington, NC, March 7.

ABC News (2007), WWAY, Wilmington, NC, May 7.

The Bible. American Standard Version.

Boggs, Wade H. Jr. (1956), *Faith Healing and the Christian Faith*, Richmond: John Knox.

Bowman, Dee (1992), Providence, *Christianity Magazine*, November, 2.

Cogdill, Roy E (n.d.), Miraculous Divine Healing, unpublished sermon delivered in Bowling Green, KY, October 5, 1952.

Cuomo, Chris (2007), *Good Morning America*, ABC, WWAY, Wilmington, NC, March 29.

Foster, R. C. (1971), *The Life of Christ: A Chronological Study of the Four Gospels*, in Gospel Studies, vol. 2, Cincinnati: Cincinnati Bible Seminary.

Hagewood, Tommy (1990), Is God Showing Me Something through My Circumstances? *Locust Light* 22, no. 10, 1–2.

Jackson, Wayne (1988), A Study of the Providence of God, *Reason & Revelation* 3, no. 1, 1–5.

Johnson, Kirk (2007), Back from the Dead, Teenager Casts Light on Shadowy Game, *New York Times*, March 28, http://web.lexis-nexis.com/universe/document.

Kuhlman, Kathryn (1975), *Dry Land, Living Waters: Las Vegas Miracle Service*, VHS, Dick Ross, dir., Kathryn Kuhlman Foundation, Pittsburgh.

Kuhlman, Kathryn (1970), *I Believe in Miracles*, Old Tappan: Revell.

Lewis, C. S. (1947), *Miracles*, New York: Macmillan.

McCarron, Gary (1987), Lost Dogs and Financial Healings: Deconstructing Televangelist Miracles, in Marshall Fishwick and Ray B. Browne, eds., *The God Pumpers*, Bowling Green, OH: Bowling Green State University Popular Press, 19–31.

Miller, Waymon D. (1956), *Modern Divine Healing*, Fort Worth: Miller.

Moorhead, Jonathan David (2004), I Corinthians 13:8–13 and Ephesians 4:11–16: A Canonical Parallel, unpublished manuscript, Dallas Theological Seminary, August 2004, 1–95.

Nolen, William A. (1974), *Healing: A Doctor in Search of a Miracle*, New York: Random House.

Pullum, Stephen J. (1988), Personal observation of Ernest Angley, Akron, February 19.

Pullum, Stephen J. (1992), Personal observation of Gloria Copeland, Nashville, October 17.

Pullum, Stephen J. (1997), Personal observation of Benny Hinn, Nashville, October 23–24.

Pullum, Stephen J. (1999), *"Foul Demons, Come Out!": The Rhetoric of Twentieth-Century American Faith Healing*, Westport, CT: Praeger.

Roberts, Phil (1975), What Is a Miracle? *The Plano Provoker*, April 17, 2–4.

Roberts, Robin (2007), *Good Morning America*, ABC, WWAY, Wilmington, NC, March 3.

Strong, James (1984), A Concise Dictionary of the Words in The Greek Testament in *The New Strong's Exhaustive Concordance of the Bible*, New York: Nelson.

Swinburne, Richard (1970), *The Concept of Miracle*, New York: Macmillan.

Turner, Allan (n.d.), Is It Possible to Interpret Providence?, unpublished manuscript, 4–5.

Vine, W. E. (1939), *An Expository Dictionary of New Testament Words*, Nashville: Royal.

CHAPTER 10

THROUGH SIGNS AND WONDERS: RELIGIOUS DISCOURSE AND MIRACLE NARRATIVES

Benjamin Beit-Hallahmi

Historians, anthropologists, and sociologists have much to teach us about the social, political, and even economic dynamics that produce and sustain miracle narratives and miracle traditions in particular cultures and communities (cf. Claverie 2003; Markle and McCrea 1994). Pyysiainen (2004) described how believing in miracles was the most efficient and least costly way of processing information in certain cultural settings, given our brain architecture. This chapter looks at the logic of belief and believers, and at the psychological process leading believers to embrace such narratives.

Explaining the general belief in miracles and/or acceptance of specific miracle narratives does not require us to use any concepts beyond those needed to explain the existence and prevalence of religious discourse in general. This chapter elaborates the notion that miracle narratives are prototypical religious fantasies. Secular fantasies may express improbable or impossible ideas, but there is always a unique element of religious ideation in all religious discourse. It has to do with the world of the spirits.

DEFINING RELIGIOUS DISCOURSE

Religious beliefs have been around for 100,000 years, or even longer, and have changed relatively little. The irreducible core common to all religions, tying humanity to the cosmos, contains the belief in spirits inhabiting an invisible world and having a relationship with us (Beit-Hallahmi 1989). All religions promote the idea of an invisible world, inhabited by gods, angels, and devils, that control much of what happens to us. Religion as a social institution is for us the mediator between the invisible supernatural or transcendent world and the visible human and natural world. That institution, with the behaviors associated with it, does not exist without the belief in the supernatural or transcendent world. Belief systems will be defined as religions only if those following them make specific references to supernatural agents or interventions. Thouless stated that what distinguished religious individuals from others is that they "believe that there is also some kind of spiritual world which makes demands on our behavior, our thinking and our feeling" (1971, 12).

The presence of the supernatural premise is the touchstone for defining behaviors as religious. What is this premise? "It is the premise of every religion—and this premise is religion's defining characteristic—that souls, supernatural beings, and supernatural forces exist. Furthermore, there are certain, minimal categories of behavior, which, in the context of the *supernatural premise*, are always found in association with one another, and which are the substance of religion itself" (Wallace 1966, 52).

Similarly, William James described the coexistence of the visible and the invisible worlds:

> Religion has meant many things in human history: but when from now onward I use the word I mean to use it in the supernaturalist sense, as declaring that the so-called order of nature, which constitutes this world's experience, is only one portion of the total universe, and that there stretches beyond this visible world an unseen world of which we now know nothing positive, but in its relation to which the true significance of our present mundane life consists. A man's religious faith . . . means for me essentially his faith in the existence of an unseen order of some kind in which the riddles of the natural order may be found explained. (James [1897] 1956, 51)

Religious utterances contain both supernaturalist and naturalist claims (Beit-Hallahmi 2001). While naturalist claims are often found in religious discourse, they are not what gives religion its unique character. While a claim such as "A man named Jesus was born in Judea under Herod" is straightforward and naturalistic, though lacking any supporting evidence, it is part of a religious narrative that is anything but naturalist, and replete with miracle stories. The naturalist, mostly fictitious, claims that religions offer us are less central and less essential than miracle narratives, which dominate religious discourse everywhere. This is the substance of religion, the discourse that makes religion attractive and is designed quite consciously and purposefully to attract believers.

Religion's most unique claim, which combines the two worlds, that of nature and that of the spirits, is the denial of death. Common to all religions is avoiding the recognition of death as the end of any individual existence, and this is one of religion's strongest compensators (Beit-Hallahmi and Argyle 1997). "Religion, whether it be shamanism or Protestantism, rises from our apprehension of death. To give meaning to meaninglessness is the endless quest of religion. . . . Clearly we possess religion, if we want to, precisely to obscure the truth of our perishing. . . . When death becomes the center, then religion begins" (Bloom 1992, 29).

Frazer described religion, with "the almost universal belief in the survival of the human spirit after death" (Frazer 1933–36, v) at its center, as resulting from the fear of the dead, which is the fear of death itself. The terror of death leads to the creation of powerful psychological and cultural mechanisms (Becker 1973; Greenberg, Pyszczynski, and Solomon 1995; Pyszczynski et al. 2004), religion being the most important. James described the function of religion as follows "Religion, in fact, for the great majority of our own race, *means* immortality and nothing else" (James 1961, 406).

The illusion of immortality, pivotal in all religions, is humanity's reaction to the inevitability of death, the universal threat to every individual human. Within the religious framework, death is not a singular event occurring only once in the history of the individual, but a transition from one form of existence to another. All religions state that dying is only a passage, a transition point in the existence of the soul, as it comes out of a particular human body.

Most humans accept the supernatural premise, and its corollary: the two-worlds assumption. The two-worlds assumption leads us to two separate modes of comprehending the physical world. The first is that of observing physical events and coping with them through much hardship, as we eat bread in the sweat of our faces, and constantly confront suffering, frustration, and injustice. The second is the notion of exceptions to hard work, frustration, and suffering in this world, which constitute miracles. For most religious people their particular tradition is experienced through routine rituals, rather than ecstasy. There are no miracles, no religious crises, and no mystical experiences in their own lives, so that any claims about exceptional events easily stand out.

DEFINING MIRACLES

Millions of miracle narratives have been circulating in human history, many obviously reused and recycled. Each one of the approximately 10,000 religions currently active on earth has claimed a few. Miracles are, for those who believe in them, natural material events that imply an intervention by supernatural forces. They are often defined as events that seem to violate our sense of the laws of nature or the order of nature, but the point of the supernatural premise is to tell us that the true order of nature includes entities and actions that transcend our mundane experiences.

Miracles are believed to take place in this world, not in the invisible world of the spirits. This is their most important characteristic in the framework of religious discourse. They are believed to occur through the intercession of benevolent spirits, but their effects are totally material, palpable, and provable to the believers, in naturalist terms. When it comes to explaining disease and cures, what is unique about miracles is not a deficient knowledge of physiology, for such can be found in many purely secular assertions, but the claimed intervention by the great spirits.

Reports of miracles deal chiefly with being saved from immanent death, either through a hostile attack or through life-threatening illness. In the Roman Catholic Church today, miracles are defined as cases of great suffering and danger, in which a physical solution is inadequate, and a special contact with a saint, such as putting his picture on the patient's body, praying to him, or making pilgrimage to his tomb, is followed by a total recovery, not explainable by the physicians involved. The only explanation then is an intercession by a saint, who, from his or her abode in the world of the spirits, chose to intervene in physiological processes occurring in this material world. To the Roman Catholic Church, the recovery must be proven with standard medical tests, including modern imaging devices.

The idea of *mana*, a powerful essence found in some objects, is reflected in common beliefs about places and persons that are imbued with the ability of causing miracles. Special miracle-making powers have been attributed to kings, saints, or sacred objects. Pilgrimages to special locations all over the world are initiated in the hope of finding miracle cures, visiting relics such as a hair from the beard of the prophet Muhammad, or tombs, places in which apparitions have been reported, or just mountains considered sacred since time immemorial.

A few years ago I visited the Oratoire Saint-Joseph du Mont-Royal and had a chance to observe hundreds of pairs of crutches hanging from the ceiling, evidence of miracle cures effected by the resident saint. Lourdes, France, is one of the best-known pilgrimage sites in the world since the nineteenth century and is the scene of numerous reported miracles (Cranston 1957). As Paloutzian (1996) pointed out, actual cure rates at Lourdes are lower than expected from what we know about spontaneous remissions of serious illness, which do occur sometimes. Sometimes the miracle-making object can come to believers who experience its power:

Eight miles from Lyesopolye lay the village of Obnino, possessing a miraculous icon. A procession started from Obnino every summer bearing the wonder-working icon and making the round of all the neighboring villages. The church-bells would ring all day long first in one village, then in another, and to little Pavel (His Reverence was called little Pavel then) the air itself seemed tremulous with rapture. (Chekhov 1915/1979, 279)

Claims about persons with special powers can be found today all over the world.

> Dan Stratton is the founder and pastor of the Faith Exchange Fellowship, a fundamentalist Christian congregation in Manhattan's financial district. His wife Ann is described as a born-again miracle worker, "whose prayers once supposedly raised a German *au pair* from the dead on the street in front of the Blue Moon Mexican Cafe in Englewood, N.J." (Chafets 2006, 21).

Ann Stratton told the congregation that, thanks to her prayers,

> A woman with brain cancer was healed, another was saved from a hysterectomy and a man came out of a seemingly permanent coma . . . a little deaf boy regained his hearing; . . . her prayers replaced a blind eye in a woman's socket with a healthy, perfectly matched green eyeball. And then, in Englewood, the *au pair* came back from the dead. . . . Today that woman's alive and well in Germany. Say, "Amen!" (Chafets 2006, 21).

Dan Stratton testifies: "She's a prayer warrior. That woman in Englewood was gone, she was dead weight; I picked her up myself. But Annie refused to give up on her until she came back to life. That happened. I saw it. Not figuratively. Literally" (Chafets 2006, 21). Despite much effort, the Faith Exchange Fellowship has had trouble finding a suitable permanent home in lower Manhattan, which proves that raising the dead can be easier than negotiating the New York City real estate market.

FOUNDATIONAL AND CONFIRMATORY REVELATIONS

Mythologies, written or orally transmitted, tell us about the creation of the cosmic order and the centrality of humans in that order. This, of course, is miraculous, and so is the revelation of the cosmic plan. All revelations, that is, the transmission of messages from the spirit world to humans, are miracles. Some miraculous events that have led to the founding of religions were individual illuminations such as Buddha's celebrated recognition of human suffering and mortality (Beit-Hallahmi 2006–2007). In addition, all mythologies offer us the stories of those saved miraculously from death through divine intervention at the right moment: Perseus, Krishna, Isaac, Hagar and Ishmael, Moses, and the baby Jesus, to name a few.

While all religions report foundational revelations, events that led to their founding, many traditions have room for confirmatory revelations, which reinforce and sustain long-held beliefs. These are apparitions in which specific messages from the spirit world are conveyed, or the presence of spirits and gods is directly felt. Most are made public, while a few remain private. One of the best-known confirmatory revelations in modern history was reported by the great mathematician Blaise Pascal. On Monday, November 23, 1654, Pascal had a vision in which he saw, in his own words: "Fire. GOD of Abraham, GOD of Isaac, GOD of Jacob, not of the philosophers and of the learned. Certitude. Certitude. Feeling. Joy. Peace." Pascal chose not to make the revelation public during his lifetime (Cole 1996).

PHYSIOLOGICAL MIRACLES

In some religious traditions, we find congregations and individuals practicing faith healing, the origin of many reported miracles (Rose 1971; Harrell 1985; Randi 1989). There have been some follow-up studies of some of those treated. Glik (1986) interviewed 176 individuals who had attended charismatic and other healing groups, and compared them with 137 who had received regular primary care. Those who had been to healing groups reported better health and subjective well-being, though their actual physical state was no different. Pattison, Lapins, and Doerr (1973) analyzed 71 cases of healings at healing services; 62 "recoveries" took place during the service, half of them suddenly; 50 had been suffering from serious illnesses.

Again there was no actual change in physical condition or life-style; what had changed was their subjective condition. They believed that they had been healed by the casting out of sin. Their MMPI (Minnesota Multiphasic Personality Inventory) profiles showed that these "recovered" individuals engaged in denial. In both of these studies the changes were improved in subjective health, and not in actual physical condition. Miettinen (1990, in Holm, 1991) studied extensively 611 cases of healings in Finland. The findings were that there was no evidence of any physical improvement, but the clients, 450 women and 161 men, of limited education and social status, experienced a subjective change, attributed to suggestibility and personal instability.

Sometimes it is claimed that in death, saintly bodies show no evidence of decay, believed to be incorruptible, thanks to the saintly qualities of the souls formerly residing in them. Testimonies about the imperishable bodies of saints are found in Christianity, Buddhism, Judaism, and Hinduism (e.g., Lenhoff 1993). In some cases the naturally mummified bodies of religious teachers became the objects of worship and pilgrimage. The mummified, well-preserved body of the Buryat Lama Itigelov, who died in 1927, can be seen at www.neplaneta.ru. His disciples claim that before dying, he asked to be exhumed. Since 2002 the body has been on display for venerating pilgrims. In the Roman Catholic tradition, the notion of the Odor of Sanctity refers to the specific scent, often compared to that of flowers, that emanates from the dead bodies of saints. St. Frances Cabrini, whose body is on display in upper Manhattan, is said to be incorruptible. In Dostoevsky's *The Brothers*

Karamazov, a saintly monk's body is expected to remain fresh after death, and its normal, mortal decomposition creates a scandal and a crisis of faith.

ESTABLISHING PLAUSIBILITY AND AUTHORITY

The first goal for every group is survival, which necessitates the creation of a common worldview. Group cohesion, created by common loyalties to imaginary beings, has great survival value. Miracle narratives, whether foundational or confirmatory, buttress and provide evidence for the validity of particular religious assertions. "These narratives are decisive proof of the truth of the group's particular religious message. The authority of Jesus was established for the early church by the resurrection, the virgin birth, and one other important group of phenomena, the miracles he performed in the course of his ministry" (Anderson and Fischer 1966, 179).

A new tradition has to establish its authority, power, and uniqueness. This leads to a valued identity, for individuals and for the whole group. The community of believers is united in accepting a particular authority, but it is naturally challenged, and this sometimes takes the form of doubting specific narratives tied to foundational beliefs.

"If Christ be preached, that he rose again from the dead, how do some among you say that there is no resurrection of the dead? But if there be no resurrection of the dead, then Christ is not risen again. And if Christ be not risen again, then is our preaching vain, and your faith is also vain" (1 Cor 15:12–14). This is a relatively modern formulation of the basic problem of all supernaturalist belief systems.

Impossible and improbable narratives are simply vital to faith. They constitute proof that those who speak for the world of the spirits are indeed in direct contact with it, and that the great spirits do intervene in mundane reality to reward those of faith and devotion. Moreover, they serve to persuade us, not about the reality of the world of the spirits in general, but about one particular belief system and one particular claim to authority. The narratives demonstrate that a particular tradition, inspired by "our" great spirits, is better and stronger than traditions based on spirits worshipped by other collectivities. "Our" miracles are clearly superior to theirs. Superiority and self-esteem are vital psychological supplies, provided by religions, and often, with less of an impact, by other ideologies.

The process of establishing religious plausibility through miracle narratives can be closely observed in the case of newly formed religions. The history of Mormonism is a case in point. This is a U.S. Christian-polytheistic millenarian group, founded by Joseph Smith, Jr. (1805–44) in 1830 in northern New York State. At age 14 Smith declared he had spoken with God. Later he had other visions, during some of which he claimed an ancient book, written on four tablets, was given to him. He claimed to have transcribed this text, which has become known as *The Book of Mormon* and has given its name to the Mormon church. *The Book of Mormon* is believed to be an ancient revelation to the inhabitants of America, written in Egyptian. This book is the movement's main scripture (Taves 1984).

The case of theosophy is similar. The Theosophical Society was founded in 1875 at 46 Irving Place, New York City, by Helena Pterovna Blavatsky (1831–91), who first attracted public attention as a spirit medium. Madame Blavtasky claimed to have spent about 40 years traveling in the East, especially Tibet, and meeting the Masters of Ancient Wisdom, or the Adepts. Actually, she was born in Russia, married General Blavatsky at 17, and a year later ran away. There is no proof of any early travels to India or anywhere else in Asia, but she is known to have founded a spiritualist group in Cairo around 1870. In 1874 she came to the United States and gained some attention as a defender of Spiritualism.

Madame Blavatsky claimed that she had been chosen by a Buddha incarnation named Tsong-kha-pa to be guided by two secret masters in the Himalayas, known as the Mahatma Morya and the Mahatma Koot Hoomi, in order to save the world. The Mahatmas are one rung in the hierarchy of perfected beings (the White Brotherhood, the Adepts, the Masters, the Mahatmas), who really supervise the evolution of this world. Blavatsky's followers reported many cases of communications from the Adepts, including written messages (Williams 1946).

Both Joseph Smith, Jr., and Madame Blavatsky took unnecessary risks by claiming physical evidence for their revelations in the form of golden tablets or written letters. This laid them open to ridicule and criticism. Some of Blavatsky's claims for supernatural powers and contacts were investigated in India in 1884 by Richard Hodgson of the London Society for Psychical Research, who denounced them as a fraudulent trickery. This was the first in a series of such denunciations.

What about exceptions to the rule that miracle narratives are vital to faith? We can think about mainstream Protestant denominations in the United States, whose austere traditions do not celebrate miracle cures or institute public displays of deserted crutches. But followers of these traditions, if they proclaim any faith, still believe in some foundational miracle narratives.

PROPHECIES AND PROMISES:
APOCALYPTIC NARRATIVES

All miracle stories are but minor variations on the great theme of victory over death. Miracles are reminders that indeed nature could be overcome by the power of the spirits. Those who can negotiate with the spirits in the right way will enjoy these minor victories. They will also remember that bigger ones are in store for each one of them individually, when they join the world of the spirits, as well as collectively, for those believers who will survive to see the coming of the *eschaton*, the end of the world.

Prophecies are promises of miracles to come, and prominent among them are apocalyptic narratives that appear in many religions. The essential ingredients of such ideas are first a total destruction of the world as we know it at present, and then a birth of a "new heaven and a new earth," for the elect, who are only a remnant of humanity. In addition to the well-known end-of-times historical traditions, there are many cases of new religious movements in which apocalyptic dreams are prominent. Even before our eventual death, we all frequently experience suffering, frustration, and failure. The eschatological vision is about eliminating both death and injustice. The promise is of overcoming the limitations and presses of the body in life and in death, as well as a victory of justice over evil. The dream is of the resurrection, Judgment Day, and the abolition of death. The profane world of the body and its demands has to be destroyed. Who can resist the wishes for a victory of justice and life over evil and death?

The *eschaton* is the time when human history ends and what we know intuitively as the laws of nature are abolished. In the apocalyptic worldview, only the true believers, a segment of humanity, have been chosen to share in the secret of total redemption and to bring it about. Eschatological dreams promise us an end to the cycle of birth and death. In addition to our cosmic victory over nature, whose laws are to be abolished, there will be a human victory of our own group of the elect over all others. With the coming eschaton, believers may be in ecstasy, because they are living at the center of history and at the heart of the cosmos. This is the climax of the universal religious drama, played out on the cosmic stage. Following rebirth through blood and fire, birth and death will disappear. There will be no body, no aggression, and no sex.

Modern religions loudly proclaiming the coming *eschaton* include not only Jehovah's Witnesses and ISKCON (Hare Krishna), but The Church of Jesus Christ of Latter Day Saints (Mormons) that promises upheavals and catastrophes that would leave only the Mormons unharmed, the Baha'i movement that promises a global catastrophe, and Osho Meditation (formerly known as Rajneesh Foundation International) that offered many proclamations of catastrophes. Only Rajneesh followers may survive. Rajneesh and his followers often discussed an expected cataclysm that would end life on earth. In 1983 Rajneesh predicted an earthquake that would devastate much of the West Coast. In 1984 he announced that AIDS was the scourge predicted by Nostradamus, and billions would die from it within the next decade, and in 1985 he predicted floods, earthquakes, and nuclear war within the next decade.

A recent version of the end-of-times fantasy is the idea of the true believers being saved by a spaceship and moved to another galaxy, following the total destruction of all life on planet earth. These ideas have been circulating for many decades and have been made famous by the often-cited, but rarely read, book by Festinger, Riecken, and Schachter (1956). This was an observational study of a religious group, founded by a "Mrs. Keech" in the early 1950s in a major U.S. metropolis. The founder claimed to have had information from a source, Sananda, that was both extraterrestrial and divine about the coming end of the world. Sananda was the Jesus of Christian mythology. She announced to the world that on a specified date, December 24, 1953, all of humanity would perish, except group members, who would be taken away in a spaceship.

A similar fantasy led to the tragedies of Heaven's Gate and the Solar Temple, in which cases the collective death ritual was intended to lead members to a rebirth on another planet (Beit-Hallahmi 2001). Heaven's Gate, first known as Bo and Peep, or the Higher Source, was a Christian-UFO group started in 1975 in Los Angeles by a former music professor, Marshall Herff Applewhite (1932–97), and a registered nurse, Bonnie Lu Trousdale Nettles (1928–85), who met in the early 1970s in Texas. The couple called themselves Bo and Peep, and were also known as Winnie and Pooh, Chip and Dale, Do and Ti, "The Him and the Her," or "The Two," in reference to a New Testament prophecy about two witnesses. The group's doctrine was known as Human Individual Metamorphosis (HIM), aiming at the liberation of humans from the endless cycle of reincarnation.

The leaders claimed that they would fulfill an ancient prophecy by being assassinated and then coming back to life three and a half days later. Following the resurrection, they would be lifted up by a UFO to the divine kingdom in outer space. Members traveled around the United States recruiting new followers and proclaiming their prophecies. They were promised immortality, androgyneity, and perfection, provided they followed the group rules. Members agreed, in preparation for the outer space journey, to get rid of most material possessions and worldly attachments, including family and work. They wore uniform clothing and identical haircuts. Marriage and sexual relations were also forbidden.

Bonnie Nettles died in 1985 of cancer, and then the group started operating in complete secrecy. Applewhite told his followers that Bonnie Nettles was actually his divine father. In late March 1997, 39 group members, including Applewhite, committed suicide in Rancho Santa Fe, California, by ingesting barbiturates and alcohol. They were found lying on bunk beds, wearing cotton pants, black shirts, and sneakers. Most of them were covered with purple shrouds. They all carried on them passports and driver's licenses, as well as small change. The victims ranged in age from 26 to 72, but 21 were in their forties. There were 21 females and 18 males. In videotaped statements read before committing suicide, members stated that they were taking this step in preparation for an expected encounter with extraterrestrials, arriving in a spaceship following the Hale-Bopp comet. It was discovered after their deaths that some of the male group members had been castrated several years before.

Making a prophecy that specifies the date of the coming apocalypse leads to unnecessary problems, because it always leads to what nonbelievers would regard as a public disconfirmation. This has not stopped scores of group leaders in modern times from making such prophecies. These prophecy failures have sometimes led to visible crisis or collapse. In other cases the prophecies have been reinterpreted or reformulated, as religious and secular belief systems are typically flexible enough to accommodate such failures (Beit-Hallahmi and Argyle 1997).

BELIEVING IN MIRACLES

Two international surveys conducted during 1991 and 1993 by the International Social Survey Program (ISSP) looked at religious beliefs in 17 countries, including data on the belief in miracles. These were the questions:

1. God: I know God exists and I have no doubts about it.
2. Afterlife: I definitely believe in life after death.
3. Bible: The Bible is the actual word of God, to be taken literally, word for word.
4. Devil: I definitely believe in the Devil.
5. Hell: I definitely believe in Hell.
6. Heaven: I definitely believe in Heaven.
7. Miracle: I definitely believe in religious miracles.

The results are shown in Table 10.1.

These findings show that belief in miracles is in most cases correlated with other religious beliefs, as it should be. The United States leads the 17 nations studied in terms of the level of beliefs in miracles, heaven, afterlife, and hell. This is consistent with what we have known for a long time about religiosity in the United States.

COSMIC OPTIMISM

Religious beliefs in general, including the belief in miracles, reflect a universal human optimism about existence and the cosmos, the material world. The experience of the past few centuries has shown that an extremely optimistic worldview is possible within an atheistic framework, but historically, religion has been the cultural institution embodying and expressing the propensity to be hopeful. This is selected by evolutionary pressures (Greeley 1981). It is a classic adaptive response to the challenges of life. It should be noted that secular optimism, as exemplified by Condorcet or Marx, is historical, rather than cosmic. It hopes for a change in the social order, but not in

Table 10.1 Believing in Miracles

Country	God	Afterlife	Bible	Devil	Hell	Heaven	Miracles	Evolution
United States	62.8	55.0	33.5	45.4	49.6	63.1	45.6	35.4
N. Ireland	61.4	53.5	32.7	43.1	47.9	63.7	44.2	51.5
Philippines	86.2	35.2	53.7	28.3	29.6	41.9	27.7	60.9
Ireland	58.7	45.9	24.9	24.8	25.9	51.8	36.9	60.1
Poland	66.3	37.8	37.4	15.4	21.4	38.6	22.7	35.4
Italy	51.4	34.8	27.0	20.4	21.7	27.9	32.9	65.2
New Zealand	29.3	35.5	9.4	21.4	18.7	32.2	23.1	66.3
Israel	43.0	21.9	26.7	12.6	22.5	24.0	26.4	56.9
Austria	29.4	24.8	12.7	11.1	10.0	20.1	27.4	N/A
Norway	20.1	31.6	11.2	13.1	11.4	23.0	17.8	65.0
Great Britain	23.8	26.5	7.0	12.7	12.8	24.6	15.3	76.7
Netherlands	24.7	26.7	8.4	13.3	11.1	21.1	10.2	58.6
W. Germany	27.3	24.4	12.5	9.5	9.3	18.2	22.7	72.7
Russia	12.4	16.8	9.9	12.5	13.0	14.7	18.7	41.4
Slovenia	21.9	11.6	22.3	6.9	8.3	9.5	13.4	60.7
Hungary	30.1	10.6	19.2	4.2	5.8	9.4	8.2	62.8
E. Germany	9.2	6.1	7.5	3.6	2.6	10.2	11.8	81.6

Source: http://www.dataarchive.ac.uk/; http://www.chass.utoronto.ca/datalib/major/issp.htm.

any laws of nature. It does not expect to conquer death, but assumes human progress in this world only (cf. Fromm 1947).

The survival value of optimism is clear (Beit-Hallahmi and Argyle 1997). In the face of death and of life's many difficulties, humanity must come up with a basic optimism, a persistent hope, that has essential survival value (Tiger 1979). This evolutionary optimism is reinforced by the experiences of infancy. Early human experience, starting with any individual conception, may be viewed as a series of miracles. An invisible hand seems to protect those of us who have survived infancy. This survival was in itself highly uncertain until recent times. We can understand why mythology and fairy tales express the idea of children under threat of desertion and extinction, and why dangers are squarely projected on parents, whose power makes them into the witches, fairies, gods, or angels of fantasy. As we grow up, we realize that powerful gods have been on our side so far, and we assume that our luck will not run out.

Hebb (1955) hypothesized that higher mammals are more vulnerable to emotional breakdown, because with greater development of intelligence, the susceptibility to imagined dangers and unreasoning suspicion is greater. Humans are protected by the protective cocoon of culture. Illusory beliefs, rituals, and art seem to have no survival value, but on reflection we realize that they play an important role in relieving anxiety and allowing culture to survive (cf. Becker 1973; Greenberg et al. 1995; Pyszczyns et al. 2004).

The content of religious beliefs may be related to a basic optimistic gullibility, displayed by humans on many occasions (mostly secular). The human tendency towards magical thinking, errors in judgment, and distortion of reality has been documented often enough. Observations of children's thinking (Piaget 1962, 1967) have noted its domination by magical notions, false causality, egocentricity, and animism. Studies of adult reasoning show it to be frequently deficient, with basic rules of evidence and logic ignored or selectively followed. Both psychoanalysis and modern cognitive psychology agree on the basic human difficulty in paying reality its due.

THE QUESTION OF REALITY TESTING

Is it possible that the belief in miracles is the result of some deficiency in the ego's capacity for reality testing? The content of many religious narratives invokes an oneiric mode of experiencing, presenting events that defy logic, and that are not just improbable but impossible and absurd. When we hear religious narratives, we often know that we are in a fairy tale mode. One may ask whether a conscious commitment to religious ideation would not undermine reality testing in general. When we listen to stories about disembodied voices coming from heaven and to fantasies about miracles and promised triumphs, we have to ask to what extent accepting such ideas affects one's negotiations with social and physical reality, and whether it does not betray a real character flaw in the believer.

The question of explaining religion within the psychopathology framework has been clearly posed: "There is no doubt that hallucinations and delusions of any sort, religious or not, are abnormal phenomena. . . . Must we accept the idea that in some of its beliefs religion is a form of collective schizophrenia, and in some of its practices a form of obsessive-compulsive psychoneurosis, different from the psychiatric syndromes because it is socially acceptable?" (Arieti 1976, 252).

Indeed, the first fact to consider in this context is that religious individuals have not invented their religion. Religious beliefs are usually acquired through social learning (Argyle 1958; Argyle and Beit-Hallahmi 1975; Beit-Hallahmi and Argyle 1997). These ideas are not private creations. The social learning of religion presents religious ideas, which may be crazy, as part of social reality.

There is no religious behavior without a prior exposure to specific religious ideas. We know that the content of mystical visions, the most intense and personal of religious acts, is wholly predictable from exposure to certain ideas, which are always learned. Visions of the Holy Virgin occur exclusively among Catholics or those exposed to Catholic ideas. It has never occurred among orthodox Muslims, and we understand why. If social learning is indeed the more important variable in creating religiosity, then social variables, rather than personality variables, should be more successful in predicting it. The question to be answered in the study of individual religiosity becomes the individual's reaction to cultural traditions.

The received social consensus may have little to do with individual dynamics. "[T]he most significant difference between a religion, as held by a person, and a state of systematized delusion resides in the element of social participation. Some people necessary to the particular person have incorporated in their several personalities approximately the same structure of transcendental beliefs and rituals . . . there is a community of assumptions. . . . It is not necessary to set up a special teaching situation in order to inculcate in the young the most consistent and constantly manifested traits of the family culture complex. Very special educative situations indeed are needed if one is to eradicate the effects of this most facile sort of acculturation. It is safe to assume that the nucleus of one's personal religion has been acquired in this automatic way" (Sullivan 1964, 81).

Social learning may imbue certain prelogical or paleological ideas with apparent immunity to critical thinking. Arieti (1956, 1976) has referred to paleologic thinking as "the foundation of many societal or collective manifestations: rituals, magic, customs, and beliefs that are transmitted from generation to generation and accepted without questions being raised as to their validity."

La Barre (1970) suggested that not only was religion the expression of impaired reality testing, but that its practices were likely to lead to greater problems. There are certainly numerous examples of catastrophes caused by religious ideas, but our observations of religious individuals and communities show that their adjustment to reality is, in most cases, quite good. One explanation is that religious beliefs are used selectively and kept marginal or compartmentalized in everyday life, and that believers know well the limits of acting on faith. It is possible to conceive of them as illustrating the mechanism of "regression in the service of the ego" (Beit-Hallahmi 1989). Psychoanalytic ego psychology has suggested that there is a natural limit to rational reality testing, and the tension of rationality is relieved by opportunities for controlled and limited regression from reality. It is this mechanism, which is not only normal but productive, that creates both art and religion.

MIRACLES AND METAMORPHOSIS

Most miracle stories relate unlikely physical events, but the domain of religious discourse includes narratives of psychological miracles, which are rare and dramatic transformations that have turned miserable humans into purposeful, happy beings. Some individuals report solitary events of experiences leading to religious conversion, which often make up a significant part of religious discourse. Beyond the dramatic, subjective "experience" we can find evidence for true changes in behavior and functioning, a true miracle cure, putting previously uncontrollable drives under control.

What characterizes the convert is an intensity of commitment, emotion, and activity. The testimonials follow a narrative formula, as the convert's autobiography is divided into Before and After. Life until the moment of epiphany is described as wasted, a total mistake, or as a providential sequence leading up to the epiphany. Every sin must be confessed so that the power of redemption is magnified (Arendt 1979).

A conscious self-transformation is openly proclaimed, as the convert relates how a past of doubt and error has been transformed into wholeness in one great moment of insight, order, and certainty. What was once fragmented and decentered is made coherent, at least in its conscious center. The new self is not just triumphant but triumphalist, expecting us to follow its example. The convert's emotional state reminds us of romantic love, which brings about exhilaration, euphoria, self-confidence, and intense energy (cf. Fisher 2004).

Offering the conversion testimonial is a real test for the new self, first because it is a public confession, exposing sins and weaknesses, and then because it is a public, self-enforcing act of commitment (bridge burning). Religious conversion has been a classical topic in the psychology of religion, starting with William James and Edwin D. Starbuck in the late nineteenth century. But both James and Starbuck were looking at converts from the out-side, with fascination, amazement, and curiosity, rather than identification. We admire converts, and some of them, especially talented or charismatic ones, become culture heroes, such as Thomas Merton (1948), but we reject, with James and Starbuck, their accounts of divine intervention.

The ability to really change is considered a major achievement and an ideal in modern culture, which promotes an imaginary triumph of an un-covered, authentic self. The common theme of reorganizing the self around a new center is modern, together with the (mostly imagined) freedom to choose or reconstruct one's identity. More recently, the search for a social utopia is being replaced by the private utopia of the reinvented self. If we cannot change the world, we are told that we can change ourselves.

THE MIRACLE OF MAX JACOB (1879–1944)

Max Jacob's story is an enigmatic story, full of contradictions, tragedies, and secrets. Fhima (2002) described Jacob's "symbiosis of paradoxical identi-ties": Jew, avant-garde artist, homosexual, convert, Catholic writer, and Jew-ish martyr. Jacob is remembered as a minor painter and a remarkable poet. A member of an explosively talented group, among whom were Pablo Pi-casso, Guillaume Apollinaire, and Amadeo Modigliani, he is immortalized in portraits by Picasso and Modigliani, and in hundreds of photographs and film clips in which he always appears next to Picasso.

In 1934 Jacob gave extended interviews (Guiette 1934) that provide us with the best source for the way in which he wanted his life to be remem-bered. What Jacob tells us about his childhood is heartrending. He was phys-ically abused by his parents and siblings, and tried to commit suicide three times. At age 13 he was taken to Paris for treatment by the great neurologist Jean-Martin Charcot. Jacob was a brilliant student, and his artistic talents were noted early. At age 19 he came to Paris with 29 francs, stolen from his mother. Trying his hand at various jobs and careers to survive, he graduated from law school, but chose painting as a career. In 1901 he met Pablo Picasso, and the two became inseparable. In 1905, the two met Guillaume Apollinaire, and made a threesome that stayed together till Apollinaire's death in 1918.

In the 1934 interview Jacob denied his homosexuality and improbably reported a love affair with a married woman, using her real name. He states that the only moments in his life he would like to relive were the first night with his lover, and the "sacred moment of God's first appearance to him, six years later" (p. 18). He reveals that he arranged to have a painting exhibited at the Salon des Independants so that his lover, Mme. Germaine Pfeipfer, would show up, only to be rebuffed by him. When she did, he was in the company of Picasso and Braque, who found her very pretty. He found her grotesque.

In 1909, in his rented room at 7 rue Ravignan, came the revelation, whose text is somewhat reminiscent of Pascal's 1654 testimonial:

> There was somebody on the wall, "Truth, truth, tears of truth, joy of truth, unforgettable truth, the Divine Body is on the wall of this poor room. . . . What beauty, elegance, and delicacy! His shoulders, his bearing! He wears a yellow silk robe with blue cuffs. He turns and I see his peaceful and shining face. Six monks bring a cadaver into the room. A woman with snakes around her arms and hair is next to me.

> *The angel:* "Innocent, you have seen God. You don't understand your happiness."
> *Me:* "Cry, Cry I am a poor human beast."
> *The angel:* "The Devil has departed, He will come back."
> *Me:* "The Devil, yes." (Guiette 1934, 254–55)

While this happened in 1909, Jacob was baptized on February 18, 1915, through the order of Notre Dame de Sion, founded by the Ratisbonne brothers (cf. James 1902). In 1921 Jacob escaped the temptations of the big city for the deserted monastery of Saint-Benoît-sur-Loire, and spent much of his time there, continuing his literary activities. He also became a supporter of L'Action Francaise, a fascist, monarchist, anti-Semitic movement. This did not help when the Nazis came, and he had to wear the yellow star. Arrested in February 1944, Jacob died the following month in the Drancy concentration camp, near Paris, on the way to Auschwitz, where most of his family died.

Jacob's conversion was not externally rewarded in any way. It was not only a negation of his family, but of his social network as well. Some of his friends thought the whole thing was a joke, another game played by a surrealistic clown. What we realize is that in the midst of all the Bohemian gaiety, Jacob was the sad clown, feeling as unloved and lonely as he did in childhood. His eyes had "all the sadness of the Jews," according to Daniel Henry Kahnweiler, the Jewish art dealer and another member of his circle (Warnod 1975, 106). The conversion created center and balance, but Jacob, by his own admission, still had all the character traits found in him before 1909. They were only differently colored.

EXPLAINING PERSONAL TRANSFORMATIONS: INTERNAL STRIFE AND INTERNAL PEACE

Conversions seem like real miracles, unplanned initiations into certainty in old or newly found beliefs. But both religious experiences and conversions are ultimately social in their sources and consequences. Sharing infrequent private revelations and conversions with the majority of believers becomes a major ritual and a source of confidence for both converts and their audiences. The dream of metamorphosis for individuals and collectivities is nourished by the example of individual, miraculous transformations.

While we are ready to believe in dramatic change, we offer secular, psychological explanations for such occurrences. When it comes to psychological miracles, we feel that we can figure out the causal processes with some (speculative) precision. The psychodynamic assumption is that both positive and negative changes mean an internal change in an unconscious system of representations (Beit-Hallahmi 1996). The source of self-reported rebirth is the resolution of conscious and unconscious conflicts, worked through a series of conscious and unconscious fantasies, to produce an attachment to a set of delusional beliefs. Every successful case of individual rebirth is the result of an internal truce among opposing personality elements.

The psychodynamic view of conversion (Freud 1928) delineates an unconscious conflict, resolved through a sudden reorganization of impulses and attachments. The ego is invested in a new love object, and this leads to higher self-esteem and a better performance of life's tasks. This internalized object may serve as a new superego, supplying the ego with an impulse control system, which has been missing.

The specific content of religious beliefs and commitments is irrelevant, and conscious religious certainty reflects the internal state of the ego. The outer peace and happiness observed in many converts is the result of an inner truce between ego and superego. What is achieved through superego victory is reconciliation with one's father and with all paternal authorities, gods included. While, on the surface, distance from the parents may be growing, the convert experiences an internal, imaginary reconciliation.

ANTECEDENTS TO METAMORPHOSIS

In both individuals and societies, religious awakening is tied to crises and anxieties. Millennial movements, Cargo Cults, and Ghost Dances have always followed catastrophes (Beit-Hallahmi and Argyle 1997); and conversion is most often preceded by personal crisis, stress, and demoralization (Beit-Hallahmi 1992; Beit-Hallahmi and Argyle 1997; Paloutzian, Richardson, and Rambo 1999; Starbuck 1899).

Parental loss is common in the early lives of converts and leaders. Muhammad, George Fox, and Ann Lee are just a few of the religious founders who were orphaned early in life. The historical founders of religions might have experienced a conversion through "creative illness," "Spontaneous and rapid recovery accompanied by a feeling of elation . . . the conviction of having discovered a grandiose truth that must be proclaimed to mankind" (Ellenberger 1970, 449–50). In a study of modern United States televangelists, an absent father, and admiration for one's mother, were uniformly reported in autobiographies. Well-controlled studies found that converts' relations with their parents are in most cases problematic.

Any desire for change must stem from dissatisfaction with the present, and a desire for radical change must stem from a radical dissatisfaction. Strozier (1994), in a study based on extensive interviews with members of apocalyptic communities, suggested that the transformation to fundamentalism, shared by millions of Americans, is a reaction to insecurity, fear, and rage. This is how the inner motivation of converts seems to be shaped. Those likely to report dramatic conversions are also likely to be socially isolated (Argyle and Beit-Hallahmi 1975; Beit-Hallahmi and Argyle 1997).

Psychological readiness, vulnerability, or individual psychopathology may be called upon to explain why particular individuals, and not others in similar social situations, have chosen, or have grown into, conversion experiences. The minority of individuals who report experiencing conversion may be regarded as being more vulnerable and more disturbed in terms of psychopathology (Olsson 1983).

Conversion has been an adolescent phenomenon, and according to Anna Freud (1966), adolescent preoccupation with religious ideas is one way of coping with instincts. The ego finds many ways of controlling them, including the neurotic, regressive solution of religious conversion (cf. Blos 1979). The vocabulary of psychopathology does not lack terms to describe those more likely to find their salvation in religion or in secular miracles: dependent and inadequate personalities, borderline personalities, hysterical tendencies leading to dissociative states, or outright psychosis. There is a parallel, noted by James (1902), between the psychological state of despair, preceding the experience of conversion or salvation, and the elation and happiness following it. One might suggest that the intensity of any salvation experience is going to be matched by the despair that preceded it. It is those disturbed individuals, often quite seriously, who are more likely to experience such sudden transformations that, in themselves, are evidence of severe pathology. The enthusiastic believers who tell us about their conversion may be covering up a deep depression.

Pruyser (1968) suggested that sudden religious conversion is an indication of a severe psychological crisis, and, at the same time, a way of warding off a total breakdown. He recommended that "sudden conversions in people whose religious traditions do not demand them . . . must be carefully evaluated in the religio-cultural background of the person" (Malony and Spilka 1991, 128). Similarly, Erikson (1968) described severe identity confusion as a serious form of pathology, from which some recover successfully and creatively (instancing William James), while others do not, sinking further into psychosis. Boisen stated that both religious experiences and psychosis are capable of producing a dramatic change in the self, whether salvation or disintegration, and described cases where a religious conversion is closely followed by a psychotic breakdown (Boisen 1945).

Preschizophrenic adolescents show a preoccupation with philosophical, religious, and metaphysical ideas (Moller and Husby 2000). In most cases, this leads to a full-blown psychosis, sometimes combined with a self-defined conversion: "The initial ineffable self-transformation is being progressively infused with content, reflected by new interests in the Buddhist thought and motivated by charismatic and eschatological concerns" (Parnas and Handest 2003, 131).

THE CONSEQUENCES OF METAMORPHOSIS

Converts want us to believe they have profoundly changed; this is part of what defines them. One change we must take seriously is self-reports about elevated self-esteem and mood. Even if what happens is a change in self-presentation, such a change is highly significant. After all, spontaneous self-presentation is what we use in diagnosing depression or schizophrenia. James (1902) and Starbuck (1899) reported a period of elation in the wake of conversion that led to higher self-esteem, and this is supported by more recent research (Zinnbauer and Pargament 1998). Ho-Yee Ng (2002) studied individuals treated for drug addiction and found that conversion led to significant positive changes in self-esteem and self-perception.

Joining a new and supportive community of believers may be therapeutic, but in many cases this cannot prevent another breakdown (Witztum, Greenberg, and Dasberg 1990). One modern observer claimed that it was easy "to discern in all the ties with mystico-religious or philosophico-religious sects and communities the manifestations of distorted cures of all kinds of neuroses" (Freud 1921, 132). In a study using converts and controls, Paloutzian (1981) found that Purpose in Life scores were significantly higher following conversion. Relief from distress has been reported in many studies (Beit-Hallahmi and Argyle 1997). On specific measures of mental health, results are more ambiguous, but conversion is helpful as a treatment for drug abuse. Despite the evidence for higher self-esteem, better impulse control, and reduction in anomie, basic personality structures do not change (Paloutzian, Richardson, and Rambo 1999), and that is what Max Jacob already told us in 1934.

One problem with psychological rebirth is its inherent instability. Individual conversion (as well as its effects) is rather precarious and susceptible to reversals. Following the dramatic events surrounding conversion, there is decline in excitement and gratification. The individual is always in danger of reverting to the old self, because of internal psychological or external reasons.

We all suffer existential anxieties, but vulnerability and deprivation, together with an openness to religious ideas, are what cause individuals to reach high levels of ego-involvement in religion (cf. Merton 1948). The painful histories and psychological triumphs of the twice-born virtuosi have made them the leaders, models, and creators of religious traditions. We in the Western world are ready to take seriously the possibility of radical transformation and renewal in the context of religious fantasies, but since the beginning of the psychology of religion in the nineteenth century, we have thought that we can offer cogent psychological, nonreligious explanations for their occurrence. We do not believe in physical miracles, but we are ready to accept claims about psychological transformations and dramatic reductions in self-destructive behaviors. We are eager to believe in the possibility of psychological change for the better, even though we are skeptical about similar physical changes in the absence of biomedical intervention.

SECULAR TRANSFORMATIONS

We can observe miraculous transformations in the absence of any religious faith or rhetoric, and we can assume that the internal dynamics are just as described above: the powerful attachment to a new/old love object. Love can transform an accursed life into a blessed one. Abraham (1925) described the case of an impostor, a young man with a criminal record, who joined the German Army in World War I, and continued his criminal career in the military, always charming, always on the run, always finding willing victims. After the war he was still a criminal telling tall tales, always being believed. Then came the great transformation in the form of real love, and the impostor became a decent human being. There was no talk of enlightenment or *satori*, but a true rebirth.

The remarkable story of Jane Edna Hunter (1940) is another case of a secular, private metamorphosis through an emotional experience of reliving her dead mother's love, which imbued a young woman in crisis with the power to become a leader. Coming from a background of great poverty, and with the help of significant personal talents, this African-American woman became a major organizer, a benefactor, and a model to others.

In secular psychotherapy we can observe a few cases of real transformation, despite the lack of evidence for its overall efficacy, and the exaggerated claims offered by advocates, which sound much like religious testimonials. What can be called psychotherapy conversions occur, first, thanks to the attachment to the psychotherapist, a powerful love object (Freud 1940), who may supersede earlier ones, and cause a new ego-ideal to be formed. In some kinds of psychotherapy the client develops a new identity, through the discovery of recovered trauma memories or even multiple personalities. The life of such clients is divided into Before and After, as they celebrate their new identity as victims of long-hidden trauma. The diagnostic label (e.g., dissociative personality disorder, PTSD) and the recovered memories of childhood events provide an identity and a meaning system: I have been victimized by monsters, and now I can take my revenge by exposing evil deeds and gaining respect in this world.

INTERPRETATION: SHADOW AND SUBSTANCE

Religion has been the dominant meaning system in human history, because it puts human existence into a framework of design, intention, and purpose. Human life is viewed not only as an integral part of a cosmic plan, but as being at the center of this plan. Clearly, this is one of the most gratifying illusion humans can ever create, and it is inextricably tied to some other gratifying illusions. Every religion in its turn brings us the good news of a great miracle, which is that humans possess an eternal soul, and thus can overcome the reality of death. Humans have been enjoying this miracle, which is the essence of religion, for countless generations.

The promise of everlasting life is to be grasped and held on to, for nothing could be more pleasing and reassuring. All supernaturalism is predicated on the notion of suspending the limitations that we all are sadly subject to in everyday life. If you start with the denial of death, other aspects of reality are likely to be ignored, and thus, in religious discourse, we are used to improbable or impossible things. Moreover, many religions tell us not only that each of us will live eternally through our souls, but that we can expect death to be eventually abolished when the end of this world comes, and those who deserve it live in a reality of bliss, justice, and eternal life right here on earth. So the good news of all religions is not the solution to individual death anxiety, but a triumph of good over evil, and all life over death. Religious assertions quite explicitly aim at going above and beyond nature, which necessarily means moving to the realm of human fantasy, guided by desire. The religious imagination is a great human triumph over nature, most directly expressed in the denial of death.

All supernaturalist beliefs are really about miracles, and all discussions of supernaturalist beliefs deal with assuming the miraculous. Victory over nature and over our natural limitations is the fantasy with which religious discourse starts. Once you accept the supernaturalist premise and the denial of death, then all reality limitations are swept away, and "all things are possible to him that believeth" (Mark 9:23). After being able to deny death, what other challenges could we have?

Supernaturalist assertions are about events, states, and prospects that are implausible, improbable, and impossible. Every religious claim is miraculous, as it denies reality and defies everything we normally experience. If we start with the supreme promise of immortality, all miracles are but small installments on the road to blissful eternity. Religion provides us fictions we are eager to embrace. A wishful, ideal solution to the human condition, religion itself is a miracle: a breakthrough in the darkness, confusion, and frustration often surrounding life. Religion in all its manifestations reflects wishes we all share, as it promises a total victory over the trials and tribulation of living and over the finality of death.

There is an obvious continuity and consistency in religious discourse uniting foundational miracle narratives and claims that may be regarded as less central and less important. Following the great denial and the great promise contained in immortality, all other denials follow, and miracles are just many small denials of pain and misery. Common miracle narratives are part of the great plot, a texture of compensations and consolations leading up to the promise of an absolute triumph. The believers can be sustained by narratives of past glories and promises of future triumphs. Miracle narratives assure us that even if the universe is not totally benign, benevolent forces are active on our side and will intervene on our behalf, if we only obey their commands. Religious devotion means pleasing the spirits, which in many cultures may mean pleasing our ancestors.

Miracles are always naturalistic claims (Beit-Hallahmi 2002) presented as evidence for the power of spirits and the power of those connected or obedient to them. Humans are subject to clear rules of reward and punishment, administered meticulously by the great spirits. Divine punishments are as vital to the religious worldview as miracles. Disasters and miracles are both part of divine plan, and the cosmic calculus is evident in both. Disasters used to play a much bigger role in religious discourse (Kelly 2005), but the discussion of natural catastrophes as evidence of a cosmic justice has become rare since the Lisbon earthquake of 1755, showing the clear impact of secularization.

Secularization means that religious discourse loses its authority and its salience in any given culture. Miracle narratives lose their status as reverence for past traditions weakens and recedes. Doubts about the veracity of miracle narratives and about the need to take them seriously have always been around, even in the Middle Ages. "It ain't necessarily so," the Gershwin brothers' 1935 song rhythmically declares. That is a modern expression of an ancient sentiment, which did not often gain public expression.

With growing secularization, which meant primarily that religious institutions were losing their political power, meaning the power to command respect and obedience, miracle stories were treated with skepticism and ridicule. Educated religionists regarded miracle narratives as an embarrassment. We can see the consequences of such embarrassment in the contemporary Roman Catholic definition of miracles, which bows to the authority of secular biomedicine and ask for its *imprimatur*. On the Protestant side, there have been the celebrated attempts to interpret miracle narratives, which are the essence of the New Testament, as demythologized, or existential parables, thus mocking and denying the experiences of untold millions of believers and readers, who have read these narratives and had no trouble deciphering their message (Anderson and Fischer 1966). Fortunately for those concerned about the survival of miracle narratives, no amount of demythologized or "existential" interpretations will affect the billions of believers eager for excitement and consolation, to relieve their quiet desperation.

Well-educated religionists will prefer their gods to remain transcendent, avoiding any entanglements with humans in ICUs. Most believers, however, still prefer extending the range of divine intervention, which means that the great spirits need to get their hands dirty, so to speak, chasing ambulances.

A fascinating religious reaction to the triumph of biomedicine can be observed in recent years in the United States, with millions of dollars being spent on studying the efficacy of prayer in helping with various medical problems. What we have here is the last and desperate stand of the sincere believers in miracles, who happen to have medical degrees and research budgets to spend. The results are expectedly pitiful (Carey 2006; Sloan and Ramakrishnan 2006). What these researchers obviously don't know is that the last word on the subject was said already in 1872 by one of the founders of academic psychology, Francis Galton (Galton 1872).

A continuing process of socialization and resocialization is essential for the maintenance of committed members and the group's survival, and this is referred to in Christianity as apologetics. A religious group can survive only when the implausible is embraced, and this must happen because without it there is no hope for immortality and cosmic salvation. Nagging doubts are always likely to come up, and confirmatory narratives and revelations allow for rejuvenation and renewed certainty.

Reik (1951) suggested that the preoccupation with dogma is a reflection of unconscious doubts. Historical struggles over the minutiae of Christian beliefs were a displacement of recurring doubts, ambivalence, and anxiety. What should be added to Reik's psychoanalytic interpretation is that doubts and anxiety about religious beliefs are not always unconscious. The same may be said of the preoccupation with miracle narratives.

REFERENCES

Abraham, K. (1925), The History of an Impostor in the Light of Psychoanalytic Knowledge, *Psychoanalytic Quarterly* 4, 570–87.

Anderson, R. T., and P. B. Fischer (1966), *An Introduction to Christianity*, New York: Harper and Row.

Arendt, Hannah (1979), *Love and Saint Augustine*, Chicago: University of Chicago Press.

Argyle, M. (1958), *Religious Behaviour*, London: Routledge and Kegan Paul.

Argyle, M., and Benny Beit-Hallahmi (1975), *The Social Psychology of Religion*, London: Routledge and Kegan Paul.

Arieti, S. (1956), Some Basic Problems Common to Anthropology and Modern Psychiatry, *American Anthropologist* 58, 26–30.

Arieti, S. (1976), *Creativity: The Magic Synthesis*, New York: Basic Books.

Becker, Ernest (1973), *The Denial of Death*, New York: Free Press.

Beit-Hallahmi, Benny (1989), *Prolegomena to the Psychological Study of Religion*, Lewisburg, PA: Bucknell University Press.

Beit-Hallahmi, Benny (1992), *Despair and Deliverance: Private Salvation in Contemporary Israel*, Albany: SUNY Press.

Beit-Hallahmi, Benny (1996), *Psychoanalytic Studies of Religion: Critical Assessment and Annotated Bibliography*, Westport, CT: Greenwood.

Beit-Hallahmi, Benny (2001) Explaining Religious Utterances by Taking Seriously Super-naturalist (and Naturalist) Claims, in *Explanation: Philosophical Essays*, G. Hon and S. Rakover, eds., Dordrecht: Kluwer, 207–30.

Beit-Hallahmi, Benny (2002), Rebirth and Death: The Violent Potential of Apocalyptic Dreams, in *The Psychology of Terrorism*, C. E. Stout, ed., Westport, CT: Praeger.

Beit-Hallahmi, Benny (2006–2007), Triggers and Transformations: Freud and Siddhartha, *Annual of Psychoanalysis*, 34–5, 151–63.

Beit-Hallahmi, Benny, and M. Argyle (1997), *The Psychology of Religious Behaviour, Belief and Experience*, London: Routledge.

Bloom, Harold (1992), *The American Religion: The Making of a Post-Christian Nation*, New York: Simon and Schuster.

Blos, P. (1979), *The Adolescent Passage*, New York: International Universities Press.

Boisen, Anton (1945), *Religion in Crisis and Custom*, New York: Harper and Row.

Carey, B. (2006) Long-Awaited Medical Study Questions the Power of Prayer, *New York Times*, 31 March, C1.

Chafets, Z. (2006), Preaching to Wall Street, *New York Times Magazine*, 17 December, 15–22.

Chekhov, Anton (1915/1979), The Bishop, in *Anton Chekhov's Short Stories*, New York: Norton.

Claverie, E. (2003), *Les Guerres de Vierge. Une Anthropologie des Apparitions*, Paris: Gallimard.

Cole, J. R. (1996), *Pascal: The Man and His Two Loves*, New York: New York University Press.

Cranston, R. (1957), *The Miracle of Lourdes*, New York: Popular Library.

Ellenberger, H. F. (1970), *The Discovery of the Unconscious: The History and Evolution of Dynamic Psychiatry*, New York: Basic Books.

Erikson, E. H. (1968), *Identity: Youth and Crisis*, New York: Norton.

Festinger, L., H. W. Riecken, and S. Schachter (1956), *When Prophecy Fails*, Minneapolis: University of Minnesota Press.

Fhima, C. (2002) Max Jacob ou la symbiose des identités paradoxales, *Archives juives*, 35, 77–101.

Fisher, H. (2004), *Why We Love: The Nature and Chemistry of Romantic Love*, New York: Henry Holt.

Frazer, J. G. (1933–36), *The Fear of the Dead in Primitive Religion*, 3 vols., London: Macmillan.

Freud, Anna (1966), *The Ego and the Mechanisms of Defense*, London: Hogarth.

Freud, Sigmund (1921), Group Psychology and the Analysis of the Ego, in *The Standard Edition of the Complete Psychological Work of Sigmund Freud*, James Strachey, ed., Vol. 18, 65–144, London: The Hogarth Press.

Freud, Sigmund (1928), A Religious Experience, in *The Standard Edition of the Complete Psychological Work of Sigmund Freud*, James Strachey, ed., Vol. 21, 167–74, London: The Hogarth Press.

Freud, Sigmund (1940), An Outline of Psycho-Analysis, in *The Standard Edition of the Complete Psychological Works of Sigmund Freud*, James Strachey, ed., vol. 23, 141–208, London: The Hogarth Press.

Fromm, Erich (1947), *Man for Himself: An Inquiry into the Psychology of Ethics*, New York: Holt.

Galton, F. (1872), Statistical Inquiries into the Efficacy of Prayer, *Fortnightly Review* 12: 125–35.

Glik, D. C. (1986) Psychosocial Wellness among Spiritual Healing Participants, *Social Science and Medicine* 22, 579–86.

Greeley, A. (1981), *Religion: A Secular Theory*, Beverly Hills, CA: Sage.

Greenberg, J., T. Pyszczynski, and S. Solomon (1995), Toward a Dual-motive Depth Psychology of Self and Social Behavior, in *Efficacy, Agency, and Self-Esteem*, M. H. Kernis, ed., New York: Plenum Press.

Guiette, R. (1934), Vie de Max Jacob, *La Nouvelle Revue Francaise*, 22, 5–19, 248–59.

Harrell, D. E., Jr. (1985), *Oral Roberts: An American Life*, Bloomington, IN: Indiana University Press.

Hebb, D. O. (1955), The Mammal and His Environment, *American Journal of Psychiatry* 91, 826–31.

Holm, N. G. (1991), Pentecostalism: Conversion and Charismata, *International Journal for the Psychology of Religion* 1, 135–51.

Hunter, J. E. (1940), *A Nickel and a Prayer*, Cleveland: Elli Kani.

James, William (1897, reissued in 1956), *The Will to Believe*, New York: Dover.

James, William (1902, reissued in 1961), *The Varieties of Religious Experience*, New York: Collier.

Kelly, J. (2005), *The Great Mortality: An Intimate History of the Black Death, the Most Devastating Plague of All Times*, New York: HarperCollins.

La Barre, W. (1970), *The Ghost Dance: The Origins of Religion*, New York: Doubleday.

Lenhoff, G. (1993), The Notion of "Uncorrupted Relics" in Early Russian Culture, in *Christianity and the Eastern Slavs*, B. Gasparov and O. Raevsky-Hughes, eds., Vol. 1, 252–75. Berkeley: University of California Press.

Malony, H. Newton, and Bernard Spilka, eds. (1991), *Religion in Psychodynamic Perspective: The Contributions of Paul W. Pruyser*, New York: Oxford University Press.

Markle, G. E., and F. B. McCrea (1994), Medjugorje and the Crisis in Yugoslavia, in *Politics and Religion in Central and Eastern Europe*, W. H. Swatos, Jr., ed., Westport, CT: Praeger.

Merton, Thomas (1948), *The Seven Story Mountain*, New York: Avon.

Miettinen, M. A. (1990), Uskonnolliset ihmeparantumiset laaketieteellis-psykologisesta nakokulmasta [Healing from a medical-psychological point of view], Series A, No. 51, Pieksamaki, Finland: Kirkon Tutkimuskeskus.

Moller, P., and R. Husby (2000), The Initial Prodrome in Schizophrenia: Searching for Naturalistic Core Dimensions of Experience and Behavior, *Schizophrenia Bulletin* 26, 217–32.

Ng, Ho-Yee (2002), Drug Use and Self-Organization: A Personal Construct Study of Religious Conversion in Drug Rehabilitation, *Journal of Constructivist Psychology*, 15, 263–78.

Olsson, P. A. (1983), Adolescent Involvement with the Supernatural and Cults, in *Psychodynamic Perspectives on Religion, Sect, and Cult*, D. A. Halperin, ed., Boston: John Wright.

Paloutzian, Ray F. (1981), Purpose in Life and Value Changes Following Conversion, *Journal of Personality and Social Psychology* 41, 1153–60.

Paloutzian, Ray F. (1996), *Invitation to the Psychology of Religion*, 2nd edition, Boston: Allyn and Bacon.

Paloutzian, Ray F., J. T. Richardson, and Lewis R. Rambo (1999), Religious Conversion and Personality Change, *Journal of Personality* 67, 1047–79.

Parnas, J., and P. Handest (2003), Phenomenology of Anomalous Self-experience in Early Schizophrenia, *Comprehensive Psychiatry* 44, 121–34.

Pattison, E. M., N. A. Lapins, and H. A. Doerr (1973), A Study of Personality and Function, *The Journal of Nervous and Mental Disease* 157, 397–409.

Piaget, Jean (1962), *Play, Dreams, and Imitation in Childhood*, New York: Norton.

Piaget, Jean (1967), *The Language and Thought of the Child*, London: Routledge and Kegan Paul.

Pruyser, Paul W. (1968), *A Dynamic Psychology of Religion*, New York: Harper and Row.

Pyszczynski, T., J. Greenberg, S. Solomon, J. Arndt, and J. Schimel (2004), Why Do People Need Self-Esteem? A Theoretical and Empirical Review, *Psychological Bulletin* 130, 435–68.

Pyysiainen, Ilkka (2004), *Magic, Miracles and Religion: A Scientist's Perspective*, Walnut Creek, CA: Alta Vista.

Randi, J. (1989), *The Faith Healers*, Amherst, NY: Prometheus Books

Reik, Theodor (1951), *Dogma and Compulsion: Psychoanalytic Studies of Religion and Myths*, New York: International Universities Press.

Rose, L. (1971), *Faith Healing*, Harmondsworth: Penguin Books.

Sloan, R. P., and R. Ramakrishnan (2006), Science, Medicine, and Intercessory Prayer, *Perspectives in Biology and Medicine* 59, 504–14.

Starbuck, E. D. (1899), *The Psychology of Religion*. New York: Scribner.

Strozier, C. (1994), *Apocalypse: On the Psychology of Fundamentalism in America*, Boston: Beacon Press.

Sullivan, Harry Stack (1964), *The Fusion of Psychiatry and Social Science*, New York: Norton.

Taves, E. H. (1984), *Trouble Enough: Joseph Smith and the Book of Mormon*, Buffalo: Prometheus Press.

Thouless, R. H. (1971), *An Introduction to the Psychology of Religion*, Cambridge: Cambridge University Press.

Tiger, L. (1979), *Optimism: The Biology of Hope*, New York: Simon and Schuster.

Wallace, A.F.C. (1966), *Religion: An Anthropological View*, New York: Random House.

Warnod, J. (1975), *Le Bateau Lavoir*, Paris: Presses de la Connaissance.

Williams, G. M. (1946), *Priestess of the Occult*, New York : Knopf.

Witztum, E., D. Greenberg, and H. Dasberg (1990), Mental Illness and Religious Change, *British Journal of Medical Psychology* 63, 33–41.

Zinnbauer, J. B, and Kenneth I. Pargament (1998), Spiritual Conversion: A Study of Religious Change Among College Students, *Journal for the Scientific Study of Religion* 37, 161–80.

CHAPTER 11

HEALING IN THE GOSPELS:
THE ESSENTIAL CREDENTIALS

Kamila Blessing

Jesus [said], "Those who are well have no need of a physician, but those who are sick; I have come to call not the righteous but sinners to repentance."

—*Luke 5:31 (NRSV)*

At least since the time when Thomas Jefferson edited his version of the New Testament (1804), deliberately eliminating miracles, Western cultures have taken for granted the idea that Jesus, as physician, is only a metaphor. Some readers assume that Jesus healed only sinners and the moral side of the person. Others assert that spiritual healing was performed only in the past, or only by Jesus. Nevertheless, in the middle of the twentieth century, significant voices began to take healing and other miracles in the Gospels seriously. Most significant is Rudolph Bultmann, universally known for his thesis that the stories of the Bible are myths. By his definition, myths are belief or creedal statements; not necessarily untrue, but if they represent some truth, it is symbolic and metaphorical. Yet even Bultmann, writing on the subject of Jesus' miracles, said this:

> The Christian community was convinced that Jesus had performed miracles. . . . Most of the wonder tales contained in the gospels are legendary . . . But . . . undoubtedly he healed the sick and cast out demons. He obviously understood his miracles as a sign of the imminence of the Kingdom [reign] of God (Lk 11:20, Mk 3:27, Mt. 11:5), exactly as his church was later convinced that it possessed the powers of the Messianic age to work miracles. (Acts 2:43, 4:9–12, etc.)[1]

Bultmann goes on to say why it must be so that miracle is central to the story of Jesus:

> God is distant, wholly other, in so far as everyday occurrences hide Him from the unbeliever; God is near for the believer who sees His activity.[2]

Bultmann was very much a part of the nineteenth and twentieth century cultural movement called scientific materialism, the theory that if we cannot humanly reproduce a certain object or result, then there is no such thing in the universe. This view reduces all of reality to what our limited minds and knowledge can produce. We should know better in this age of the Hubble Space Telescope and the discovery by physicists of black energy, which supposedly fills what used to be considered empty space in the universe. Today, that old theory of empty space is increasingly shown to be inadequate to explain the universe, or even the natural healing ability of the human body.

For this reason, even the medical community is today beginning to look at the spiritual side of healing. For this reason also, we must take another serious look at healing and other miracles in the Gospels. The task of this chapter is to explore and describe the Gospel stories of healing and their theological import.

THE GREAT PHYSICIAN

Some scholars think that the stories of healing in the Bible are simply part of a traditional ancient hero story. However, the fact is, there was an actual Jesus. He was a historical figure, mentioned in the works of Josephus, a Palestinian Jew who worked as a historian for Caesar in Rome in the first century. Josephus wrote:

> At this time there appeared Jesus, a wise man. . . . For he was a doer of startling deeds, a teacher of people who receive the truth with pleasure. . . . and when Pilate . . . condemned him to the cross, those who had loved him previously did not cease to do so. . . . And up until this very day the tribe of Christians, named after him, has not died out.[3]

Several writers of the early second century, such as Roman historians Tacitus, Lucian, and Suetonius, confirm various facts about Jesus despite their prejudice against the Christians. Finally, the Jewish law book that is part of the Talmud, known as Sanhedrin, which is very much opposed to Jesus and the Christians, also confirms certain major tenets of the Gospel story, albeit through negative statements. The Talmud was written in the third or fourth century, but reflects the Jewish reaction to Jesus very near to the time of his earthly life. In general, these negative sources converge upon two points:

- Jesus was a teacher (Josephus, Sanhedrin 43a)
- Jesus did in fact work wonders (Josephus, Sanhedrin 43a, Lucian)

The Gospels of course tell us firmly that Jesus did heal, and we have no historical records to contradict that assertion. Just as important, at the end of Mark's Gospel, we are told that it was not all in the past. In Mark 16:17–18, Jesus says: "These signs will accompany those who believe: In my name . . . they will place their hands on sick people, and they will get well." The epistle of James commands the church to carry out spiritual healing (Jas 5:13–16). Clearly, Jesus and his disciples held that the task of healing was to be a major aspect of Jesus' mission, and also the mission of the incipient church.

In fact, the Gospels present healing as the whole point of Jesus' coming, the changing of people's lives at all levels of existence. Four times in the Gospels, Jesus refers to himself as physician in the context of healing sinfulness. However, his healing ministry was far wider than that reported in the biblical text. To see this, we need only to think about the word, salvation; in Greek, *sozo*, to save, to heal, to deliver from illness. English derivatives include save, salve, salvage, to bring about the literal salvation of something. It is intrinsically connected with healing, to save from being sick, death-ridden, or destroyed materially, physically, emotionally, and spiritually.

The Gospels do not present Jesus as one who came to bring only an ethereal, invisible afterlife. There is no place in the Gospels where it says Jesus came to save people's *souls*. The Gospels proclaim a total healing of the whole person.

Why the Misunderstanding?

The misunderstanding about the nature of healing in the Gospels persists for historical and philosophical reasons. We are heirs of Greek culture and of a Western, rational mode of thought that has been superimposed upon the teachings of Jesus. Ancient Greek philosophers, particularly Plato and Aristotle (fourth century BCE), wrote that the physical and the spiritual are essentially different and separate from one another. Plato said, in essence, that the human being was a spirit trapped inside a body. Aristotle softened this proposition by making it subtler, but still, the physical person was a pale reflection at best of true humanity. For Christians and Jews, this position means that if we were made in the image of God, we are still so distant from God's nature that we are essentially incompatible with the spirit.

Beginning sometime in the first century, certain early Christian groups held a view parallel to that of Plato and Aristotle: that the physical and earthly were actually negative or evil and a spirit, particularly the Spirit of God, would never stoop to become one with its material or physical container. For them, Jesus could not be both divine and human in his earthly presence. Therefore, the Spirit of God could not enter into a person's physical body to heal it. These views were later solidified and promoted by a group called Gnostic Christians.

This negative dualism denied the Incarnation, God become human. Though the resurrection is the miracle that launched Christianity, without the Incarnation there is no Jesus, no God-as-flesh to be resurrected. For this reason, the birth of Jesus is recorded in Matthew and Luke. "The Word became flesh" (John 1:14), is John's once-for-all pronouncement of the incarnation and its theological import. It is also John's birth story for Jesus. If the Incarnation is denied, then Jesus' healing can be denied; in fact, the entire Gospel story falls apart.

It is for these reasons that the Gnostic denial of Jesus' dual nature was later condemned as a heresy. Jesus, as truly human and truly divine, is central in the Nicene Creed and in Christian theology generally. However, a negative form of dualism crept back into Christian theology during the Middle Ages when Plato and Aristotle were rediscovered in Europe. These philosophers' work became the basis of the most influential theology of the Middle Ages. The body was again seen as a temporary and imperfect representation of personhood or God-likeness. Healing of the body by means of prayer went out of fashion. These attitudes toward healing persist today. As a result, some Christians believe that the miracles in the Gospels did occur, but those things no longer happen, a stance called "cessationism." Others believe that even the miracles in the Gospels are simply the product of uneducated believers presenting Jesus as a mythical hero.

Excursus: The Resurrection of the Body and the Denial of Healing Miracles

Since this chapter is devoted to the Gospels, we cannot go deeply into systematic theology. However, a sketch of what became of the doctrine of bodily resurrection in theology is appropriate. The resurrection of the body was maintained by most of the church as a doctrine. This is important because it directly contradicted the denial of miracles. Yet it went largely unnoticed that the body is either holy to God or not, and therefore worth saving or not, and cannot be both.

The greatest theologian of the Middle Ages, Thomas Aquinas (1200s) rejected Plato's absolute division between the physical and spiritual, and accepted Aristotle's more subtle argument that the physical is the temporal and limited expression of a spiritual essence, for instance, of humanity. Thus Acquinas distinguished between the physical and spiritual while maintaining the doctrine of the resurrection of the body. However, notably Acquinas did not support the healing of the body in his theological works. Some modern theologians have maintained the doctrine of bodily resurrection, although Bultmann did not. More recently, even some Roman Catholic theologians have rejected the resurrection of the body (directly refuting Catholic doctrine), notably eminent Catholic theologian Hans Küng (in *Eternal Life? Life after Death as a Medical, Philosophical, and Theological*

Problem, Doubleday, 1984). Influential Episcopal bishop John Spong also denies the resurrection of the body.

However, one of the greatest biblical theologians of the modern era, N. T. Wright, has written a massive investigation of the meaning of resurrection in the Bible and its contemporaneous cultures (*The Resurrection of the Son of God*). In it, he shows that our only evidence (the Gospels) do credibly maintain that Jesus was in fact resurrected. He thus effectively refutes new theologies that reject all physical resurrection as irrational or as revisionist history.

Other theologians argue the issue of when the body is resurrected—immediately or at a final moment in natural time when God resurrects the faithful from the dead. To this Karl Barth answers "immediately"; others say that this conclusion goes beyond the text of the New Testament. Certainly Jesus' body is represented in the Gospels as resurrected immediately. It is possible that the resolution lies in the fact that God created natural time as he created all other things and therefore can dispose of it as he wishes.

Nevertheless, the great creeds of the historic church maintain the doctrine, specifically the Apostles' Creed ("I believe in . . . the resurrection of the body"). To deny this doctrine is tantamount to denying the whole fabric of the New Testament (and the Old) because without the resurrection of the body we deny Christ's resurrection and therefore the whole basis and impetus for Christianity. Bodily healing was offered by Jesus and through his believers as evidence of this greater miracle; therefore the two things go together. This fact is made explicit in the Gospels where resurrections of the dead were among Jesus' healings.

It is notable that other religions often consider the body to be of no further use after death, unless it is given back to nature. *The Tibetan Book of the Dead,* an ancient "guide" for the soul of the dead and for the mourners, is an example of this very different take on the holiness of God's creation that is the body.

Now let us return to the subject of the denial of miracles.

Modern Arguments over Biblical Miracles

Some argue against miracles because some strata of the New Testament (NT) text are late, but the entire New Testament was written by the beginning of the second century, and our oldest complete manuscripts are from the fourth century. We have to take the Bible on its own terms; it is the text around which the church grew and flourished. D. Moody Smith's, *John Among the Gospels* (2001, Columbia: University of South Carolina Press, Second Edition), indicates how complex the development of the texts of the Gospels was, and sets the question of strata dates in context

There is a valid question whether a passage appears to have characteristics that mark it as part of the oldest stratum of the story of Jesus as opposed to a later interpretation by someone with an interpretative agenda. N. T. Wright has shown the originality and reliability of the greatest miracle, the resurrection.[4] Some argue that the Gospels differ from each other and therefore some part of them must be incorrect. Every Gospel has the aim of telling the story as faithfully as possible, addressing the issues that faced particular communities of believers, with slight differences. All were written within a century of Jesus' life and death, by those who had heard the witness of the apostles and had been transformed by the story to which they witnessed. All the Gospel writers present a concept of the human being that is different from the Western idea, one in which healing by miracle is fully logical and, indeed, necessary to their message. In the Gospels, the incarnation says firmly that the body is holy to God, and in the resurrection, the ultimate healing has incipiently been fulfilled. Therefore the healings and miracles in the Gospels must remain valid, or the message is seriously damaged.

The Whole and Indivisible Person

There is a specific reason Jesus' healing by means of prayer is perfectly sensible to the Gospel writers. The Hebrew notion of personhood is that of a unitary entity. Paul's letters seem to take a Greek view of body, spirit, and soul. However, in the Judaic perspective, persons are characterized by integrated and unified personhood. To put it another way, Hebrew thought is aspective, not partitive: we can speak of physical, spiritual, and other *aspects* of the person, but not of those things as distinct and separate from one another. In the Greek New Testament, as in English, there simply were not words that could express the total unity of the human being and make the intention clear. But to Jesus, Paul, and the other writers of the Bible, the inseparability of the human being was an unquestioned reality. Persons are made in the image of God, body, heart, brain, mind, spirit, genitals, and all (Gen 1:27).

The impact of Jesus' resurrection upon the apostles and disciples was the immediate reason for spreading their belief in Jesus and the one reason to write down the accounts of Jesus' life later in the first century. The resurrection is the reason we have the NT. This ultimate teaching of the NT contains within it what is implicit in creation: that the physical body is holy to God and to be honored as the *instrument*, not merely a disposable container, of our spirituality, our relationship with God. The resurrection of Christ, as presented in the Gospels, puts back the holiness of the entire creation, including its physical aspect.

The concept that the essential aspects of a person cannot be separated is confirmed by the resurrection. It does involve a paradox. Surely, the physical body disintegrates after our death. Paul makes an analogy with a grain of wheat. The seed has in it the entire wheat plant. When planted a tall plant grows; a living thing. It is the whole of the plant. Notably this resurrection is not resuscitation. The original seed is not dug up and dusted off[5] but is as a whole transformed.

Another analogy to resurrection is that of a fine perfume. I am told that among professional perfumers, there are people called *noses* who can take a complex perfume and identify every type of flower, spice, or other scent in it. A really good *nose* can tell you exactly where the flowers were grown. The flower, in its original physical form, is no longer visible. In fact, to our human eyes, it has been destroyed. However, the essential identity of the specific flower is still intact.

An individual person dies and the body is gone, but God knows that person in his or her individuality, just as surely as we would know a friend if she came back in her original body. That is the basic Christian understanding of salvation. Paradoxical as it seems, Jesus came to save the whole, essential self of each one of us, not just a part of us. In the Gospels, Jesus gave to people a foretaste of the healing of the total self, in the form of the healing of illness or injury. He also thereby showed that God's plan is to redeem the entire creation, not only an invisible spiritual part of it.

MIRACLES: GOD'S DEMONSTRATION PROJECT

In fact, Jesus deliberately used his healings and miracles as an audiovisual aid to show people what more God has to offer them. Ancient people were not necessarily superstitious or naïve, as we tend to think. The Jews knew that the Messiah would be able to perform such saving acts. Imposters were stoned. In the Gospel stories, most of the witnesses treated the miracles of Jesus as invitations to a new kind of understanding. Jesus performed a miracle, and the crowds followed him, listening to his teaching. They saw the miracle before they came to believe in him (Jn 2:11). The healings were his way of getting people's attention and demonstrating God's power, the presence of God's reign. Thus Jesus did not heal all the sick, but just a paradigmatic few.

For the above reasons, one-fifth of the verses in the Gospels are devoted to healings. Over one-third of the Gospels address healing, apart from the accounts of the incarnation and the resurrection. This is not a minor matter.

What Healings?

All in all, by the count of the *Thomson Chain Reference Bible's* "Chain Index," where repetitions of the same story have been consolidated, Jesus performed 18 physical healings, four resurrections including his own, five exorcisms, each of which included some physical and psychological healing, and 10 other miracles. About 20 times, the Gospels refer to Jesus healing all who came, or to God's healing in general. Of the 10 other miracles, seven are miracles of provision, feeding, or nurture, also a form of healing because it sustains the life of the receiver. These miracles include turning water to wine at the marriage in Cana, feeding the 5,000, feeding the 4,000, provision of tribute money in the mouth of the fish (Mt 17:27), the catch of fish in Luke 5, the second catch of fish in John 21, and the resurrection appearances. The appearances provide for the life of the incipient Christian community and sustain them emotionally and physically as they begin to go out into all nations (Mt 28:19).

The other three miracles are the stilling of the storm, walking on the sea, and the cursing of the fig tree, all demonstrations of the power and presence of God in the world. These miracles signify provision for improved life in this world and the next.

The Essential Credential

In performing these miracles, Jesus deliberately invoked what was, for the Messiah, the essential credential. John the Baptist sent some people to ask: "Are you the one who was to come?" (Mt 11:3). By this, John meant, "Are you the Messiah?" Jesus replied: "Report to John what you hear and see: The blind receive sight, the lame walk, those who have leprosy are cured, the deaf hear, the dead are raised, and the good news is preached to the poor" (Mt 11:4–5; see Lk 4:16–21). That is the one proof Jesus needed, and the only qualification he offered. This list of types of healing comes from Isaiah 61:1–2, the accepted list of the credentials of the genuine Messiah. Jesus gave a similar testimony in Luke 4. At the synagogue in Nazareth, he read aloud that passage from Isaiah. When he finished, he said to the congregation: "Today this scripture has been fulfilled in your hearing" (4:21).

Such was Jesus' claim. Much of the reason the Gospels give for believing Jesus' claim comes, paradoxically, from the circumstances of the crucifixion. We need only to look at the last of the plots to kill Jesus. The occasion was the raising of Lazarus. In John 11, the stated reason was specifically the miracles. When Lazarus had been raised, some people "went to the Pharisees and told them what Jesus had done" (Jn 11:46). The immediate result is recorded in John 11:47–48: "The chief priests and the Pharisees called a meeting of the council, and said, 'What are we to do? This man is performing many signs. If we let him go on like this, everyone will believe in him, and the Romans will come and destroy both our holy place and our nation.'" They had to kill Jesus, precisely because his miracles could not be disproved. Jesus' worst enemies acknowledged his miracles.

Finally, Jesus made it clear that his followers were to do the same kinds of healing. He never once sent out his disciples to preach without also telling them to heal; and they did so. The story of the formation and growth of Christianity after the resurrection, found largely in the book of Acts, shows the continuation of healing miracles in the church. The disciples continued to use miraculous healing as evidence of the truth of Jesus' promise of salvation, just as Jesus himself had done. Healing was their essential credential, too.

One among Many? About Ancient Healers

Some scholars believe that the stories of Jesus' healing simply are a Christian parallel of the ancient pagan literature about spiritual healing and healers. Or they believe Jesus was just one of many wonder-workers of his time. In the pagan literature, the healings were the entire point. In the Gospels, the healings were all about ministry to the suffering, with the exception, perhaps, of John 9 in which Jesus manipulates and exploits the suffering of a blind man to make his own political-theological point about the superficiality of Jewish legal constraints. The miracles pointed to the divinity of Christ, the completion of salvation, and the unique and ongoing relationship between the believer and God.

The truly important thing in understanding healing in the Gospels is that Christianity was brought about by Jesus, and then by the disciples demonstrating the power of God on this earth, through healing. The miracles stunned Jews and pagans alike, and some of each were transformed forever by the direct and indirect action-in-the-world of this healer and savior, Jesus. That Jesus healed and therefore demonstrated and promised a genuine salvation was the point of the Gospels. In short, the healings and miracles are presented as the *essential credential*.

WHAT KIND OF HEALING?

What kind of healing did Jesus do? He did the kinds that are still today the most difficult. In general, there are three kinds of healing: physical, including functional and organic; emotional; and ethical. In functional physical illness, something in the body does not function correctly, but the function can be restored. In organic illness, part of the body is defective, and more is needed than restoring its function. The emotional is what we would call psychological healing. Ethical relates to change of character and behavior. In all of the Gospels, there are only two ethical healings, the woman at the well (Jn 4),[6] and Zacchaeus, who decided to stop extorting money from people (Lk 19:2–9).

Many of the healings by Jesus were the kinds that are still a mystery for modern medicine: the organic, and the psychological. For example, Jesus healed the paralytic (Mt 9). We do not know if his bones were deformed, which would be an organic illness; otherwise, it was a functional illness. The healing of the man with the withered hand (Mt 12:10) is definitely in the organic category of physical healing.

What about psychological healing? While on the cross, Jesus presented his mother and his disciple John to each other as a new mother-son family.

That was in the category of emotional healing, even though the text does not tell us how they felt afterward. We do know that the terrible fear felt by the disciples after the crucifixion was replaced by joy and confidence when they saw the resurrected Jesus. His statement to them was a healing of the emotions and of the spirit: "Jesus said to them again, 'Peace be with you. As the Father has sent me, even so I send you.' And when he had said this, he breathed on them, and said to them, 'Receive the Holy Spirit'" (Jn 20:21–22). Though the resurrection itself is the focus of the story, we should not overlook the fact that an emotional healing of enormous proportions had also taken place.

Now let us consider actual mental illness, that is, emotional illness that is severe enough to interfere with a normal life. It is common knowledge that mental illness is often impossible to cure. Clinically ill people are frequently recidivist. Alcoholics and addicts are even more so. Jesus' healing of the young boy in Matthew 17:14–18 is described as an organic disorder, epilepsy, and a psychological disorder. Jesus cast out a demon. Both probably refer to the organic disorder of seizures. However, Jesus is described as performing a number of exorcisms, all of which were likely some serious form of psychopathology. The ancient cultures thought that evil spirits could be one source of a tormented mind, and so there is a connection between exorcism and psychological healing. One thing we know: the Gospels tell us that those who had been possessed, and all of the others who were healed by Jesus, were totally healed (Mk 1:23–26).

Healed persons never returned to Jesus for another cure of the same thing. In one healing (Mk 8:22–25), a man who had been treated by Jesus for blindness returned to say the healing was not yet complete: "I see people like trees walking" (v 24). Jesus gave him another treatment and his healing was complete. The Gospel writers did not cover up this instance. In fact, this odd detail of the story sounds a lot like an eyewitness account of the event. Clearly we have here a careful attempt to preserve the accurate history of the miracle.[7]

The critical point is: Jesus successfully carried out the most difficult of all healings. He most pointedly took on the worst sickness of all, our mortality. Jesus resurrected three people: Jairus' daughter (Mk 5:21–24, 35–43; Lk 8:41–42, 51–56); the son of the widow of Nain (Lk 7:11–17); and Lazarus (Jn 11:1–44). Such was the demonstration project of healings and miracles confirming the incipient presence of the reign of God's grace that works and love that heals.

Jesus' Approach to the Sufferer

Jesus, apparently, never turned anyone away. The point is made strongly in the story of the man who, in asking for the healing of his son, makes it clear that he has little confidence in Jesus. He says to Jesus, "If you are able to do anything, have pity on us and help us" (Mk 9:22). Even after Jesus' assurance, he is still uncertain. However, being desperate, he says, "I believe; help my unbelief!" (Mk 9:24). In this case, his desperation was what brought him to Jesus in the first place. He would have tried anything. Of course, Jesus did heal the son of the man. The father's lack of faith was no barrier to healing.

Likewise, Jesus never told anyone, apparently, that he was too sinful to be healed. In certain specific instances, he healed the person and then said "sin no more" or "your sins are forgiven." In those healings, notably that of the paralytic (Mt 9:2; Mk 2:3; Lk 5:18), forgiveness is a healing unto itself. Jesus used the healing to demonstrate to the onlookers that he possessed God's power to forgive sin. In any case, and in every case where sin was involved, he healed first, and only then commanded holiness. Though Jesus acknowledged that sin can be a cause of suffering, he also made a point (Jn 9) that sin may have nothing to do with the affliction. More important, however, is the overall theological issue: if Jesus was to be true to his own purpose in coming, the message of salvation and its audiovisual aids, the healings, could not depend upon people's limitations. This is the doctrine of grace, unearned mercy from God, which is central in the Christian worldview. In this, Jesus contradicted one entire stream of OT theology that maintains that suffering is always God's punishment. Jesus represents the other stream of OT belief, namely, that God is only good and brings his people only good, and out of his loving–kindness grants healing in a broken world.[8]

In fact, Jesus promised that prayers in his name would be answered (Jn 14:13). He did not say when or how. However, the act of asking for healing, that is, one type of prayer, may itself be a sort of healing, of the relationship between the person and the Lord. Thus in the healing of Mark 9, the son was healed of possession and the father was also healed by being brought into relationship with God through a personal interaction with Jesus.

THE THEOLOGICAL PURPOSE OF HEALING IN THE GOSPELS: A VIEW FROM THE GREEK

A great deal of the significance of Jesus' miracles is carried in the Gospels through the choice of specific Greek words. Several Greek terms are used for one concept such as healing or miracle. When there are many occurrences of any one of those terms, or if different groups of people used one *versus* another, we know that the writer was trying to convey more than what occurred factually. He was making a specific theological point or interpretation by his choice of Greek words.

Further, as with body, spirit, and soul, there are often no English words that are precisely equivalent to the intended meaning of a Greek term. Various Greek terms are often translated by just one English word such as healing. In such a case, as indicated in the work of Laato and Koskenniemi in this volume, the biblical writer's intended connotations are lost. Thus translations often dilute meaning of the text, hiding it from the modern reader.

For example, in John 11:12, most translations say something like, "if he [Lazarus] is sleeping, he will get better." Actually, the last word is a form of *sozo*, he will be saved. The theological meaning of the healing of Lazarus is thus obscured in translation.[9] For these reasons, let us explore the terms for two central concepts: healing; and miracle or mighty work. There are three terms for healing, and three for miracle.

Terms for Healing: Salvation in Nuce

The Gospels contain 52 uses of the term *to heal*. This English term actually represents three different Greek terms, as shown in the following Table 11.1.

Let us begin with *sozo* because we have already talked about its meaning. The four instances of its use for healing occur in Matthew 9:21; Mark 5:23; Luke 8:50; John 11:12. The use in John refers to Lazarus. The other uses are *not* repetitions of a single saying from one Gospel to another but occur in the context of other, distinct healings. Thus there are four distinct witnesses, three of them in the mouths of people who were looking for healing and received it. These witnesses are saying to the reader: healing is a sign, foretaste, and guarantee of the greater salvation. Here is the explicit message that the healing we see, in itself, is not the entire point. The Gospel writers are distinguishing Jesus from other healers and instituting the reign of the God of Israel, signified by Jesus' kind of healing.

Table 11.1   Greek Terms for Jesus' Healing Actions

Greek Term	Pronunciation	Principal Meaning	Gospel Usage
Therapeúo and therapeía	Thera-pew'-o (long o) Therapy'-a	Total healing emphasizing the direct action of God	27 times together
Iátro	Ee-at'-ro ("at" as in English; long o)	"Heal" with emphasis upon the Great Physician (NT: Jesus; OT: the LORD).	20 times
Sózo	So'-dzo (long o's)	1. "Heal" as a sign of the availability, through Jesus, of personal relationship with God. 2. "Save" as in salvation per se	4 times[i] 7 times[ii]

[i]There is one use of one other term with which we will not deal here.
[ii]These seven are not among the 52.

Therapeúo (a verb) and *therapeía* (a noun) bear meanings in the Gospels that are distinct from their use in other ancient literature. The original root meaning in classical Greek was *to serve*, as a servant serves his master, but also as a human being serves or worships God. The verb implies devotion to and advancement of the good of the one served. Classical writers, specifically Plato, also used it to mean *to care for the sick*. In the Gospels it is used pointedly to mean *causing the wholeness of*:

- Persons (for example, Lk 9:11) or
- The nations (that is, Gentiles, see Rev 22:2).

The latter signifies that God is going to bring the nations to worship and be accepted by the God who raised Jesus from the dead (Rom 4:24). These healings are represented as the direct action of God in the world, taken in the name of Jesus and by the agency of the Holy Spirit of God. This message is the essence of the Gospel, embodied in Jesus and acknowledged by the persons who gave the original witness to Jesus.

Iátro emphasizes the role of the spiritual physician. In the Gospels, the focus is on the great physician, Jesus. In the Septuagint, the Greek translation of the OT, *iátro* is used to translate the Hebrew word *raphah*, to heal. In Hebrew, the Lord is called, among other titles, *Adonai Ropheh*, the Lord the Healer. The understanding in the Gospels, as in the OT, is that the Father in heaven is the ultimate healer. The healing itself is never the point, but rather, a demonstration of God's reign breaking in upon the world. *Iátro* in the Gospels particularly keeps before the reader one point, namely, that central in every healing is the person of Jesus present with the one who is healed.

SUMMARY: THE MEANING OF HEALING

Thus the three terms for healing, all mixed together in English, actually make a series of theological statements and promises. Healing is accomplished by God's direct intervention for the person on this earth, intending to restore wholeness of the entire person. The personal presence of Jesus is central in the act of healing and, of course, in salvation. Finally, a personal relationship with the healer is offered to everyone, no matter who they are. In ancient Judaism, it was unthinkable that God would include pagans in salvation, even though Isaiah and others prophesied that the Gentiles would all worship God, and that in fact, Abraham's original blessing was in part for the "healing of the nations" (*goyim*). The book of Acts depicts Paul's mission to the Gentiles. These Greek terms, taken together, anticipate that God intended to extend his healing reign to all ethnic groups and persons.[10] The Gospels intend to propel the reader to these conclusions. The promises in English pale compared with what the writers of the Gospels intended to say.

Miracle: God's Power on Earth

The terms for *miracle* are also theologically significant. There are three major words, shown in Table 11.2. In understanding these terms, it is useful to know the distinction made by scholars between John and the first three Gospels, Matthew, Mark, and Luke (Synoptics—seen as similar). *Dýnamis* (power, mighty work), *semeíon* (sign), and *érgon* (a work), are used somewhat differently by the Synoptics than in John. All of the usages, however, specifically invoke the power of God as manifested in the OT. Their use in general conveys one message: the Jesus of the Gospels is fulfilling the promises of the OT prophets that God intends to restore his creation. The principle term for Jesus' wonder works in the synoptics is *dýnamis*, power or act of power, hence also miracle or great work. The use of this term to refer to Jesus' mighty works, however, is limited to the Synoptics. The Synoptics put a strong emphasis on Jesus' coming to destroy evil, and proclaim God's reign on earth.[11] *Dýnamis* perfectly expresses this double purpose, particularly in connection with exorcisms.

Sign in the Synoptics

Semeíon ("Sign") Is Used in Three Ways

1. In an eschatological (end of the world) setting. This usage stems from the prophetic and apocalyptic parts of the OT such as Daniel 4:2.
2. When nonbelievers demand a miracle as proof.
3. As a simple description of the miracles of Jesus and the apostles.[12]

Matthew, Mark, and Luke use *sign* in the pejorative context. An example is Matthew 12:38: "Then some of the scribes and Pharisees said to him [Jesus], 'Teacher, we wish to see a sign from you.' But he answered them, 'An evil and adulterous generation asks for a sign, but no sign will be given to it except the sign of the prophet Jonah.'" He was referring to the Jonah story in which he was in the belly of the fish for three days, and then was saved. Jesus' burial for three days and rising again would be a sign to all. The Synoptics also use *semeíon* in phrases such as *the signs of the times* (Mt 16:3, an eschatological usage) and *signs from heaven* (Mt 16:1, a simple designation of the miraculous).

Sign in John

John's use of *semeíon* is unique and very deliberate. Except for the summary in 20:30, John uses *sign* only in chapters 1 to 12, hence the term *the book of signs* applied to those chapters. In John, s*emeíon* is used by other people to describe Jesus' works; Jesus himself uses *érgon* ("work"). It has been said that *sign*

Table 11.2   Jesus' Power in Action

Greek Term	Pronunciation	Principal Meaning	Gospel Usage
Dýnamis	Din' - amiss	"Power," "a mighty work"	Used in this way only in Matthew, Mark, and Luke; signifies Jesus' specific work of defeating the devil and evil in the world
Semeíon	Sem – eye' - on	"Sign"	Usage unique to John signifying the oneness of Jesus and the Father; implication is that the reign of God on earth has already begun. In John, signs are the evidence of the present fulfillment of OT promises, rather than an anticipation of a future "coming."
Ergon	Erg' - on	"A work"	17 times in John, by Jesus, denoting his oneness with the Father; twice in the synoptics

expresses the human viewpoint about the miracles (who is that fellow?); while *work* expresses the divine viewpoint (salvation fulfilled "in your hearing").

The most characteristic Johannine use of *sign* is as a favorable designation for a miracle, similar to the third usage above, but with a punch. For example, 2:11 says: "This [changing water to wine], the first of his signs, Jesus did at Cana in Galilee, and manifested his glory; and *his disciples believed* in him" (emphasis mine). The reader is given to know that there will be a series of demonstrations of the Lord's power (the first of his signs), of his oneness with the Father whose power it is since such signs cannot be performed by a mere human, and therefore of God's glory. These signs will create the unique relationship between Jesus and his disciples, and they believed in him. All of this is contained in the term *semeíon* in the context of that sentence.

John is usually said to recount seven signs, each of which demonstrates these same theological points. The seven are:

- healing the official's son (4:46–54)
- the multiplication of loaves (6:1–15)
- walking on water (6:16–21)

These three have parallels in the Synoptics; the next two of the seven are:

- healing the paralytic (5:1–15)
- the man born blind (9).

These are similar to healings in the Synoptics, but from different sources; and finally:

- changing water to wine at the marriage in Cana (2:1–11)
- the raising of Lazarus (11:1–44)

which have no Synoptic parallels. In fact, there are eight signs, not seven, the last being the resurrection of Jesus. The number eight signifies the beginning of the new creation, seven and the Sabbath (seventh [day]) symbolizing the completion of the original creation. The seven miracles explicitly named signs in John signify that the old creation is complete in the sense of having fulfilled its purpose and being ready for a resurrection *in toto.*

Each sign is accompanied by a verbal exposition of its meaning. For example, in John 6:1–15, Jesus miraculously fed the 5,000; this event is followed by the discourse wherein Jesus proclaims "I am the bread of life" (6:35).[13] Jesus is thus compared with both Moses and manna. Whereas Moses was an earthly leader, though appointed by God, and manna could sustain only earthly life, John makes the point that Jesus was able to sustain life eternal, through the direct action of God (6:32–33).

The Oneness of Jesus with God

John places tremendous emphasis on the oneness of Jesus and the Father. For example, in John 8:28–29: "Jesus said, 'When you have lifted up the Son of Man, then you will realize that I am he, and that I do nothing on my own, but I speak these things as the Father instructed me. And the one who sent me is with me; he has not left me alone, for I always do what is pleasing to him'" (see also Jn 5:30; 12:50; 14:10). In this connection, John often uses *sign* in a way that is analogous to the second Synoptic usage. In John, faith may be based on signs, but it is an incomplete faith because it fails to focus specifically upon the relationship between Jesus and the Father.

Sign and Evil: The Reign of God Now Present

Unlike the Synoptics, John does not emphasize Jesus' mission against evil per se. (In fact, John records no exorcisms.) His emphasis is upon the miracles as revelation—as signs—inextricably connected with salvation. *Sign* pointedly evokes the signs and wonders of the Old Testament, particularly related to salvation and liberation from bondage, as in Exodus 3:12: "[God] said, 'I will be with you; and this shall be the sign [*semeíon*] for you that it is I who sent you: when you have brought the people out of Egypt, you shall worship God on this mountain.'" In John, such physical restoration is always a sign of spiritual life granted by God (see Jn 11:24–26).

In John, the new spiritual life is *already* granted. Where the Synoptics look for a second coming of the Lord in which judgment and salvation will finally

take place (Mk 10:30), John looks at Jesus' physical presence as well as his resurrection appearances as the realization of God's reign on earth. It is incipient
but nevertheless already victorious. Thus he can write (Jn 1:12), "to all who
received him, who believed in his name, he gave power to become children of
God." It is significant that in Greek, the verb "he has given" is a continuing
past tense; it is already a done deal for believers in general and it is ongoing.
God has continued to give this power to new believers in the time since the
Gospel was written. The end of John complements the beginning: unlike the
Synoptics, Jesus' last words are "It is finished" (19:30), signifying that the entire task of salvation has been completed. See also John 17:4 where Jesus prays
and says to God that he has completed the work God gave him to do.

The reader can see the two different views of salvation as complementary.
The Gospel of John was written later than the Synoptics and had greater
signs and wonders continuing in a later decade—to which John witnesses.
Also, the kingdom is not fully come; John's point is that we need not be in
suspense; it is promised. It is a done deal.

Johannine signs parallel the prophetic actions of the Old Testament.
Jesus performs an action at God's command like, for example, Isaiah 20:2;
Jeremiah 13:1–11; Ezekiel 12:1–16. As with the prophets, the action (sign)
points beyond itself. The signs point to a present spiritual life and foretell a
spiritual life that is to be attained without the necessity of signs after Jesus'
resurrection. However, there is a difference between Jesus' signs and those of
the prophets. With Jesus, the sign itself is intrinsically valuable and directly
changes the lives of those who are healed, fed, or given a view of the reign
of God (as in changing water to wine). The prophets' signs are followed by
a prophecy in words, but the words often foretell something fearful such as
invasion by the Babylonians. With Jesus, the people sometimes do not want
to hear what he says in explaining the signs, but the prophetic word is always
an invitation to salvation.

Work in John

I have already introduced the third term, *érgon*, work. *Érgon* is used by
Jesus of his miracles 17 times in John, many of them powerful statements of
the relationship between Jesus and the Father. As an example: Jesus said, "Do
you not believe that I am in the Father and the Father is in me? The *words*
that I say to you I do not speak on my own; but the Father who dwells in me
does his *works*. Believe me that I am in the Father and the Father is in me; but
if you do not, then believe me because of the *works* themselves. Very truly,
I tell you, the one who believes in me will also do the *works* that I do and, in
fact, will do greater [works] than these, because I am going to the Father"
(John 14:10–12) (emphasis mine). *Érgon* is used with this meaning only twice
in all of the Synoptics, in Matthew 11:2 and Luke 11:28.

In these verses, as elsewhere, *word* and *work* are closely related, and the Father's words and works are the sole source of the words and works of Jesus. The word *work* in brackets represents a place in Greek where the word is not literally present, but is implied. John clearly means us to hear *works* four times, emphasizing their importance. Note that if it is by their fruits that we are to know people, it is much more so with the Son of God.

In John, *érgon*, unlike the other two terms for miracle, represents the entire mission of Jesus. The term has a special function that is augmented by *semeíon:* it very deliberately and pointedly echoes the mighty acts (works) of God on behalf of his people in the OT. Most importantly, *érgon* and *semeíon* are prominent in the accounts of creation and of the exodus. In the creation story, there is a special connection between *work* and *word* because God accomplishes creation by the word alone. In the Gospels, as Raymond Brown writes, "*Word* reminds us that the value of the miracle is not in its form but in its content; the miraculous *work* reminds us that the word is not empty, but an active, energetic word designed to change the world."[14]

SUMMARY: MIRACLE IN THE FOUR GOSPELS

All of the Gospels proclaim the continuation and fulfillment of God's promises as recorded in the OT. However, the miracles in John are fewer than in the Synoptics. The Synoptics, taken together, emphasize a future kingdom, the defeat of evil and the reign of God to be completed after a second coming of Christ on the clouds of heaven. John, on the other hand, dwells most upon God's reign already incipiently granted, the oneness of Jesus and God, and the relationship of Jesus and the believer. The significance of the difference between John and the Synoptics, regarding miracles, is this: *In the Synoptics, miracles are demonstrations of the reign of God returning through Jesus Christ. By the later time of John, the signs had been accepted as the backbone of all that Jesus was and is; in themselves, they constitute the definitive statement of the Gospel and thus the salvific work of God in the world.*

Reactions to the Signs: The Man Born Blind

In the Gospels, the people who witness the healings and other signs respond in several different ways. These are most clearly delineated in John but occur in all of the Gospels. There are four general categories of response:

1. Refusal to see the sign with any faith (Caiaphas, Jn 11:47)
2. Regarding signs as wonders and believing in Jesus merely as a wonderworker: Jesus refuses to accept this response, for example, in John 2:23–25; 3:2–3; 4:45–48; 7:3–7.
3. John 10:38 regarding signs as evidence of Jesus' oneness with the Father, particularly after the resurrection (Thomas in Jn 20:28: "My Lord and my God!")

4. Believing in Jesus without seeing signs (Jn 20:29; compare 14:12), based on the word of those who were with Jesus when he was present on earth.[15]

John and the Synoptics all propel the reader to one conclusion, specifically through the stories of healing and the ultimate healing, the resurrection: the faith of the apostles is available to God's people even in the present age. The gospels charge the believer to take to heart the word of the apostles' testimony and to ask for healing for themselves and others. The healing includes a relationship with Jesus, though that relationship may come after healing. The believer is then to pass on the healing and the relationship to all nations.

The point is brought home forcefully in John 9, when Jesus was about to heal the man born blind. The disciples asked Jesus, "Who sinned, this man or his parents, that he was born blind?" Jesus answered, "Neither this man nor his parents sinned, but this happened so that the work of God might be displayed in his life." Look carefully at what this must mean. It cannot be that God wanted the man to be blind. What Jesus was saying, and what he then acted upon very forcefully by healing the man, was this. First, the man's sin did not cause the blindness. Second, in this man's body, the glory of the Lord God will be known. The healing of blindness, regarded as something only the Messiah could do, will be accomplished. With the repetition of Jesus' statement, "I am the light of the world" (Jn 9:5, echoing 8:12), the onlookers are given to know that genuine knowledge of God in the world will be given to anyone who is open to it.

All four types of reaction to the miracle occurred in this healing. The rulers of the synagogue refused to see the healing as a work of God at all. The man's parents apparently acknowledged the wonder work but did not acknowledge Jesus as one with God's own person and power: "His parents answered, 'We know that this is our son, and that he was born blind; but we do not know how it is that now he sees, nor do we know who opened his eyes'" (9:20–21). The man himself, with crushing and ironic simplicity, testified to the oneness between Jesus and God. Responding to the Pharisees' refusal to believe in the divine origin of the miracle, "the man answered, 'Here is an astonishing thing! You do not know where he comes from, and yet he opened my eyes. . . . Never since the world began has it been heard that anyone opened the eyes of a person born blind. If this man were not from God, he could do nothing'" (9:30–33). It is evident from this text that the reader of a later era is also to see the entire miracle as evidence of Jesus' oneness with the Father and of his ability to bring about the ultimate salvation.[16] Indeed, the irony of this last statement makes the reader feel totally idiotic if he does not agree with the statement of the healed. That is John's style.

Finally, the man, having been excommunicated by the rulers of the synagogue, met Jesus again. John strongly implies that Jesus came specifically to show him that with God, he was still a participant in the covenant, synagogue or no synagogue. The man, evidently healed of the powerful social and religious rejection he had just suffered, turned to Jesus and said, "'Lord, I believe.' And he worshiped him" (9:38). At this juncture, Jesus also rebuked the establishment, in another of John's ironies, by referring to the Pharisees as blind. Overhearing, "some of the Pharisees near him . . . said to him, 'Surely we are not blind, are we?' Jesus said to them, 'If you were blind, you would not have sin. But now that you say, *We see*, your sin remains.'" The roles were reversed; the blind saw and the seeing were theologically blinded. In John 9, then, the essential credential has been demonstrated, the credential that states that Jesus is one with God and that he is salvation come in person.

CONCLUSION

Healing in the Gospels thus represents the entire message of the Gospel writers and of Jesus himself as they remembered him. With the incarnation, Jesus reclaimed the human body as holy, prophesying the restoration of creation. The defeat of the final enemy, death, is promised. With the resurrection of Jesus' body, his whole self, he became the fulfillment of that promise. In between, the healings and other miracles each present the promise and the incipient victory of God's reclamation of the world.

The Gospels, particularly John, leave the reader with a challenge. Put in modern terms it is this: does the reader choose to be Thomas Jefferson or Thomas the Apostle? With Jefferson, idealizing Jesus' ethical standards but denying the miraculous and God's presence in him? Or with the apostle, realizing the unique nature of Jesus and the immediate presence in him of "My Lord and my God!" (Jn 20:28)?

Certainly, the Gospels were written to propel the reader to the latter revelation. However, it is not just an aspect of the Gospels, a literary style, or a superstition superimposed upon a reforming Jewish prophet. The miracles are the very substance of their message. The medium *is* the message, as McLuhan declared! Without the miracles, the promise of eternal life and salvation is reduced to a mere ethical proposition, a speculative philosophical statement that can be put aside if the reader so chooses. As Bultmann wrote, "Everyday occurrences hide Him [God] from the unbeliever; God is near for the believer who sees His activity. . . . Undoubtedly he [Jesus] healed the sick and cast out demons . . . as a sign of the imminence of the Kingdom of God."[17] With the miracles, then, the Gospels proclaim the renewed dominion of the God of history, the one who can, truly and directly, be known.

NOTES

1. Rudolph Bultmann (1958), *Jesus and the Word*, L. P. Smith and E. Lantero, trans., New York: Charles Scribner's Sons, 172.

2. Bultmann, *Jesus and the Word*, 178.

3. Josephus, Flavius (1996), Testimonium Flavianum, *Antiquities* 18.3.3, quoted in Luke Timothy Johnson, *The Real Jesus: The Misguided Quest for the Historical Jesus and the Truth of the Traditional Gospels*, San Francisco: HarperSanFranciso. Josephus also confirms the historical existence of John the Baptist and James the brother of Jesus. Luke Timothy Johnson's book analyzes the work of the Jesus Seminar and contends that their methods are arbitrary and unscholarly, such as in their method of voting on the historicity of Jesus' sayings as recorded in the gospels. Many scholars conclude, however, that the reference to Jesus in Josephus is a late Christian interpolation. Moreover, Johnson seems to have missed the point that the voting on the part of the Jesus Seminar was an agreed upon method, among the scholars participating, of expressing consensus, to the degree that it existed among them, and not a method for asserting absolute truth.

4. N. T. Wright (2003), *The Resurrection of the Son of God*, Minneapolis: Fortress.

5. This expression of what does not happen to the seed is from N. T. Wright, *The Resurrection of the Son of God*, 342.

6. The woman at the well in John 4 is usually assumed to be a sinner because she had had many husbands. However, in the ancient Judaic world, women often did not have a choice about marriage. Her questionable status is that she was a Samaritan, and thus was not accepted by the Jews. Nevertheless, there may be an ethical healing in her. Instead of remaining alone and keeping her knowledge of Jesus to herself, she began to talk to all of the townspeople and thus reoriented her own and their entire thinking about the Messiah.

7. There is also the account of Jesus in Nazareth (Mk 6:5–6), where "he could do no deed of power there, except that he laid his hands on a few sick people and cured them. And he was amazed at their unbelief" (see also Lu 4:14–30). If these potentially embarrassing episodes are preserved faithfully, we have no reason to think that the rest of the account hides any failure of power against suffering. The theological point is in fact positive: Jesus did not do his work against the will of the persons who were invited to experience the incipient Kingdom of God.

8. The book of Job argues these points graphically and comes to the conclusion that Job did not sin; his afflictions were caused directly by the fact of evil in the world (represented by Satan); and God loves him and honors his undaunted faithfulness by healing him. *Nota Bene*: "Satan" means "false accuser." Job is not about God allowing Satan his way, but about God's awareness of the falseness of the accusation of the sufferer. It also attests to God's personal intervention and restoration of the accused sufferer.

9. One place the meaning of *sozo* is not obscured in translation, but nevertheless is misunderstood, is James 5:15: "The prayer of faith will save the sick, and the Lord will raise them up." *Save* here is *sozo* with all of its meanings, and "raise up" means exactly that—a literal and/or prophetic resurrection by divine healing. Together, these two terms are unambiguous.

10. As in Mark 9:24, "Immediately the father of the child cried out [to Jesus], 'I believe; help my unbelief!'"

11. John does not emphasize Jesus destroying the work of the devil as do the Synoptics; but consider 1 John 3:8, thought by many scholars to be the work of the same author as the Gospel of John.

12. Raymond Brown (1966), *The Gospel According to John* (2 vols.), Garden City: Anchor Bible Series, 527. Acts 2:22 equates all three of the terms discussed here, citing threefold the miraculous deeds of Jesus to demonstrate that he is the Messiah.

13. "I am" sayings are unique to John; there are seven of them, loosely connected with the seven signs.

14. Raymond E. Brown (1996), *The Gospel According to John*, 527.

15. Ibid., 530–31. A more complete categorization of stages of belief in Jesus— and relationship with him—is documented in Blessing (2001), John, *Women's Bible Commentary*, Westmont, IL: InterVarsity Press.

16. A more thorough exploration of the way in which the miracle and John's text work to include the reader in a full relationship with Jesus is presented in Kamila Blessing (2004), Family Systems Theory as Hermeneutic, *Psychology and the Bible: A New Way to Read the Scriptures*, vol. 1, ch. 13, J. Harold Ellens and Wayne G. Rollins, eds., Westport, CT: Praeger.

17. Bultmann (1958), *Jesus and the Word*.

REFERENCES

Beyer, Hermann W. (1965), Therapeúo; and Therapeía, *Theological Dictionary of the New Testament (TDNT)*, Vol. 3, 128–32, Gerhard Kittel and Gerhard Friedrich, eds., Geoffrey Bromily, trans., Grand Rapids: Eerdmans.

Blessing, Kamila, (2004), Family Systems Theory as Hermeneutic, in *Psychology and the Bible: A New Way to Read the Scriptures*, J. Harold Ellens and Wayne G. Rollins, eds., Vol. 1, ch. 13, Westport, CT: Praeger.

Brown, Raymond E. (1966), *The Gospel According to John*, Garden City, NY: Doubleday.

Brown, Raymond E. (1979), *The Community of the Beloved Disciple*, New York: Paulist Press.

Bultmann, Rudolph (1958), *Jesus and the Word*, L. P. Smith and E. Lantero, trans., New York: Charles Scribner's Sons.

Kung, Hans (1984), *Eternal Life? Life after Death as a Medical, Philosophical, and Theological Problem*, Garden City, NY: Doubleday.

Lewis, Clive Staples (1947), *Miracles*, Revised edition issued by the publisher in 1960, San Francisco: HarperSanFrancisco.

Oepke, Albrecht. (1965), Iáomai, *Theological Dictionary of the New Testament (TDOT)*, Vol. 3, 194–215, Gerhard Kittel and Gerhard Friedrich, eds., Geoffrey Bromily trans., Grand Rapids: Eerdmans. This article contains a thorough and fascinating explanation of *iátro* and a lengthy discussion of the differences between pagan and New Testament accounts of divine healing.

Wright, N. T. (2003), *The Resurrection of the Son of God*, Minneapolis: Fortress Press.

CHAPTER 12

WHAT WE CAN LEARN FROM MIRACULOUS HEALINGS AND CURES

Patrick McNamara and Reka Szent-Imrey

While theologians have long debated what could be learned about God from the study of miracles, we consider in this chapter what might be learned about human health from a close study of miracle cures. We think the traditional scientific approach to reports of miracles has all too often been concerned merely with debunking these reports and events rather than with learning from them. The assumption seems to be that if the events can be debunked then nothing can be learned from them. Or rather, given that miracles cannot occur, it follows that the only thing to be learned from them is that people are gullible and easily fooled. There apparently is no end to the boundless credulity of human beings.

We believe this debunking approach to reports of miracles is unfortunate because it neglects real study of these events. While debunking may have a constructive role to play when it urges ill and vulnerable people to not neglect consultation with medical experts, it all too often is merely a destructive and triumphalist enterprise that leaves these ill and vulnerable people feeling tricked and demoralized rather than empowered and focused. In the standard debunking scenario the hero-scientist runs to the side of the individual whose cancerous lesions have suddenly receded and informs him that there really is no cure and no chance that he will escape death;. that instead he is gullible, stupid, and still has the cancer and that therefore he is just buying into an illusion;. and that finally our hero the scientist should be thanked for providing this information to the unfortunate man.

In the zeal to debunk all miracle cures, there is a tendency to eschew careful study of the facts. We believe that extraordinary healings do occur and that they indicate normally unrealized healing resources within persons. Weil (1996) points out that an elaborate healing system exists in the body, a system that repairs wounds, renews bone and, most important, corrects mistakes that creep into our DNA blueprint and, if uncorrected, could result in cancer or other disease.

RELEVANT DATA

Our biology, apparently, can promote remarkable cures, given the right circumstances. This is the stark and extraordinary lesson to be learned from miraculous healings, yet it clearly has not been learned by the scientific community. There is no concerted effort by the biomedical community to investigate reports of miraculous healings, spontaneous remission, or to investigate potential physiologic correlates of these healings. Yet reports of spontaneous healings and spontaneous remissions of chronic diseases, like the cancers, regularly appear in the medical literature.

Unfortunately very little is known about these spontaneous healings. We could find no reviews of the literature and no controlled epidemiologic studies of incidence of spontaneous remission in any of the major diseases. According to the Institute of Noetic Sciences (http://www.noetic.org/research/sr/main.html), the number of spontaneous remissions from chronic disease may be 10- to 20-fold greater than previous and poorly documented estimates of one in 60,000 to 100,000 cases.

Aside from the well-known but poorly documented phenomenon of spontaneous remission and healing there is the well-documented but poorly understood phenomenon of the placebo response. With respect to the placebo response there is a better, more intensive research effort, but once again, this research effort is not strongly supported by the larger biomedical community nor are there many laboratories dedicated to exploring and understanding the placebo response.

Benedetti, Mayberg, Wager, Stohler, and Zubieta (2005) suggest that the placebo response is a psychobiological phenomenon that can be attributed to the patient's subjective expectation of clinical improvement on the one hand and to classical mechanisms of Pavlovian conditioning on the other. The best-documented placebo effects have been in the field of pain and analgesia, but there are recent indications of strong placebo effects in the immune system, in motor disorders like Parkinson's Disease, and in depression. Benedetti's review of neuroimaging studies of placebo effects revealed increased activation of a large set of frontal regions with concomitant decreased activation in the amygdala.

The frontal cortical networks are known to inhibit subcortical limbic sites that mediate emotion and impulses and further that the amygdala is known to mediate aversive emotional states. Benedetti, therefore, suggested that one facet of the placebo responses involved a powerful suppression of negative emotions. While this suggestion is undoubtedly true it can only be a partial explanation of the placebo effect. A huge part of the placebo response of course involves the expectation that relief is on the way as well as faith and belief in the efficacy of the cure. In order to adequately understand the placebo response therefore we will need a full account of the role of emotion, expectancy effects, belief, and finally of faith. Certainly faith and hope are the major psychological factors involved in miracle cures.

Miracle cures go way beyond mere placebo effects. While placebo effects can temporarily relieve distress, a miracle cure is a cure or a reversal of a severe illness or impairment. In contradistinction to placebo effects, the psychology of expectation and the effects of expectation on health seem much more promising avenues for understanding miraculous healings—yet funding for this research is hard to get and journals only rarely accept papers on expectation effects. Even expectation effects, however, are not rich and powerful enough to capture the phenomenon of miracles. Indeed we know of no models that have yet been able to capture the complexity of miraculous healings. That is because there are no detailed scientific models of faith. What is faith? Who has it? How does one acquire it? While there are theological answers to these questions, scientists routinely ignore the theological accounts of faith and hope. At a minimum, however, faith is a religious trait and hope is a spiritual virtue. Yes, it is true we speak of faith in doctors and scientists, and the like, but when we speak of the active ingredient in miraculous healings we speak of religious faith.

Faith, of course, is connected to and dependent upon religion or at least a religious or spiritual context. The context for most miraculous healings is typically religious. Religion and religious belief, in turn, is extraordinarily complex. Religious belief at a minimum involves a history of acquisition or education in the belief system; current emotional and personality makeup, participation in public rituals, practice of private rituals of devotion, and the like. There is something about religious belief and practice that facilitates miraculous healings in certain individuals. That apparently involves faith. Thus a rational approach to the study of miraculous healings should include both a study of the impact of religious practices on healing, the biology of the healing itself, and the wild card factor: faith.

One recent theoretical approach to the relationships between religion and healing is McClenon's ritual healing theory (McClenon 2002). McClenon argues that the development of human religious rituals functioned in part to facilitate healing and it was their efficacy in doing so that promoted the evolutionary rise of religion among human beings. According to McClenon, early hominids practiced repetitive, therapeutic rituals based on dissociative processes. These rituals, practiced over many millennia, provided survival advantages to those with genes promoting dissociative psychological

processes and the ability to go into hypnotic and trance like states. Rituals fa-
cilitated biologically based forms of unusual experience: trance, apparitions,
paranormal dreams, and out-of-body experiences. These episodes created recurring patterns within folk religion, generating beliefs in spirits, souls, life
after death, and magical abilities. These beliefs are the foundations for shamanism, humankind's first religious form. The ritual healing theory argues
that ritual healing practices shaped genotypes governing the human capacity
for dissociation and hypnosis, allowing modern forms of religiosity.

While clinical studies indicate that hypnosis and trance is particularly
effective in alleviating pain, asthma, warts, headache, burns, bleeding, gastro-
intestinal disorders, skin disorders, insomnia, allergies, psychosomatic disorders, and minor psychological problems (Bowers and LeBaron 1986), there
is no evidence that suggests that the placebo response depends on the ability
to go into dissociative psychological states like trance. Nor is it clear why
dissociation should facilitate any kind of healing. Certainly manipulation of
attention can distract a person for a little while from the feeling of pain, but
the placebo response as described above is related to expectancy and belief
and faith, not merely to distraction.

Because the ritual healing theory of religion and religious healings
depends so decisively on the ability to go into dissociative states it cannot explain miraculous healings. That is because most reports of miraculous healings have not involved reports of dissociative or ecstatic states of any kind.
Instead what seems to be the most important factor is this thing called faith
and its accompanying virtue, hope.

Let us look at concrete examples (Leuret and Bon 1957, 94–98).

Cure of Pierre Bouriette (1858) (Traumatic Blindness)

Pierre Bouriette was a quarry worker on de Pic du Jer. It was his job to set
off the blasting charges, which produced stones for the quarry men. Twenty
years before the apparitions of Mary at Lourdes, in 1838, his right eye had
been injured by an explosion. For twenty years this organ had been a blind,
red, oozing sore. One day he came to a Dr. Dozous and asked whether he
should go to Lourdes, stating that he understood that "Bernadette's water
cured people."

Three days after his interview with Dr. Dozous, Bouriette washed his blind
eye in the still muddy spring water. He did not really have much faith in the
water's powers; curiosity rather than hope was the driving force behind his
action. He was quite taken aback when he realized that, when he had washed
his eye, he could see with both of his eyes. It might be thought that his immediate reaction would have been to thank the Lady of the Apparitions, or
Bernadette, who happened to be there at the time. He actually did what not a
few still do, he rushed to the physician, to have his cure properly verified.

Dr. Dozous did in fact verify the cure, the first such medically verified cure at Lourdes. Bouriette evidenced no signs of going into a dissociative or trance-like state. Instead he simply had faith in the curative quality of Bernadette's waters. But is faith really the curative factor? What about cases of healings in children or people without any religious faith at all? Perhaps the most difficult case for the view that religious faith is the key ingredient in miraculous healings is the phenomenon of healings of sick infants. The second historically recorded cure at Lourdes involved an infant and was medically verified by Dr Dozous. This is the case of Louis-Justin Bouhohorts.

Cure of Louis Bouhohorts (1858) (Osteomalacia and Febrile Wasting)

Louis Bouhohorts was 18 months old. He lay quite still in his cot, for he had not moved since birth. He suffered from a syndrome characterized by fragility of his bones—then given the name of osteomalacia. He never had moved, nor sat, nor stood up—nor, obviously, had he ever walked.

In addition to this he suffered from a febrile wasting disorder which had at that time brought him to death's door. As he lay in extremis in his cot, his father remarked to his mother, still stubbornly nursing him, "Let him be; it's obvious he's nearly dead." At which he left to fetch a neighbor to sew his shroud—who soon arrived with the necessary material. But his mother snatched the child from his cot and wrapped him hurriedly in the first thing that came to hand—a kitchen cloth. Running to the grotto, she covered the last fifty yards on her knees. This part was then rough and stony, unlike the smooth modern pathways. Making her way through about 40 curious people standing at the foot of the grotto she arrived to find Bernadette praying and Dr. Dozous awaiting events.

There was a small pool, roughly five feet by two, dug by quarry workers of the Pic du Jer in thanksgiving for their fellow worker Bouriette's cure. Into this icy water (48°F) she plunged young Louis-Justin to his neck. She kept him there for fifteen and a half minutes (timed by a concerned Dr. Dozous). When she took him out, he was stiff and blue, which was hardly to be wondered at.

His mother, rather ashamed of what she had been doing, wrapped him, still stiff, in his kitchen cloth, took him into her arms, returned home and put him in his cot. When his father saw him in this condition, he felt no anger but simply said to his wife, "Well, you should be happy anyway, you've managed to kill him off." He turned away with tears in his eyes while the child's mother remained in prayer beside the cot. After some moments she tugged at her husband's coat. "Look—he's breathing." Which in fact, he was. He fell asleep now and spent a quiet night. He woke gurgling next morning and took his breakfast—this, despite his age, at his mother's breast. According to her he had a good meal. She put him back into his cot and went into the next room to do her household chores. Leaving him alone did not worry her—he had never moved. A little later she heard behind her the patter of feet. On looking around there was Louis-Justin—cured of all his suffering, the osteo-malacia, the wasting illness, which had almost carried him off. Furthermore, he could walk—without having learned to walk.

While Bouriette's cure might be ascribed to a simple faith or to some extraordinarily potent placebo effect or more likely some sort of expectation effect, surely the infant's cure cannot be accounted for in these terms. Given that the child was only 18 months old it seems unlikely that the cure could be ascribed to faith, trance, or belief effects. A child of that age does not believe in anything. Thus, neither our emphasis on faith nor science's emphasis on the placebo effect nor the ritual healing theory described above can explain the cure.

In short we have no explanation for the miraculous healing of an infant. At most the current state of science might help to explain miraculous heal-ings in adults. For the rest of this essay we will therefore focus on healings in adults and ask what might science and medicine learn from these extraor-dinary healings.

For a religious person no special explanation is needed for these miracu-lous cures, but for the scientist some sort of explanation must be attempted, not in order to debunk the religious explanation but in order to learn from the cures. What sort of naturalistic explanation might help?

COSTLY SIGNALING THEORY, CST

We situate our approach to understanding illness phenomenology and ill-ness recovery within an evolutionary theoretical framework concerned with communication between people or between animals or organisms of any kind. This communications theory is known as Costly Signaling Theory (CST; Bliege-Bird, and Smith 2005; Bradbury and Vehrencamp 1998; Grafen 1990; Maynard-Smith and Harper 2003; Zahavi 1975; Zahavi & Zahavi 1997). CST is concerned primarily with understanding animal signaling behaviors. The basic idea is simple: for signals between two parties to be workable or believ-able by both parties they must be reliably unfakeable. Only signals that can-not be faked can be trusted to carry honest information. Unfakeable signals are those signals that are metabolically, motorically, or behaviorally difficult to produce (costly). Their production costs or costliness is their certification of honesty.

Costly signals are preferred by animals under conditions in which the animals are capable of deception but require reliable and honest signaling between the parties, for example, between the two sexes during mating sea-son. Many of these costly signals have come to be known as handicaps. For a signal to classify as a handicap the net benefits for displaying the signal (ill-ness in our case) must be higher for a high-quality individual than for a low-quality individual (or the costs of an illness must be higher for low-quality individuals). Thus a low-quality signaler must be able to send a signal sug-gesting high quality; must be able to fake high quality. The signal must be costly to fake but not impossible to fake. The handicap principle asserts that low-quality signalers generally do not send false signals because it simply does not pay; the net costs are too high.

We suggest that in some cases an illness, after it has passed the acute phase, can function as a signal. That is because illnesses carry information about the genetic qualities of the ill individual. At a minimum if the illness is severe and the individual survives the illness, then the individual displays resilience and good genes. This is the kind of information that CST claims is crucial for devel-opment of cooperation between two parties. In the human context people want to partner, in a marriage or a business or for a hunt, with reliable, resilient, intel-ligent, robust, trustworthy individuals. To identify such individuals they need to find reliable, unfakeable sources of information. Surviving an illness is one such source of reliable information. It is not the only source but it *is* one source and thus illness behaviors are scrutinized by others whether we like it or not.

So the questions we need to ask ourselves when considering illness as a signal bearing important information about an individual's genetic quality are the following: (1) Do people use illness to signal others? and (2) Is illness correlated with genetic quality? We answer each of these questions in turn and then turn to a summary about how CST might treat miraculous healings in religious adults.

Do People Use Illness to Signal Others?

Humans, of course, engage in a range of signaling behaviors, but can ill-ness plausibly be considered one of them? Human signaling behaviors include everything from speech and language exchanges to emotional displays; body language such as clothes, postures, tattoos, and gestures; and other nonver-bal behaviors. Our basic claim in this paper is that illnesses can function as signals. Illnesses, for example, can function to facilitate signaling when they produce some effect such as an emotion or a mood or a bodily posture or a behavior that communicates a message to an observer. An ill person typically behaves differently than a healthy individual. Many illnesses create back-ground moods and behavioral dispositions that linger long after the illness has passed. Showing an illness to another gives the other a direct window onto recent brain/mind activity, and thus a direct window into the quality of the individual sharing the illness.

Like many other costly signals, illnesses are considered to be involuntary physiologic, cognitive and emotional experiences and thus less fakeable than voluntary signals. We contend that many of the signals produced by a person who is ill can be and should be construed as costly signals, emotions or behaviors that are costly to the individual. The informational and affective content of the illness creates a mental set in the individual that signals other people concerning the qualities of the individual who is ill. For example, an ill or impaired person is very obviously handicapped.

People use information concerning the health of an individual when considering interactions with that individual. Among other things an illness is interpreted as a signal to remove the acutely ill individual from social circulation. During acute phases of an illness the person is removed from daily interactions and obligations and allowed to rest. After the acute phase of the illness has run its course however, the individual is treated differently. Depending on the strength and vitality of the recovered individual, he or she may be treated with greater respect and deference, even if the illness becomes chronic. As long as he or she survives the illness he or she will attain to greater prestige and status. If on the other hand the illness becomes chronic and increases in severity he or she may be shunned and stigmatized.

The opposite social effects, enhanced prestige versus stigmatization, that follow the opposite outcomes of an illness demonstrate the capacity of an illness to be interpreted as a signal bearing enormously consequential information. An individual who has recently been ill may find either that he is shunned and left to die or that his social prestige is considerably enhanced. An illness is therefore treated as if it bears reliable unfakeable information about the quality of an individual. Illnesses thus satisfy the primary condition to function as a costly signal within the framework of CST.

What information regarding quality will an individual send with an illness? First it may be information concerning resilience. If I have survived an illness I may be able to survive another illness and therefore I will be a valuable member of the tribe. Another signal or piece of information that an illness might carry concerns an individual's *character*. Let us back up a step to explain how the issue of character fits in with CST.

For cooperation to evolve, the problem of the free-rider, the faking ill person, must be overcome. A free-rider is someone who takes the benefits of cooperation without paying any of the costs associated with cooperation. They are cheats and exploiters. One way to handle this problem of the free-rider is to impose stringent membership conditions for participation in the cooperative group. These membership requirements can serve as hard-to-fake tests and ultimately signals, when the individual adopts them, a person's willingness and ability to cooperate with others. What kinds of signals could serve such a role? CST theorists (Irons, 1996, 2001; Sosis, 2003, 2004) have pointed out that a number of religious behaviors, like restrictive diets, participation in rituals and rites, ascetical practices, and altruistic giving might be such signals as these behaviors are both costly and hard-to-fake. It is precisely the costliness of these behaviors or traits that render them effective since individuals incapable of bearing such costs could not maintain the behavior or trait. Free-riders would find it too expensive to *consistently* pay the costs of religious behavior and thus could be winnowed out of the cooperative group. Most people, even free-riders, can sustain a restrictive diet or attendance at ritual services for a short period of time, but few free-riders would be willing to engage in such costly behaviors over long periods of time.

Since group members cannot measure directly a person's willingness to inhibit free-rider behavioral strategies, they will need a different measure of willingness to inhibit free-rider tendencies. Willingness to perform costly religious behaviors for relatively long periods of time can function as reliable signals of willingness to inhibit free-rider strategies and ability to commit to cooperation within the group. Included in such costly religious behavioral patterns are the hard-to-fake *virtues and character strengths*, as free-riders would not be willing to incur the costs in developing and practicing such virtues. Sustaining virtuous behavior is, to say the least, difficult. That is why character and virtue cannot be faked, at least over the long term. Character therefore can serve as a signal of quality (Steen 2003). Just as ritual and religious practices, *when practiced consistently over time*, help winnow out free-riders from the group, so too will development of hard-to-fake character strengths. To act generously and altruistically consistently over time is a convincing indicator of character as it requires the ability to consistently inhibit short-term gratification of selfish impulses. We suggest that coping with a long illness over time can be a particularly potent revealer of a person's character. Given that is the case it follows that individuals who potentially interact with that individual will use the illness as a way to study that person's character.

It is extremely important to remember that we are dealing with the so-called environment of evolutionary adaptation in which people lived in relatively small groups of no more than 200 people. The average life span was 40 years with sickness and illness a frequent event. While reputation and prestige certainly were used in estimations of a person's character, it is reasonable to suggest that a person's behavior during an illness was used as well. If tribal members observed a person's behaviors during an illness then it follows that the ill person would use the opportunity to signal concerning his quality and his social intentions (willingness to cooperate) to these others.

Though there is no guarantee that an illness will be used by an individual to signal information concerning social intention, illness certainly functions that way. An illness can allow the person to advertise quality and thus honesty in communicative interchanges, and so the long-term results of a strategic illness are improved social interactions for the individual and thus increased fitness. It may seem odd to us that the way Mother Nature defeats free-riders and achieves cooperative interchanges among her creatures is to have them develop and display handicaps, or to have them use an illness and its associated negative emotions to signal willingness to cooperate. After all, negative emotionality and illness is, on the face of it, not too attractive, and many handicaps, like the paradigmatic peacock's tail, works precisely because it is attractive to peahens. So how can illnesses serve a handicapping strategy if most of what they produce is content containing a lot of negative emotionality?

Negative emotions can be powerful signals when used as leverage in social interactions (eliciting sympathy/empathy from conspecifics; Frank 1988; Hagen 2003; Sally 2005). When used in this way they enhance social ties or alliances. In any case at least 30–50% of the population exhibit and report a chronic experience of negative emotionality (Kessler et al. 2005; Riolo, Nguyen, Greden, and King 2005; Watson and Clark 1984). Negative emotionality treated as a trait evidences moderate to high levels of heritability (Bouchard 2004). Evidently people who exhibit high negative emotionality are considered attractive enough to at least a portion of the general population as they marry mates and produce offspring who inherit the disposition for negative emotionality.

Current evolutionary approaches to negative emotionality, and game theory simulations of the evolution of cooperation in human groups, predict that some portion of the population will exhibit high levels of negative emotionality as negative emotionality performs several different signaling and social functions. These include indicating the presence of cheats or free-riders in the population; indicating withdrawal or voluntary abstention from social bargaining processes; indicating resilience against adversity, that is, character strength; and eliciting sympathy or empathy from conspecifics. These enhance social ties and alliances (Fessler and Haley 2002; Hagen 2003; Neese 1998; Sally 2005). It is not for us to solve the problem of the existence and widespread prevalence of negative emotionality. The available evidence however indicates that it is widespread and it can function as a signal and be attractive to others.

Can Illness Signal Genetic Quality?

The short answer to this question is *no:* illness does *not* signal inferior genetic quality. *Surviving an illness,* however, can signal genetic quality as it suggests resilience. It will be recalled that the conditions for the evolutionary or game-theoretical stability of costly signaling (Grafen 1990), in the realm of illness effects, were that individual differences or variation in illness effects must be correlated with some value or quality, such as genetic quality, of the individual who uses illness to send signals to some observer. Or more precisely, the cost or benefit to the signaler of illnessing must be quality dependent, namely, the marginal cost or marginal benefit of illnessing is correlated with the signaler's quality.

Illness is a perfect medium for the signaling of quality. Depending on previous mental and physical health, individuals differ in their abilities to bear the cost associated with a new illness. Some individuals experience little or no long-term effects of illness, while others suffer severe mood and cognitive changes including psychotic hallucinations. Many illnesses leave scars and sometimes these scars are worn as badges of honor. An individual who carries scars from these illnesses reveals something of his history and quality. The scars reveal that he is a survivor.

How Then Might CST Account for Miraculous Healings in Religious Adults?

First recall that we are agnostic on the supernatural origins of miracles. Our task here is the more modest one of trying to present one naturalistic approach to these phenomena so that medicine may learn from them. If illness can signal crucial information about genetic quality and social intention in individuals who unconsciously use illness that way, then once the signal is sent and verifiably received by the intended receivers the information-bearing function of the illness is completed. At that point our version of the CST approach to miraculous healing would predict a miraculous healing. The scenario is roughly this: an individual gets sick. He goes through the acute phase. He survives the acute phase and now the illness begins to be a candidate for taking on a signaling capacity. If the individual finds himself in a social situation where he needs to signal *convincingly* that he is a quality individual and is not a free-rider; that he is truly interested in cooperating and that he is trustworthy and resilient; he will begin to use the chronic phase of the illness to signal this information to significant others. The greater the need to convince others that the signal is unfakeable and trustworthy the more dramatic the illness symptoms will be. Once the individual is convinced that the message has been received and believed, then the purpose of the signaling behavior has been fulfilled and there is no further need for the illness. At that point conditions for a miracle cure are present and that is when CST predicts they will occur.

If we are correct, miracles can teach medicine a great deal. First and foremost miracles tell us that an innate biology exists that can reverse an illness and that this innate healing system can be accessed and activated under social, communicative, and contextual conditions described and captured by costly signaling theory.

REFERENCES

Benedetti, F., H. S Mayberg, T. D. Wager, C. S. Stohler, and J. Zubieta (2005), Neurobiological Mechanisms of the Placebo Effect, *Journal of Neuroscience* 25, no. 45, 10390–402.

Bliege-Bird, R., and E. Smith (2005), Signaling Theory, Strategic Interaction, and Symbolic Capital, *Current Anthropology* 46, 221–48.

Bouchard, T. (2004), Genetic Influence on Human Psychological Traits: A Survey, *Current Directions in Psychological Science* 13, no. 4, 148–51.

Bowers, K. S., and S. LeBaron (1986), Hypnosis and Hypnotizability: Implications for Clinical Intervention, *Hospital and Community Psychiatry* 37, 457–67.

Bradbury, J., and S. Vehrencamp (1998), *Principles of Animal Communication*, Sunderland, MA: Sinauer Associates.

Fessler, D.M.T., and K. J. Haley (2003), The Strategy of Affect: Emotion in Human Cooperation in *Genetic and Cultural Evolution of Cooperation*, 7–36, P. Hammerstein, ed., Cambridge: The MIT Press.

Frank, R. (1988), *Passions within Reason: The Strategic Role of the Emotions*, New York: Norton.

Grafen, A. (1990), Biological Signals as Handicaps, *Journal of Theoretical Biology* 144, no 4, 517–46.

Hagen, E. H. (2003), The Bargaining Model of Depression, in *Genetic and Cultural Evolution of Cooperation*, 95–124, P. Hammerstein, ed., Cambridge: The MIT Press.

Irons, W. (1996), Morality, Religion, and Human Nature, in *Religion and Science: History, Method, and Dialogue*, 375–99, W. Richardson and W. Wildman, eds., New York: Rutledge.

Irons, W. (2001), Religion as a Hard-to-Fake Sign of Commitment, in *Evolution and the Capacity for Commitment*, 292–309, R. Neese, ed., New York: Russell Sage Foundation.

Kessler, R. C., O. Demler, R. G. Frank, M. Olfson, H. A. Pincus, E. E. Walters, P. Wang, et al. (2005), Prevalence and treatment of Mental Disorders, 1990 to 2003, *New England Journal of Medicine* 352, no. 24, 2515–23.

LeDoux, J. (2000), The Amygdala and Emotion: A View through Fear, in *The Amygdala*, 289–310, J. P. Aggleton, ed., Oxford: Oxford University Press.

Leuret, F., and H. Bon (1957), *Modern Miraculous Cures*, New York: Farrar, Strauss and Cudahy.

Maynard-Smith, J., and D. Harper (2003), *Animal Signals*, Oxford: Oxford University Press.

McClenon, J. (2002), *Wondrous Healing: Shamanism, Human Evolution and the Origin of Religion*, DeKalb: Northern Illinois University Press.

Neese, R. (1998), Emotional Disorders in Evolutionary Perspective, in *Evolutionary Approaches to Psychopathology*, special issue, *British Journal of Medical Psychology* 71, no. 4, 397–415.

Riolo, S. A., T. A. Nguyen, J. F., Greden, and C. A. King (2005), Prevalence and Treatment of Mental Disorders, 1990 to 2003, *American Journal of Public Health* 95, no. 6, 998–1000.

Sally, D. (2005), A General Theory of Sympathy, Mind-Reading and Social Interaction, with an Application to the Prisoner's Dilemma, *Social Science Information* 39, no. 4, 567–634.

Sosis, R. (2003), Why Aren't We All Hutterites? Costly Signaling Theory and Religious Behavior, *Human Nature* 14, 91–127.

Sosis, R. (2004), The Adaptive Value of Religious Ritual, *American Scientist* 92, 166–72.

Steen, T. (2003), *Is Character Sexy? The Desirability of Character Strengths in Romantic Partners*, unpublished dissertation, University of Michigan.

Watson, D., and L. A. Clark (1984), Negative Affectivity: The Disposition to Experi-
    ence Aversive Emotional States, *Psychological Bulletin* 96, no. 3, 465–90.
Weil, A. (1996), *Spontaneous Healing: How to Discover and Enhance Your Body's Natural
    Ability to Maintain and Heal Itself,* New York: Ballantine Books.
Zahavi, A. (1975), Mate Selection—A Selection for a Handicap, *Journal of Theoretical
    Biology* 53, 205–13.
Zahavi, A., and A. Zahavi (1997), *The Handicap Principle: A Missing Piece of Darwin's
    Puzzle,* New York: Oxford University Press.

CHAPTER 13

ARE MIRACLES ESSENTIAL OR PERIPHERAL TO FAITH TRADITIONS?

Louis Hoffman and Katherine McGuire

Miracles are reported in all the major world religions. This seemingly universal embrace of miracles in religion, in itself, seems to suggest there is something very important about the role of miracles in faith traditions. However, there are many ways to interpret miracles, and the placement of miracles varies greatly. For example, in Buddhism, the role of miracles is typically much more peripheral than in many of the theistic traditions, which will be our primary focus in this chapter. Perhaps that is understandable since Buddhism is essentially an ethical philosophy and psychology rather than a faith system with a divine figure or force at the center.

Kathryn Tanner, in her exploration of cultural influences on theological beliefs, asserts that within Christianity there is nothing that all Christians agree upon.[1] Although this is a bold position that initially seems hard to defend, there is a logical rationale behind it. If taken in broad strokes, there are many things that arguably all Christians agree upon, such as the centrality of the historical Jesus in the Christian tradition. Few would claim Jesus as nonessential to Christianity. However, to claim agreement on what the centrality of Jesus in Christianity means is a very different proposition. In other words, *even if all of Christianity can agree on essential content, they are not able to agree upon the meaning of this content*. This principle could be applied to all major world religions.

A challenge to this supposition is that there is no one entity that retains the power to determine what Christianity is. Many who identify as Christians would define Christianity more narrowly, excluding others who would consider themselves Christians. Tanner states,

Social solidarity . . . can only be ensured through common concern for
very vague, or one might say, very condensed, symbolic forms and acts.
Just to the extent that they remain ambiguous, amenable to a variety of
interpretations, are they able to unify a diverse membership, to coordinate
their activities together in the relatively non-conflictual way necessary for
a viable way of life.[2]

Miracles can unite or divide faith traditions, and they can enhance or challenge individual faith. Thus, the role of miracles should be considered in
terms of *the practical consequences of miracles in the faith tradition* as well as the
theological necessity of miracles.

Tanner goes on to state that theological *investigation* into issues of shared
concern can serve to unite, but the requirement of *agreement* divides.[3] Faith
traditions can agree upon the central concern of the role of miracles and this,
arguably, could be considered essential to the faith communities. However,
agreement on what miracles mean or what constitutes a miracle is nonessential and potentially divisive or destructive to the faith community.

THE ROLE OF MIRACLES IN FAITH

Throughout history, scientists, philosophers, and theologians have grap-
pled with the elusive nature of miracles and their relation to myth. Debate
over the occurrence, attribution, interpretation, and significance of these extraordinary events has been particularly evident within the Christian faith,
where miracles are often considered central to belief. For this reason, we
briefly discuss the role of miracle in other monotheistic faith traditions, but
have chosen to concentrate primarily on the roles of miracle and myth and
their impact on faith in the Christian tradition. Much, although not all, of
what we discuss in terms of Christianity has parallels in other monotheistic
traditions.

Defining and Explicating the Extraordinary

The word *miracle* is often bandied about in the vernacular and has come to
mean anything in the normal course of events that causes astonishment. Earlier nuances of the term *miracle*, however, typically implied the intervention
of a supernatural force in the natural world, the result of which was an extraordinary and seemingly unexplainable event.[4] For purposes of our work,
we define *miracle* as an anomalous event caused or influenced by some type
of external metaphysical reality, such as God or an ultimate being. However,
in order to understand better the authentic meaning of the word miracle,
its relationship to myth and how the term *miraculous* is interpreted within
monotheistic faith traditions, we should examine its roots.

The word miracle derives from the Latin *miraculum*, which means to wonder. Similarly, in the original Greek texts of the Bible, the most commonly used word for miracle was *terata*, meaning wonders. In the Christian faith, many of the wonders heralded through oral tradition and subsequently chronicled in the Bible were those extraordinary acts performed by Jesus that seemed to defy nature. One such act was Jesus' transformation of ordinary water into wine at the wedding feast of Cana. The transformation was seen as extraordinary because it appeared to operate outside the realm of the natural world.

A miracle produces a sense of wonder precisely because its cause is hidden and unexplainable in natural terms. Appearing to operate outside the ordinary course of events, a miracle is often interpreted as a sign of the connection between the supernatural and our world. St. Thomas Aquinas defined a miracle as something outside the order of nature.[5] He saw miracles as events that we admire with some astonishment because we observe the effect but do not know the cause. Specifying cause, the contemporary Christian writer, C. S. Lewis, also defines miracle as the interference with nature by supernatural power.[6]

In examining the difference between the ordinary course of nature and the extraordinary occurrence of a miracle, it is helpful to examine the terms normally used by Christian theologians when describing miracles. These terms help to separate the miracle occurring in the broad sense, such as justification of the soul, from a miracle occurring in the strict sense, that is, an occurrence that is grasped by the senses. Three delineations for extraordinary miracles specify whether the events occur *above*, *outside*, or *contrary to* nature. A miracle is said to be *above nature* when the effect produced is above the native powers and forces in creatures for which the known laws of nature usually prevail. An example of a miracle occurring *above nature* would be raising a dead man to life. Other examples of this type of miracle involve human beings who levitate or demonstrate bilocation. Alternatively, a miracle is said to occur *outside of nature* when natural forces may have the power to produce the effect, but could not have by themselves produced it in the way it occurred. An example of this is the sudden healing of diseased tissue. Indeed, diseased tissue has the potential to heal over time; however, a sudden healing can sometimes defy scientific explanation. Lastly, a miracle is said to occur *contrary to nature* when the produced effect is contrary to the natural course of things.

The Miracle within Monotheistic Faith Traditions

Within Christianity it has been customary to chronicle miraculous events and equate them with proof for the existence of God and a divine power. In doing so, Christianity has laid claim to some of the most renowned miracles.

Nonetheless, the concept of miracle also exists within other faith traditions. People of all creeds, including agnosticism, experience miracles. In the Jewish tradition, believers distinguish between the so-called hidden miracle and the revealing miracle.[7] In rabbinic thinking, a hidden miracle is an occurrence that is so mundane that its wondrous nature is overlooked. Hidden miracles may include the rising and setting sun and the beauty of creation. In Judaism, these ordinary miracles are more significant than revealing miracles that appear to occur outside nature, for through ordinary miracles, God is viewed as constantly renewing the miracle of his creation. While Judaism does not emphasize, as central to the faith, the miraculous in the sense of extraordinary intervention, it still does not discount the extraordinary, revealing miracle. Rather, while acknowledging that God can and does intervene in an extraordinary fashion, such as he often does in Old Testament (OT) stories, Judaism suggests these miracles are not the bedrock of Jewish belief.[8]

Similar to the Jewish perspective, the Islamic stance on miracles does not view these extraordinary occurrences as central to the faith in the way that the miracles of Jesus are important to the Christian tradition.[9] Nonetheless, the Qur'an is considered miraculous, per se, and miracles are also regarded as signs and wonders. The miraculous may include all of creation, much like the Jewish concept of the ordinary or hidden miracle, or it may include the wondrous workings of The Prophet, Muhammad. Interestingly, it is recorded that The Prophet declined to perform miracles whenever he was asked to do so. Nevertheless, many miraculous events are attributed to Muhammad. Some of these reported miracles include his miraculous feedings of large numbers of people when food supply was very scarce, the instantaneous creation of wells when there was no source of water available, and his uncanny ability to predict future events. These miracles of the revealing nature are not always woven into a consistent narrative of his life, but are simply listed in some texts as a way to show that The Prophet did perform miracles like other prophets before him. As opposed to the almost didactic manner of miracle reporting in the Bible, the Islamic referencing of miracles is not necessarily intended to illumine points of doctrine.[10] Overall, the purpose of the miracle within the Islamic faith is to show how Muhammad was the agent for Allah, who allowed him to change the ordinary course of events. In this manner, the Muslim belief about miracles is similar to that held by most Jews and Christians: miracles occur because of interference by the supernatural, and in the case of an extraordinary miracle, such interference demonstrates a disruption in the ordinary course of nature.

Upon examining the different faith perspectives on miracles, we can correctly conclude that while various religions may disagree on their concept of God, they collectively attribute miracles to the working of a divine presence that intervenes in nature. Furthermore, in many faith traditions, miracles are viewed as symbols embodying a divine message. Protestant theologian Paul

Tillich views symbols as participating in the reality for which they stand. He distinguishes symbols from signs, stating signs bear no resemblance to that to which they point.[11] Hence, miracles may function in a mode similar to that of myths, since both contain an element that we humans recognize individually and collectively to be true.

Miracles as Producing and Enhancing Faith in God

When writing of Christ's miraculous ascent into heaven, St. Augustine said the books of the Bible record "not merely the attesting miracles, but the ultimate object of our faith which the miracles were meant to confirm. The miracles (a)re made known to help men's faith."[12] Miracles, therefore, can be thought not only to confirm the supernatural character of God, but also to enhance the faith of believers.

Miracles contribute to faith by providing tangible evidence for their human audience. The result is inevitably the provocation of awe, wonder, or a deeper belief in that which is unseen yet nonetheless believed. In this sense, miracles encountered through lived experience may initiate belief or strengthen the faith of believers. Likewise, miracles using others as conduits to enhance a deeper belief in the divine presence are also effective in this way. As an example of this, we will consider an apparition story of the Virgin Mary. While Catholics do not consider Mary as an equal to her son, she is still viewed as one through whom the power of God is revealed. In the miracle of Our Lady of Fatima, Mary appeared to three innocent Portuguese children in 1917. The children testified that during the apparitions, she appeared as a radiant woman standing among the leaves of a small oak tree. She instructed the children to pray for world peace and an end to war. Several prophecies the lady made to the children were realized. In her last appearances, a crowd of nearly seventy thousand onlookers, believers and skeptics alike, observed the dark and clouded sky suddenly clear and reveal the sun, which reportedly spun like a pinwheel, with yellow, blue and violet rays streaming from its rim. The three children to whom Mary had appeared earlier reported seeing Mary within the sun. The sun purportedly stopped whirling and appeared to zigzag toward the earth, while the crowd cowered in fear. Extraordinarily, the earth and the clothing of all present went from a state of dampness due to the rain, to instant and complete dryness. Was this truly a miraculous event? This question has been debated for nearly a century as skeptics employ astrophysics to explain the phenomena of the spinning sun, along with behavioral science to explain the collective perception by the nearly seventy thousand people, of an extraordinary event. Meanwhile, some believers accept the apparition simply on faith. While Marian apparitions are not considered central for belief in the Catholic faith, which takes a sober view of miracles, for some believers, the effect of the miracle provides a sense of wonder and awe at the possibility of divine presence and supernatural intervention in human affairs.

Miracles, whether directly experienced or passed on through word of mouth, become part of what Smith, in *The Meaning and End of Religion*, calls the cumulative traditions of religion.[13] That is to say, past miracles become part of the myths and narratives that, along with other elements, inform and awaken present faith. Indeed, the miracles chronicled in the New Testament have served as evidence to bring some people to faith just as the miracles reportedly did during the life of Christ. In the New Testament (NT), there are numerous accounts of Christ's direct intervention in the natural course of things. In the Gospel of John (11:1–44), for example, Jesus commands Lazarus to come out from the tomb and the dead man emerges, tied head and foot with burial bands. By biblical report, this caused many of the Jews who witnessed the event to believe in Christ and his divine power. Others, however, did not believe and turned Jesus in to the Pharisees.

DISBELIEF

In our entertainment of the miracle phenomena, we shall not presume that the possibility of miracles is accepted by all. Throughout history, some have remained so convinced of the uniformity and sovereignty of nature that they are compelled to deny the probability and even the possibility of miracles, or to explain them away. The skeptical view of extraordinary miracles, held by philosophers, behavioral scientists, and theologians alike, ultimately depends on the assumption that the material universe alone exists. As the eighteenth-century philosopher David Hume proffered in *Enquiry Concerning Human Understanding*, "A miracle is a violation of the laws of nature, and as a firm and unalterable experience has established these laws, the proof against a miracle from the very nature of the fact, is as certain as any argument from experience can possibly be imagined."[14] Hume's denial of miracles has been echoed by many others throughout the history of scientific and even theological thought.

Relying on the fundamental premise that whatever happens is natural and whatever is not natural simply does not happen, the controversial Protestant theologian, David Friedrich Strauss, introduced the concept of biblical miracle as myth in his 1835 work *The Life of Jesus: Critically Examined.*[15] In disagreeing with the two warring factions of the nineteenth century, the rationalists and supernaturalists, Strauss shocked his contemporaries by asserting that biblical miracles, such as the multiplication of the loaves and fish, are actually mythical in nature. According to Strauss, the miraculous feeding of nearly 5,000 people by Jesus should not be taken as a literal occurrence. That this astonishing multiplication of food may have taken place is, in Strauss' view, not even the point. What was of more importance to him was the figurative truth contained in the myth/miracle: Jesus is the Bread of Life who nurtures his followers. Strauss's mythical sense of the Gospel stories, once considered highly controversial, has now become an accepted way of viewing the miracle stories for many contemporary Christian believers. Nevertheless, this is not to say that the occurrence of extraordinary events is always impossible.

Other more contemporary thinkers have totally discredited the notion of miracles, those occurring in the biblical context as well as those occurring in quotidian experience. Robert R. Funk, biblical scholar and founder of the very controversial Jesus Seminar and Weststar Institute, is one such scholar. Funk has stoutly maintained that the notion of God interfering with the order of nature from time to time, to aid or punish, is no longer credible. He states that "miracles are an affront to the justice and integrity of God, however understood."[16] He views miracles as conceivable only as the inexplicable; otherwise they contradict the regularity of the order in the physical universe.

In other disciplines, such as psychology, the miraculous event has been explained in various ways. Carl Jung's explanation for visions and apparitions centers on his psychological theory, which posits that the unconscious psyche has "an indeterminable number of subliminal perceptions, [and] an immense fund of accumulated inheritance factors left by one generation of men after another."[17] According to Jung, these psychic inheritances, also called archetypes, are universal patterns and motifs, coming from the collective unconscious, and are often the basis for religions and myths. To Jung, individual apparitions, much like dreams, involve psychic content from the unconscious that is forced into our conscious life. The experienced vision is then interpreted in a religious context.[18]

Other psychological theories explaining the causes of extraordinary events include mentalistic theories, which identify a specific mental state like stress, anxiety, despondency or mental illness, as being responsible for miracles like conversions, apparitions, stigmata, inedia, bilocation, and levitations. It must be noted however, that mentalistic theories cannot account for certain extraordinary occurrences taking place after death. Specifically, the state and functioning of the mind cannot possibly account for the extraordinary condition of Incorruptibles, those saintly people whose bodies remain totally preserved without human intervention, for years after their deaths.

Other relatively recent research in the field of psychology addresses the connection between attachment style and spirituality. This research suggests that some experiencing of extraordinary miracles, such as sudden religious conversion, which is often attributed to the intervention of the Holy Spirit, may be linked to the attachment style of the individual.[19] Attachment style, first studied by psychiatrist John Bowlby and developmental psychologist, Mary Ainsworth, stems from the early interactions of a child with the primary caregiver and is often determined by the feedback the child receives from the caregiver. These interactions are said to create an internal working model that can persist throughout an individual's lifetime and deeply affect future relationships.[20] Four identified attachment styles include: *secure attachment*, which is exhibited in those individuals who have received a caregiver's true attention; *avoidant attachment*, which is apparent in those who have experienced coldness and rigidity from their caregivers; *anxious-ambivalent attachment*, which is often demonstrated by those who have experienced a highly inconsistent primary caregiver; and *disorganized/disoriented attachment*, which was differentiated by Main and Solomon and indicates an individual who tends to display very paradoxical, chaotic "come here/go away" behavior.[21] These individuals have usually experienced "frightened, frightening or disoriented communication with their primary caregivers."[22]

According to Kirkpatrick, research on attachment styles and religious experience suggests that adult religiosity, particularly in the form of sudden religious conversions and highly emotional religious experiences, is associated with insecure childhood attachment.[23] These results may imply that those with insecure attachment have a negative internal working model of attachment relationships and thereby seek to avoid intimacy, closeness, and love. Among those who do experience a religious conversion, however, something dramatic happens to cause a sudden change in perception. To someone with an insecure history of attachment, this sudden awareness of God as a warm, forgiving, and compassionate figure would undoubtedly lead to a more intense conversion or religious experience, something falling outside the realm of the normal experience. Indeed, we venture to say it may appear to be miraculous for the individual experiencing the conversion. In addition to conversion, there is some evidence that individuals with insecure attachments may also have a predisposition for other types of intense religious experience.[24]

MIRACLES AS PRODUCTS OF FAITH

Thus far, our examination of miracles, believers, and skeptics raises interesting questions about the existence of God and the relationship between miracles and faith. Therefore, in our discourse on miracles, we would be remiss if we avoided a very obvious point, which is that faith is essential for belief in miracles, even if miracles are not essential for faith. C. S. Lewis wrote, "Unless there exists, in addition to Nature, something else we may call the supernatural, there can be no miracles."[25] Indeed, it is logical to assume that faith in a supernatural power must precede the acceptance of miracles.

Paradoxically, Christians would find it difficult to accept the tenets of their faith if they did not believe on some level in the miraculous, for Christianity is predicated on several pivotal and miraculous events: the virgin birth, the resurrection of Christ, and his ascension into heaven. For many, these events are understood in the figurative rather than the literal sense. However, merely believing in that which is not seen (God) is a leap into the abyss of the unknown requiring suspension of natural disbelief. Faith, according to Hebrews 11:1, "is the realization of what is hoped for and evidence of things not seen." Specifically, the very nature of faith implies that one makes the choice to believe in that which is not clearly revealed through the sensory intelligences. On the other hand, faith in the unseen does not necessarily entail the intervention of a miracle.

Throughout history, both believers and nonbelievers alike have posited the basic question: Does God exist? This question is fundamental to all of human existence; for even when one is uncertain or does not believe in God or a supernatural force that interfaces with human existence, the question still becomes unavoidable as an individual searches for the significance of his or her personal existence.

If we do suppose God exists, then how do we know this? Admittedly, our ways of knowing the existence of God are imperfect. In *Belief and Unbelief*, Michael Novak suggests that since God is basically incomprehensible to any human intellect, no creature can attain to a perfect way of knowing God.[26] The age-old question then follows: Is it even possible to know anything beyond what we perceive with the senses? The history of humanity's epistemological search for ultimate meaning or a creative force, like the Unmoved Mover, is well documented, and early philosophers, such as Aristotle, did not question that human knowledge is primarily derived from the senses. The theologian and mystic Theresa of Avila suggested that the miraculous event offered internal and external proof of the existence of God: "If God is a knowable object, He is such on the basis of man's experience, both of the invisible world and interior world."[27]

General acknowledgement of extrasensory truths does not mean the existence of God has been readily accepted, in a literal or mythical sense. Despite the fight of church authorities in the eighteenth century to denigrate the rise of scientific knowledge, the positivist mentality that was initiated in the late eighteenth century has led to disbelief of unempirical matters; this mentality has largely prevailed. Positivism may be seen as a methodology or philosophy of suspicion wherein the concept of *god* has lost its prior meaning. Positivists question whether human beings are capable of knowing anything beyond what is perceived by the senses or quantified empirically. Therefore, human reason is completely subjected to scrutiny of the senses and to the laws of empirical validation. While this mentality has undoubtedly led to greater developments in technology, as well as in the natural and biological sciences, it has rendered the concept of *god* seemingly useless to many.

In spite of the pervading positivist mentality, the desire to know God or some supernatural force persists in modern times. Many still ask the question and seek for signs of a supreme being's existence, which appears to indicate an internal, existential motivation in the form of a search for meaning. Pascal provocatively offered, "We do not seek God nor attempt to prove Him if we have not already found him."[28] Pascal also asserted that either God exists, or He does not, and human beings would do well to make a wager in favor of God's existence without the benefit of certainty. In the Pascalian sense, then, miracles are peripheral to whether God actually exists. On the other hand, if God does exist, anything is possible, including miracles.

Thomas Merton, the twentieth-century Trappist monk and social activist, also suggested that by our nature as intelligent beings, we tend to have a simple and natural awareness of the reality of God, without which the mere question of his existence could not arise in our minds.[29] As this pertains to the question of miracles, Merton's assertion supports the concept that faith in a supernatural force who intervenes in human affairs must logically precede one's acceptance of the veracity of miracles. That is to say, faith in God or a supreme being, either realized or unrealized, is essential for sustaining belief in miracles. A noteworthy example of unrealized faith informed by miracle is the conversion of St. Paul of Tarsus. While on the road to Damascus with the express purpose of hunting down the disciples of Christ, he was struck by a light coming from the sky. The light knocked him off his horse and rendered him blind. At that same time, a voice with an unexplainable origin was reportedly heard by Saul and others. The voice, thereafter identified as Jesus, rebuked Saul and commanded him to cease persecution of Christians and do as he was instructed. While the conversion story of St. Paul illustrates the rapid trajectory from disbelief to belief, we do not wish to suggest this is the normal course of events for most believers. Miraculous conversion stories notwithstanding, the acceptance of miracles appears to be secondary to an initial belief in a supreme being.

LACK OF MIRACLES AS A BARRIER TO FAITH

For some, not experiencing miracles can be interpreted as not having faith, especially when the source attributed to miracles is a god-figure. The spirit of human competition and the quest to measure oneself against another are, arguably, natural human tendencies. Because the human relationship to a god-figure often metaphorically assumes the role of parent and child, we humans can sometimes feel like the overlooked offspring whose siblings are more favored by the father. This is especially true whenever we hear of another's miraculous experience, but have yet to experience our own. On a very unconscious and insecure level, we may think, "If only I were a better son or daughter, I might win more favor with my father." On a more conscious level, we may find ourselves saying, "Because I do not have enough faith, or I am not worthy enough, God does not choose me as an object for his revelation." Sometimes, the lack of tangible proof of the existence of God may render some persons so insecure about their relationship to God that they denigrate the very possibility of God's existence. In this sense, the lack of experienced miracles becomes a barrier to faith.

In her work, the visionary St. Theresa of Avila leaves her readers under no illusions about the matter when she states that for most people, visions and direct intervention by God are deemed unnecessary to faith.[30] She also states that there are many saintly people who never experience a single vision, while others receive these gifts and are not saintly. It follows, therefore, that visions and extraordinary events are not a secure basis for judging one's position in the spiritual life.

Nevertheless, numerous theorists, from Freud to the present, suggest the phenomenon of an internalized God-image that helps to determine our security or insecurity over our relationship with God. God-image is determined by both self-concept and parent/child relationship and an individual's personal image of God.[31] Undoubtedly, images of God as wrathful, controlling, or uninvolved are associated with self-esteem, as are personal images of God as loving, close, and nurturing. Those individuals embracing the wrathful image of God undoubtedly feel more distanced from and disfavored by God. According to Rizzuto, belief in God or its absence depends upon the conscious identity that is established as a result of the God-representation of a given developmental stage, such as that of a parental figure, and its relationship to that person's self-representation.[32]

Based on research in the area of God image, we feel strongly that a person's perceived experience of God, coupled with his or her self-image, impacts that individual's perception of the miraculous, as well. Nevertheless, both believers and nonbelievers alike feel the power of a presence that they invent. In this way, faith is rather like myth. It is our human capacity for myth, faith in an "I believe" construct, perhaps regarding a supernatural force, that ultimately allows us to entertain the possibility of miracle.

MIRACLES AND MYTH

To speak of miracles is not without controversy; however, much of this controversy is more related to terminology than to the underlying ideas. The idea of myth has undergone a significant transformation since the earliest conceptions of this term. Today, most people speak of myth as a falsehood. However, as Rollo May states, "There can be no stronger proof of the impoverishment of our contemporary culture than the popular—though profoundly mistaken—definition of myth as falsehood."[33] When faith traditions that emphasize the importance of miracles interpret the label of miracles as myths as implying that they are false, they rightly become defensive. However, as we will illustrate, labeling miracles as myths does not discredit them, but rather has the potential to enhance the power of miracles.

As implicitly illustrated in May's statement, definitions of certain terms, such as myth, are a product of culture that often reflects important aspects about the culture. Postmodernism reflected a shift in the understanding of language. In the modern period, language was often assumed to have a true or correct definition. It was seen as always being propositional and specifically denotive. However, in postmodern times, language is understood as socially constructed.[34] Given this, the evolution of the definition of words often reflects important changes in cultural understandings. In the ancient Greek understanding, myths were intended to reflect meaning, but were not necessarily intended to be interpreted literally.[35] However, through the modern period, truth came to be understood differently and the emphasis shifted to literal truths, or scientific truths. Myths, therefore, were either literally true or simply fantasy. The modernist epistemology, or theory on the nature of truth, shifted the meaning of myth to falsehood. In fact, myth is more true and more truth than empirical data. Myth is an "I believe" statement that conveys a core truth, together with the interpretation or claim regarding its meaning. These creedal statements of meaning, proximate and ultimate, are much more important to us as truth than is mere empirical or logical data.

May believed the shift in the understanding of myth in itself was dangerous and destructive. When science replaced myth, meaning changed with it. Meaning became head knowledge, whereas mythical knowledge is more holistic; myth grips the entirety of a person. As knowledge became more one-dimensional and concrete, meaning shrank; the most powerful and productive meaning systems were devalued and miniaturized. But the definition is only the beginning of the story.

Rollo May and the Cry for Myth

A prophetic tone is evident in much of May's writing. Scholars throughout history have always been drawn to making predictions about the future. What is remarkable about May's predictions is the accuracy they prove to have over time. This was not due to any claimed psychic or miraculous abilities, but can be attributed to his being deeply aware of human nature and very observant of trends in culture.

May, writing during a time that represents the early transition from the modern to the postmodern period, was very aware of the costs of such a transition, even though he did not utilize the language of modernism or postmodernism very often. For May, it was not so much that postmodernism or modernism were good or bad, but rather, that the transition from one period to the next brought cultural upheaval. While others were discussing the intellectual validity of postmodernism and the new ideas reflected therein, May was observing how the transition impacted meaning systems. Here we can identify a second concern May had about myths in his time.

As noted earlier, May was concerned about the tendency for modernism to reinterpret myths as false. This was compounded by deconstruction of myths associated with the transition from modernism to postmodernism. May states,

> I speak of the *Cry* for myths because I believe there is an urgency in the need for myth in our day. Many of the problems of our society, including cults and drug addiction, can be traced to the lack of myths which will give us as individuals the inner security we need in order to live adequately in our day. . . . This is especially urgent as we seek to give meaning to our lives; in our creativity, our loves, and our challenges; since we stand on the threshold of a new century. The approach of a new period in history stimulates us to take stock of our past and to ask the questions of the meaning we have made and are making in our lives.[36]

The transition from one period to the next requires a critiquing and deconstructing of the previous period, including the meaning systems of the previous period. In part, this occurred because the modernist project failed, and it failed in areas where it made its strongest promise: to end war, end disease, and offer opportunities at a utopian lifestyle. Although its failure opened the door to new opportunities in the postmodern period, it came with the cost of a loss of myths.

The Nature of Myth

May understood myths as belief or meaning systems that could not be proven to be true.[37] Belief, in this sense, is contrasted with knowledge. Knowledge, regardless of its accuracy, tends to be one-dimensionally rational. It involves one part of our subjective experience. Conversely, myths, because there is always an element of uncertainty in them, includes anxiety. Belief takes courage because it is inclusive of anxiety; conversely, knowledge is easy. *Many individuals seek the comfort of knowledge instead of the meaning of myth.*

The power of myths lies in their connection to the innate existential drive for meaning. Speaking from the existential tradition, May argues that myths as meaning systems are more powerful and holistic than science or rationalism. This is not to say that science and rationalism are bad; they are just incomplete. Science and reason are reflective of a basic need for security, but security without meaning is rather dull. Anxiety, although often uncomfortable, requires courage and brings in the affective dimension of knowledge, therefore making it more holistic.

Mythic and Miracles

If miracles are understood as myth, their power lies not in their literal truth or validity, but in the truth of their meaning. Paul Tillich, one of May's influential mentors, connected miracles to a sense of wonderment or awe. Indeed, this sense of wonderment is closely connected to Tillich's approach to identifying a genuine miracle:

> A genuine miracle is first of all an event which is astonishing, unusual, shaking, without contradicting the rational structure of reality. In the second place, it is an event which points to the mystery of being, expressing its relation to us in a definite way. In the third place, it is an occurrence which is received as a sign-event in an ecstatic experience. Only if these three conditions are fulfilled can one speak of a genuine miracle.[38]

The reality of a miracle, as such, is measured at least in part by the response it is able to produce. Miracles, then, serve to connect us with the inscrutable, with the very mystery of being.

That miracles cannot be proved should not be seen as a threat to the nature or purpose of a miracle. Conversely, as Tillich illustrates, if a miracle were to enter into the realm of the known or explainable, it would lose part of the very essence of a miracle and would cease to be a miracle. In revisiting the basic question of this chapter, whether miracles are essential to faith traditions, we can provide a different answer in light of myths. If miracles serve the purpose of drawing one closer to God, the mystery of being, or the ground of being, then they are necessary insofar as they are the means to accomplish this purpose. Whether the miracles exist is not as relevant as the purpose that belief in them serves. The corollary to this asks if miracles remain essential if there are other means to draw people to God. The answer, it seems, is no.

A story from the NT illustrates this principle. In Luke 16:19–31, Jesus tells a parable about a rich man who neglected the suffering and needs of a poor man named Lazarus. When both had died, Lazarus was in heaven while the rich man was suffering in the fires of hell. The rich man begged for relief, even in the form of Lazarus dipping his finger in water and cooling his tongue. His requests were refused. Then the rich man asked to have Lazarus sent to warn his brothers so they would not end up in eternal suffering like the rich man. The response came stating, "If they do not listen to Moses and the prophets, neither will they be convinced even if someone rises from the dead" (Luke 16:31, NIV). One interpretation of this story would be to state that the rich man requests a miracle, Lazarus returning from the dead, to warn his brothers. In response, God tells them that even a miracle would not create faith, so there is no need for it. In other words, miracles are intended to promote faith, but there are many other media to accomplish this same task. Furthermore, without the seeds of faith, miracles are not powerful enough to produce genuine faith.

MIRACLES AND COMMUNITY

Thus far, we have focused on the role of miracles in the lives of individuals. Now we shift the focus to miracles and community, or cultural, contexts.

Miracles and Myths in Culture

Miracles and myths are always interpreted in a cultural context and cannot be understood apart from this. Furthermore, myths tend to be more powerful when they are shared. There is an interesting paradox in this, however: Myths are always a product of culture, but belief in myths is a highly personal act. A reinterpretation of Tillich can provide a frame of reference for dealing with this paradox. In Tillich's thought, myth can be understood as a special type of symbol, and the power of the symbol is that it allows people to participate in that toward which the symbol points. In other words, there is a transcendent element to symbols that help a person participate in something beyond his or her own personal boundaries.[39] This could be expanded to state that myths help people transcend their personal boundaries to participate in community on a deeper, more transcendent level.

Several important applications emerge from this theme that are relevant for contemporary culture. When myths are understood as knowledge or as factual, they become divisive, often leading to conflict.[40] Facts are not humble; faith contains greater space for a more modest perspective. In other words, by returning to an understanding of myth, many divisions, arguments, and even wars may be prevented. It is excessive confidence in what is believed, or too much faith, that is dangerous. When believing in miracles, or even recognizing more contemporary miracles, becomes part of the standard for considering oneself a member of a religious group, harm occurs. On a personal level, this may emerge in forms of spiritual abuse in which members are admonished for their lack of faith. On a broader social level, this can be used as a justification for manipulative, coercive, or even violent evangelism techniques. In other words, requiring a certain understanding of miracles in faith communities is not only nonessential, but it is potentially destructive. However, this does not mean miracles are not important.

Walter Truett Anderson, in conceptualizing the transition from modernism to postmodernism, states, "We are in the midst of a great, confusing, stressful and enormously promising historical transition, and it has to do with a change not so much in *what* we believe as in *how* we believe."[41] This is instructive in distinguishing between destructive and constructive usage of miracles. The distinction is not about the content of *what is believed*, but rather it is *how the content is believed and utilized*. When miracles are believed in as faith, they are constructive; when they are believed in as literal empirical truth, they are destructive.

Constructing Myths

For May, myths are a natural product that emerges from culture as part of a collective wrestling with the existential condition and the search for meaning. In a sense, cultures cannot help but create myths; they can not survive without them. Communities spontaneously develop bodies of belief. However, at the same time, not all myths are healthy or sustaining. In *The Cry for Myth*, May explores a number of typical Western myths including *Faust*, *The Great Gatsby*, and the Frontier Myth in the United States. These stories reflect underlying meaning systems in our culture, and they represent examples of the way people live. Furthermore, they help people recognize meaning and bring meaning to their own personal stories.

Myths emerge from a cultural unconscious, so to speak. They often are best articulated in various forms of art, such as literature and movies. What artists do when they articulate myths is put forward an understanding or meaning that has been in the cultural unconscious but that has been unidentified. They bring the meaning into a symbolic format that people can interact around, even if they cannot clearly articulate it. By making the cultural unconscious into symbolic form, and potentially conscious meaning, they serve to unite people.[42] Artists give communities a set of images and a language in which to realize and recognize their belief systems.

Miracles as Unifying

May stated, "Myths are our self-interpretation of our inner selves in relation to the outside world. They are narrations by which our society is unified."[43] We have discussed this idea several times already in the chapter, but it is worth restating. Although not intended to be an exhaustive list, two important, constructive roles of miracles have been identified: (1) increasing individual faith, and (2) uniting people with shared beliefs. Miracles, as important myth systems, provide solidarity among members of a faith tradition, as well as the broader culture. Several reviews of the literature have indicated that it is the relational or communal factor of being religious that has the most powerful benefits for physical and psychological health.[44] Even if they are not literally true, miracles can serve the purpose of uniting and increasing psychological and spiritual health for the individual, the faith community, and the culture.

CONCLUSION

In this chapter we have tried to present a complex, multilayered answer to this question regarding whether miracles are essential to faith. There are many ways in which the requirement of a certain type of belief in miracles has been destructive. Because of this, we hesitate in stating that miracles are essential. Yet, at the same time, miracles have historically served to unite and inspire members of a faith community. Therefore, we do not want to discount the value of miracles.

If forced to resolve the pros and cons of miracles we would say that miracles are necessary for most faith traditions, but that there remains a tremendous amount of ambiguity about what a miracle is and what constitutes belief in it. This ambiguity is good. Miracles can range from the process theology viewpoint that miracles are God working within and being limited by natural laws; to a more fundamentalist view that belief in the literal occurrence of all the miracles in the sacred scriptures is necessary to be beliefs as reported in these texts. In the former sense, they are not miracles at all according to some definitions; though nonetheless miraculous.

This is a complex issue deserving serious consideration for everyone. Each of us must come to terms with how the question of the apparently miraculous in life illumines our sense of meaning and ultimacy. The benefit of this quest for greater meaning is more helpful when carried out as a dialogue between persons, experiences, and insights; rather than in the desire to conjure, craft, or create dogma.

NOTES

1. Kathryn Tanner (1997), *Theories of Culture: A New Agenda for Theology*, Minneapolis: Fortress.

2. Ibid., 122.

3. Ibid.

4. Note, however, that this does not necessitate working against the laws of nature. Although some definitions of miracles necessitate breaking, violating, or overpowering laws of nature, other viewpoints, such as process theology, understand miracles as working within the laws of nature. See David L. Wheeler (2000), Confessional Communities and Public Worldviews: A Case Study, in John B. Cobb, Jr., and Clark H. Pinnock, eds., *Searching for an Adequate God: A Dialogue between Process and Freewill Theists*, Grand Rapids: Eerdmans, 97–148.

5. Thomas Aquinas (1948), *Summa Theologica*, Fathers of the English Dominican Province, trans., New York: Benzinger Brothers, 520.

6. Clives Staples Lewis (1952), *Miracles*, New York: Macmillan.

7. Ronald Isaacs (1997), *Miracles: A Jewish Perspective*, Northvale, NJ: Jason Aronson.

8. Ibid.

9. Kenneth Woodward (2000), *The Book of Miracles: The Meaning of Miracle Stories in Christianity Judaism Buddhism Hinduism Islam*, New York: Simon and Schuster.

10. Ibid.

11. Paul Tillich (2001), *The Dynamics of Faith*, New York: Perennial.

12. Aurelius Augustine (1958), *City of God*, New York: Image Books, 513.

13. Wilfred Smith (1963), *The Meaning and End of Religion*, New York: Macmillan.

14. David Hume (1993), *An Enquiry Concerning Human Understanding*, Eric Steinberg, ed., Indianapolis: Hackett.

15. David Freidrich Strauss (2006), *The Life of Jesus: Critically Examined*, George Eliot, trans., New York: Continuum International.

16. Robert Funk (1998), The Coming Radical Reformation: Twenty-one Theses, *The Fourth R* 11, July–August, 4.

17. Michael Grosso (1983), Jung, Parapsychology, and the Near-Death Experience: Towards a Transpersonal Paradigm, in Bruce Greyson and C. P. Flynn, eds., *The Near-Death Experience: Problems, Prospects, Perspectives*, Springfield: Charles C. Thomas, 176–214.

18. Phillip Weibe (1997), *Visions of Jesus: Direct Encounters from the New Testament to Today*, New York: Oxford University Press.

19. Lee Kirkpatrick (2005), *Attachment, Evolution, and the Psychology of Religion*, New York: Guilford.

20. John Bowlby (1969), *Attachment and Loss*, vol. 1, *Attachment*, New York: Basic Books.

21. M. Main and J. Soloman (1990), Procedures for Identifying Infants as Disorganized/Disoriented during the Ainsworth Strange Situation, in M. T. Greenberg, D. Cicchetti, and E. M. Cummings, ed., *Attachment in the Preschool Years: Theory, Research, and Intervention*, Chicago: University of Chicago Press, 193–246.

22. Daniel Siegel (1999),*The Developing Mind*, New York: Guilford.

23. Lee A. Kirkpatrick (2005), *Attachment, Evolution and the Psychology of Religion*, New York: Guilford. See also Lee A. Kirkpatrick (1997), A Longitudinal Study of Changes in Religious Belief and Behavior as a Function of Individual Differences in Adult Attachment Style, *Journal for the Scientific Study of Religion (JSSR)*, 36, 207–17; Christopher S. M. Grimes (in press), God Image Research: A Literature Review, in Glen Moriarty and Louis Hoffman, eds., *The God Image Handbook for Spiritual Counseling and Psychotherapy: Theory, Research and Practice*, New York: Haworth Pastoral Press.

24. Glen Moriarty, Louis Hoffman, Christopher S. M. Grimes, and Jay Gattis (March 25–28, 2004), *God and Attachment: Using Integration Techniques to Change Working Models*, unpublished paper presented at the International Conference of the Christian Association for Psychological Studies, St. Petersburg, Fla.

25. Lewis (1952), *Miracles*.

26. Michael Novak (1994), *Belief and Unbelief, a Philosophy of Self Knowledge*, New York: Mentor Omega.

27. Theresa of Avila (1980), *The Collected Works of St. Theresa of Avila*, Kevin Kavanaugh and Otilio Rodriguez, trans., Washington, DC: ICS.

28. Blaise Pascal (1966), *Pensées*, A. J. Krailsheimer, trans., Baltimore: Penguin, 150.

29. Thomas Merton 1963), *Life and Holiness*, New York: Herder and Herder.

30. Thomas Dubay (1989), *Fire Within*, San Francisco: Ignatius Press.

31. James Jones (2007), Psychodynamic Theories of the Evolution of the God Image, in Glen Moriarty and Louis Hoffman, eds., *The God Image Handbook for Spiritual Counseling and Psychotherapy: Theory, Research, and Practice*, Haworth Pastoral Press.

32. Rizzuto, Ana Marie (1979), *The Birth of the Living God*, Chicago: University of Chicago Press.

33. Rollo May (1991), *The Cry for Myth*, New York: Delta, 23.

34. Nancey Murphy (1996), *Beyond Liberalism and Fundamentalism: How Modern and Postmodern Philosophy Set the Theological Agenda*, Harrisburg: Trinity Press International

35. May (1991), *The Cry for Myth*.

36. Ibid., 9–10.

37. Ibid.

38. Tillich, Paul (1951), *Systematic Theology*, vol. 1, Chicago: University of Chicago Press, 117.

39. Tillich (2001), *Dynamics of Faith*.

40. This parallels Tanner's ideas from the beginning of the paper.

41. Walter Truett Anderson (1995), Introduction: What's Going on Here? in Walter Truett Anderson, ed., *The Truth about the Truth: De-confusing and Re-constructing the Postmodern World*, New York: Tarcher/Putnam, 1–11.

42. By putting the cultural unconscious into myths, they are not necessarily making it conscious. Herein lies a difference with the traditional psychoanalytic idea of making the unconscious conscious as part of healing. From an existential perspective, making the unconscious conscious is one form of healing or growth. However, many deep meanings remain elusive to concrete understanding. By putting them in a symbolic or mythic form, people can interact with them and benefit from them experientially, even if they do not fully understand them.

43. May (1991), *The Cry for Myth*, 20.

44. See Betty Ervin-Cox, Louis Hoffman, Christopher S. M. Grimes, and Steve Fehl (2007), Spirituality, Health, and Mental Health: A Holistic Model, in Ilene Serlin,ed., *Whole Person Health Care*, vol. 2, *Psychology, Spirituality, and Health*, Westport, CT: Praeger, 101–34.

REFERENCES

Aquinas, Thomas (1948), *Summa Theologica*, Fathers of the English Dominican Province, trans., New York: Benzinger Brothers.

Anderson, Walter Truett (1995), Introduction: What's Going on Here? in *The Truth about the Truth: De-confusing and Re-constructing the Postmodern World*, Walter Truett Anderson, ed., New York: Tarcher/Putnam.

Augustine, Aurelius (1958), *City of God*, Gerald G. Walsh, trans., New York: Image Books.

Bowlby, John (1969), *Attachment and Loss: Vol. 1, Attachment*, New York: Basic Books.

Dubay, Thomas (1989), *Fire Within*, San Francisco: Ignatius Press.

Ervin-Cox, Betty, Louis Hoffman, Christopher S. M. Grimes, and Steve Fehl (2007), Spirituality, Health, and Mental Health: A Holistic Model, in *Whole Person Healthcare: Vol. 2, Psychology, Spirituality, & Health*, Ilene Serlin, ed., Westport, CT: Praeger.

Funk, Robert (1998.), The Coming Radical Reformation: Twenty-one Theses, *The Fourth R* 11, July–August, 4.

Grimes, Christopher S. M. (In press), God Image Research: A Literature Review, in Glen Moriarty and Louis Hoffman, eds., *The God Image Handbook for Spiritual Counseling and Psychotherapy: Theory, Research, and Practice*, New York: Haworth.

Grosso, Michael (1983), Jung, Parapsychology, and the Near-Death Experience: Toward a Transpersonal Paradigm, in *The Near-Death Experience: Problems, Prospects, Perspectives*, 176–214, Bruce Greyson and C. P. Flynn, eds., Springfield, IL: Charles C. Thomas.

Hume, D. (1993), *An Enquiry Concerning Human Understanding*, Eric Steinberg, trans. and ed., Indianapolis, IN: Hackett.

Jones, James (In press), Psychodynamic Theories of the Evolution of the God Image, in *The God Image Handbook for Spiritual Counseling and Psychotherapy: Theory, Research, and Practice*, Glen Moriarty and Louis Hoffman, ed., New York: Haworth.

Isaacs, Ronald (1997), *Miracles: A Jewish Perspective*, Northvale, NJ: Jason Aronson.

Kirkpatrick, Lee A. (1997), A Longitudinal Study of Changes in Religious Belief and Behavior as a Function of Individual Differences in Adult Attachment Style, *Journal for the Scientific Study of Religion (JSSR)* 36, 207–17.

Kirkpatrick, Lee A. (2005), *Attachment, Evolutions, and the Psychology of Religion*, New York: Guilford.

Lewis, Clives Staples (1952), *Miracles*, New York: Macmillan.

Main, M., and J. Soloman (2005), Procedures for Identifying Infants as Disorganized/Disoriented during the Ainsworth Strange Situation, in *Attachment in the Preschool Years: Theory, Research and Intervention*, 193–246, M. T. Greenberg, D. Cicchetti, and E. M. Cummings, eds., Chicago: University of Chicago Press.

May, Rollo (1991), *The Cry for Myth*, New York: Delta.

Merton, Thomas (1963), *Life and Holiness*, New York: Herder and Herder.

Moriarty, Glen, Louis Hoffman, Christopher S. M. Grimes, and Jay Gattis (March 25–28, 2004), *God and Attachment: Using Integration Techniques to Change Working Models*, unpublished paper presented at the International Conference of the Christian Association for Psychological Studies, St. Petersburg, Florida.

Murphy, Nancey (1996), *Beyond Liberalism and Fundamentalism: How Modern and Postmodern Philosophy Set the Theological Agenda*, Harrisburg: Trinity Press International.

Novak, Michael (1994), *Belief and Unbelief, A Philosophy of Self Knowledge*, New York: Mentor Omega.

Pascal, Blaise (1966), *Pensées*, A. J. Krailsheimer, trans., Baltimore: Penguin.

Rizzuto, Ana Marie (1979), *The Birth of the Living God*, Chicago: University of Chicago Press.

Siegel, Daniel (1999), *The Developing Mind*, New York: Guilford.

Smith, Wilfred (1963), *The Meaning and End of Religion*, New York: Macmillan.

Strauss, David Freidrich (2006), *The Life of Jesus: Critically Examined*, George Eliot, trans., New York: Continuum International.

Tanner, Kathryn (1997), *Theories of Culture*, Minneapolis: Fortress

Theresa of Avila (1980), *The Collected Works of St. Theresa of Avila*, Kevin Kavanaugh, trans., Washington, DC: ICS.

Tillich, Paul (1951), *Systematic Theology*, Vol. 1, Chicago: University of Chicago Press.

Tillich, Paul (2001), *The Dynamics of Faith*, New York: Perennial.

Weibe, Phillip (2007), *Visions of Jesus: Direct Encounters from the New Testament Today*, New York: Oxford University Press.

Wheeler, David L. (2000), Confessional Communities and Public Worldviews: A Case Study, in *Searching for an Adequate God: A Dialogue between Process and Free Will Theists*, John B. Cobb, Jr., and Clark H. Pinnock, eds., Grand Rapids: Eerdmans.

Woodward, Kenneth (2000), *The Book of Miracles: The Meaning of Miracle Stories in Christianity, Judaism, Buddhism, Hinduism, and Islam*, New York: Simon and Schuster.

CHAPTER 14

RELIGIOUS AND SPIRITUAL MIRACLE EVENTS IN REAL-LIFE EXPERIENCE

Russ Llewellyn

According to a 2006 survey by the Pew Forum on Religion and Public Life, "29 percent of Americans say they have witnessed 'divine healing.'" This is an increase from another poll three decades ago that found only 10 percent of Americans believed in divine healing. The belief in divine healing increases to 62 percent among Pentecostals and 46 percent among Charismatic Christians.[1] Contrast that with a 2006 Rice University Study of 750 professors of natural sciences where only about one-third believe in God. In the general population in America, only about one in 20 (5%) do not believe in God. A Virginia Commonwealth University study found that 87 percent think that scientific developments actually make society better. Among those respondents who believe that, 87 percent describe themselves as religious. In a *Time* magazine poll, 81 percent say that "recent discoveries and advances" in science have not significantly impacted their religious views. Only 4 percent have said that science has made them less religious.[2]

So, between the scientific community and the general population, including that of Evangelicals, exists a large gap in convictions about a core belief regarding the existence and behavior of God. The evangelical community has representatives that express reluctance to believe in miracles and the supernatural. Mainstream Evangelical writer Philip Yancey describes himself as a skeptic. He cites Christians who roll around in wheelchairs and others with stumps for amputated limbs, as people who are prayed for and yet are unhealed. For them, "divine healing feels like the cruelest joke of all." He says he never read of a healing of pancreatic cancer, cystic fibrosis, or ALS. Nor does he think there are verified instances of AIDS being healed. He says the "church has had to change its message from 'Simply believe you'll be healed' to a more difficult message of preaching against risky behavior, caring for the sick and dying, and looking after the millions of orphans resulting from the disease."[3]

So, we have the dilemma of scientists who do not believe in God, let alone miracles and the supernatural, and many Christians who have grown skeptical of miracles, healing, and supernatural experience; contrasting with many in the general public who say they have witnessed a divine healing.

PERSONAL INTRODUCTION TO THE QUESTION ABOUT RELIGIOUS AND SPIRITUAL MIRACLES

I come with a decided bias to this question of whether religious or spiritual miracle events are real in our experience. I believe I am one. So, for me, the matter of religious or spiritual miracle events being real in our experience is full of concrete meaning. I believe I have experienced many such events. I believe I know of many. When I say that I am one, I am not talking about the ordinary miracle of birth. I am talking about a number of things. First, my father at age 5 in the year 1915 had four various potentially fatal illnesses at once: brain fever, spinal meningitis, mastoiditis, and pneumonia. The doctors told my grandparents that if he lived, he'd be a vegetable. The nuns at the Pittsburg hospital prayed and the people at the Baptist Church prayed. My father, Lewis, was healed and recovered and referred to afterward by the nuns at the hospital as the "Miracle Boy."

A second event to which I refer is the improbability of my parents meeting or marrying even though they lived only 80 miles apart in Pennsylvania. Neither was an impulsive adult. Both were committed to major obligations. My father owned a printing shop and my mother had just finished a one-year commitment to look after her father following her mother's death. She had been pre-enrolled at Juniata College. Both my parents came from different Protestant traditions and both, in unique circumstances, left home to attend Bryan University in Tennessee as soon as they heard of it instead of continuing with their original plans. There they met and married. I am the firstborn child of that marriage.

My mother had multiple sclerosis (MS), which required that she use a wheelchair by the time I was 19. She received many prayers for her healing from MS, including one in which a shorter leg from childhood polio was lengthened, but she received no cure from MS. She did, however, live until she was 86 years old, unusual for someone with MS. Could not her remission from increasing attacks of this disabling illness come as the result of prayer?

WHAT ARE RELIGIOUS OR SPIRITUAL
MIRACLE EVENTS?

I will be using the term *miracle* to mean a supernatural event. Our culture often uses the term applied to nature, such as the miracle of conception or childbirth. Some natural phenomena are breathtaking and awesome and are so improbable in design as to suggest a creator. Any event, including physical events or natural phenomena, may be considered a miracle event because of the spiritual or religious meaning and interpretation of the person viewing the event. But these are not what I refer to as a miracle; I refer rather only to those things that would not occur within the natural order and laws of nature.

The difference between what is religious or spiritual has to do with the nature of the event and its interpretation. If it is religious in nature, it would fit within a person's faith or belief system. These systems of belief or ritual are often organized as institutional religions. Something spiritual may be considered religious as well; but in our Western culture, people often distinguish themselves as spiritual but not religious. Spiritual means, of the spirit. The nature of the event deals with the spirit. To be spiritual may mean to be supernatural, or it may be natural, meaning of the human spirit or some other spirit in nature. Religious meaning comes from human interpretation of events, or the interpretation of those who have a role within religious systems to construe meaning. A religious miracle event is one that a person holding a particular religious faith position interprets as being a supernatural occurrence. Spiritual miracle events are those we are compelled by our faith position and experience to interpret as coming from a spiritual source or process. The spiritual source or process may be an energy. It is not materially substantial or physical.

If we say there is a possibility of spiritual or religious miracles, it's because we have a set of assumptions about the nature of reality. We assume that there is a world of the spirit. We also assume that this spirit world can interact with our world of sensory experience and observation. The worldview of scientists may be either completely naturalist, or moderately naturalistic, but neither focusing upon nor excluding the supernatural, or supernaturalist, believing in the possibility of both natural and supernatural phenomena.[4] Vitz argues that scientists should declare their supernaturalist or antisupernaturalist assumptions. All worldviews begin with a set of assumptions about God, truth, nature, and humanness, and these assumptions form the beginning place of scientific inquiry. The worldview of the scientist deals with what he believes are true scientific assumptions, and how that truth may be known in scientific inquiry.

Reality of Miracles in Our Experience

Throughout church history, there have been people who have experienced divine visions, supernatural experiences, visitations, miracles. Julian of Norwich (c. 1342–1416) was thought to be lying on her deathbed as a young woman at age 30, but had a series of visions of Jesus and the meaning of the cross. In 1373 she recovered to write about these visions and the revelations she received and the meaning they had.[5] The twentieth century has had numerous people who have identified themselves as Christian and have reported visions and revelations. Many of them have been healers who have left a legacy of evidence of divine power at work. Some known for healing are Smith Wigglesworth, John G. Lake, A. A. Allen, Maria Woodsworth-Etter, William Branham, Derek Prince, Kathryn Kuhlman, and Oral Roberts.

The twenty-first century has seen such prophetic people of stature as Bob Jones, Rick Joyner, James Goll, Cindy Jacobs, Nita Johnson, Chuck Pierce, and Graham Cooke. And it has seen healing evangelists like Reinhardt Bonke, Benny Hinn, Heidi Baker, and Todd Bentley.[6] In addition, the Healing Rooms Ministries have prayer rooms around the world currently numbering 623. There have been many people who have reported visitations from Jesus, or experiences in which they visit heaven, such as Nita Johnson, Shawn Bolz, Kathie Walters, or Choo Thomas.[7]

WHERE DO WE LOOK FOR DATA?

An antisupernaturalist scientific bias has made data collection difficult because it eliminates categories. The word *miracle* is not used in any of the journals we searched. Even though there are many healings that medical science cannot explain, the category of unexplained healings doesn't exist in professional journals. Categories, constructs, and naming are necessary in order for data to be gathered and conclusions drawn.

What Are the Scientific Assumptions?

Christians who are scientists often have some different assumptions about the nature of reality and of God than do their secular counterparts. Religious or spiritual miracles have to do with the interpretation of observations or experience. In other words, it has to do with meaning. Scientific bias restricts data and skews results. Empirical science had skepticism built in as an assumption. Unless something is proved to be true, it is assumed not to be true. The scientific assumption is that something is assumed not to exist until it can be proven to exist.

In a scientific way, God can be neither proved nor disproved; but Christians and other theists begin with a set of assumptions that God exists and is knowable. Christians who are scientists do not denigrate secular science but are open to the option that phenomenological data and heuristic argument might well urge that the data confirms their assumption, when the search is conducted with that possibility in mind. Scientific measurements have mapped the ocean depths; but science has not been able to directly observe whether there is life at the bottom of the ocean or what its nature is. At every level where we have been able to get submersibles and take pictures, fish and other marine life exist, varieties and kinds that had not been seen before. It may be a reasonable conclusion to believe that life exists at the deepest levels of the oceans that we have not yet observed; but science does not conclude that hypothesis until it is tested and proven. What do people believe in the meantime? Do we believe that exists life at the bottom, or do we assert that it does not exist? We all believe it is highly probable though it has not yet been proven. The phenomenological data and heuristic perception militates in favor of its existence.

The Knowability of Reality

Science makes assumptions based on beliefs about the knowability of reality. This philosophic approach is called epistemology, how we can know what we know. There are different beliefs about whether human beings can know something outside themselves in a one-to-one correspondence, or whether we can know only approximately. Science has made assumptions about whether we can know—probability. The assumption is that we can know something only with a certain degree of certainty called probability. So our statistics, the mathematics in science, describe a degree of knowability of a certain reality as a probability: the higher the degree of probability, the higher the likelihood that something is true. Science by its nature approaches certainty and truth, but by the nature of its assumptions cannot arrive at an absolutely certain truth. Yet, we human beings build our lives on the degree of certainty we do have both from the conclusions we have made from science and from what we have concluded is true from other sources of experience and perception than science.

Science also makes assumptions about the difference between subjectivity and objectivity. It assumes that humans can assume an observer role in which there is a disinterested or detached interest in the outcome of scientific inquiry. Since all inquiry comes out of assumed positions about the nature of God and reality, one's bias is always in the assumptions. Science has an inherent problem in handling subjective data that cannot be independently verified. For example, the process of thinking can be independently verified, but the content of the thought cannot. Thus, spiritual content that is a part of one's consciousness and subjective awareness cannot be independently or scientifically verified. We are left with an objectifying of subjective content, calling it self-report. Because of the objective nature of science, it has limitations in dealing with all the data of reality, especially subjective data. Supernatural and spiritual data are often subjective.

The Mind–Brain Bias

Many scientists make the assumption that the mind cannot exist without the brain, that human consciousness is not possible without brain functioning. This is at heart a materialistic assumption and presupposition. Pim van Lommel, a retired cardiologist from the Rijnstate Hospital, followed 344 survivors of cardiac arrest; 18 percent reported having NDE's (near death experiences) while their brains showed no wave activity. This observation conflicts with current assumptions which van Lommel states as: "according to our current medical concepts it's impossible to experience consciousness during a period of clinical death."[8] I believe that one place where the mind-brain bias is most evident is in the understanding of the out-of-body experience. Some clinicians describe this as dissociation, giving no validity to this out-of-body viewpoint.

Supernaturalist or Naturalist Assumptions

Empirical science makes assumptions about the nature of reality and God as the cause of the worlds of nature and of the human and animal kingdoms. Secular science often holds the position that God is a possibility, but is unknown, or irrelevant. Deists think of him as unknowable or distant: God set the universe in motion according to certain laws and does not intervene in his creation. Christians who are scientists are likely to have a supernaturalist world view. To the Christian, God is the creator who can and does reveal himself in and to his creation. The Christian interpretation of the data of science affects the interpretation of meaning of spiritual experience. Christian do not usually have trouble with the data of scientific observation; but do have problems with the presupposition that truth is knowable only through empirical scientific inquiry. A Christian takes the position that "all truth is God's truth," whether delivered to us by secular or by faith-based science.

When scientists make the assumptions that God is nonexistent or irrelevant, they conclude that God is an imagined creation of human beings based on their needs; and that God is a human projection. Such assumptions in the construction of psychological personality inventories can lead scientists to conclude mistakenly that a person who believes that God communicates with him is necessarily psychotic. While that belief is a possible psychotic indicator, most Christians believe that God can and does ordinarily reveal himself to people. So one's assumptions about God affect one's interpretation of the data.

The mechanical or physical nature of the universe is now understood in terms of time and energy. Quantum physics posits that the largest part of the observable universe is not matter but energy. String theory asserts the possibility of other dimensions of reality than those observable to our senses. When we begin to think that other realities are possible, simultaneous with our observable and measurable realities, we have the possibility of a spiritual world and reality that exists simultaneously with our contemporary observable, measurable, or sensory reality. The Christian worldview assumes that these spiritual realities are not only possible and probable, but that they are observable with another sensory capacity, a spiritual sensory capacity.

The Bible contains hundreds if not thousands of spiritual revelations including interpretations of natural events. The Christian believes that the Bible could not exist if it were not for the possibility of revelation, communication from God to human beings. The Bible explains that people are not only given spiritual sensory capacities that parallel the natural human sensory abilities. Here is an example from Matthew chapter 13: "Though seeing, they do not see; though hearing, they do not hear or understand. In them is fulfilled the prophecy of Isaiah: 'You will be ever hearing but never understanding; you will be ever seeing but never perceiving. For this people's heart has become calloused; they hardly hear with their ears, and they have closed their eyes. Otherwise they might see with their eyes, hear with their ears, understand with their hearts and turn, and I would heal them.'"[9]

PSYCHOLOGICAL OR PERSONAL EXPERIENCES CAN BE SPIRITUAL IN NATURE

The Bible also teaches that spiritual maturity enables us to exercise sense organs of perception and train ourselves to distinguish between good and evil thereby (Hebrews 5:14). NT writers constantly invest the emotions people have with a spiritual meaning. For every sensory capacity, there is a corresponding spiritual sensory capacity. For every human emotion, there is a corresponding spiritual emotion. I believe that in our Western culture, *spiritual* has come to mean an attitude, value, belief system, or interpretation that someone holds. To the Christian, it is more than this. Spiritual is a dimension of reality that is different from natural reality, but exists simultaneously with natural reality. In biblical terms, the world of nature and the world of the spirit are different but overlapping worlds. The world of the spirit is the larger world, and includes the world of nature.

The derivation of the word *psychology* comes from the Greek word psyche, meaning *soul*. So the meaning of psychology was the study of the soul. The biblical teaching about soul, or our earthly human nature or personality, includes the spirit. "The soul is the temporal expression of the spirit. The soul deals with life in the physical body. The soul is the expression of the spirit in the physical and material world with its finite and temporal limitations. Our soul is the creative outworking of our spirit through our life in the world, blending the finite and the visible with the eternal and invisible."[10]

One of the areas of overlap between the soul or psyche and the spirit has to do with our worth or value, self-esteem or esteem by others, our honor.

A biblical perspective differentiates between the temporal and the eternal in this most important human and spiritual value.

By our living for God's glory, a glory that is beyond this life, we receive a worth that is spiritual—of His Spirit—infinite and eternal. Our worth comes from the very heart of God's love and Spirit, the infinite nature of God himself. Our soul is the container and translator of infinite worth, carrying the things of time and the material world into the world of the spirit, which by its very nature is eternal.

The destination of all things in time, including the soul, is eternity. The nature of being, in that place, is spirit. Both soul and spirit as the nonmaterial part of the self are eternal. At times, the Bible refers to the unseen part of the person as soul, and at other times as spirit. Depending on the author and the context, soul and spirit are sometimes used interchangeably. When that occurs, the likeness or similarity between them is being emphasized. At other times they are differentiated. God, for example, is often referred to in the Bible as Holy Spirit. Spirit describes the essence of God's being and existence. Human beings are also described as having a spirit. The following Scripture talks about the human spirit: "For this is what the high and lofty One says—He Who lives forever, Whose name is holy: 'I live in a high and holy place, but also with him who is contrite and lowly in spirit, to revive the spirit of the lowly and to revive the heart of the contrite'" [Isa 57:15].

In this passage, heart and spirit are parallel words. Heart is used to mean the innermost being of the person, the sensitivity to what is most cherished and prized; it probably expresses the central emotional and affective meeting place of the person's soul and spirit. To love God with our whole heart, mind and strength and our neighbors as ourselves is a union of both soul and spirit as one. One set of emotions the self has gives us a picture of the overlap that can occur between the soul and spirit. Some emotions occur simultaneously in both soul and spirit because they are both temporal and eternal. They belong to both soul and spirit, and are perceived in our spirits as well as with our soul through our bodily senses.

The example comes from the Apostle Paul who says: "These three remain: faith, hope and love. But the greatest of these is love" [I Cor 13:13]. We may experience love in our hearts, the place through which our spirits flow 'our innermost beings.' Or we may experience love in our emotions, feeling loyalty, affection or solidarity with family, friends or other people—the way we feel in our souls. Or we may experience love in our passions experienced in and generated from our bodily feelings which may be expressed through a hug, a touch or a kiss. Or we may feel any combination of these feelings simultaneously, merging together spirit, soul, or body as one.

Let me use a metaphor of a house. If the house represents the body, the person living in the house represents the spirit. All that's done while the person lives in the house represents the soul. In this metaphor, all the person does, good and bad, become the furnishings of the house. Human consciousness, thoughts, and personal identity comprise part of our soul, just as do our emotions and actions. Think about the person in the house. He is spirit. He has a personality. All that happens to him, all he is, thinks, intends and does becomes a part of him, his soul. As he expresses himself, even his house takes on the character of his personality, his spirit. As long as the person is alive they all function together as one person: body, soul and spirit.[11]

In human personality, many things are subject to the eternal and spiritual or the supernatural dimension of reality. Since the past is a part of eternity, it is not just past, but in eternal dimension is accessible as present. This has great potential impact in the transformation and healing of trauma from the past. The parallel notions of soul and spirit mean that the supernatural power that is available through God's Spirit, not just the human spirit, can be available in the healing process. The human capacities of mind, will, emotion, and judgment can be subject to the eternal kingdom of God or the temporal kingdom of humankind. Roles and attitudes we take regarding ourselves can be expressions of our human nature acting either toward or against itself. This capacity to be for or against ourselves, God, or others I take to be an essential capacity of human beings and is the spiritual capacity for good or evil.

Some of the Kinds of Spiritual/Supernatural Events

Dreams

A Christian may believe that dreams (1) can be more than the processing of unconscious material, containing communication from spiritual beings, (2) can be information from God, (3) can give spiritual meaning to past experience, or (4) can be predictive of future events. People's dreams can be accessed by spiritual beings from both God and Satan. One such dream came to Bilquis Sheikh, a Pakistani Muslim, a vivid dream of Jesus that became a revelation to her that led her on a journey to believe in Jesus as the Savior of the world.[12]

Visions

Spiritual visions are more than imagination or personal creativity. They can be revelations from a spiritual being. Phillip Wiebe did careful interviews of 28 people who had visions of Jesus, the Christ, which they thought were from God. He documents these in his book.[13] Some of the kinds of spiritual and supernatural events include:

Prophesies
Knowing something that has not been naturally disclosed
Angelic and demonic beings
Answers to prayer

Many Christian people who are functional and not delusional have reported visitations from Jesus and being taken to heaven: Anna Roundtree,[14] Todd Bentley,[15] Shawn Bolz,[16] Kathie Walters.[17] One of the most extensive reports of visitations to heaven and conversations with Jesus comes from Choo Thomas.[18]

I asked God many years ago, "Are you still doing miracles of healing today?" Within the week of my asking that question, three people told me about miracles that had happened in their lives. One was a good friend who had done a summer missions experience on one of the Alaskan islands when he was 19 years old. He and other teens were playing in a volleyball area when one of the girls tried to put ice down his shirt. In running away from her he tripped in a ditch. He thought he had broken his ankle because his foot was flopping around and it hurt badly. His ankle swelled. Because they did not have a hospital on the island he went on a ferry with a missionary to another island to have the injury treated. As they rode on the ferry, the missionary had her hand on his back and was praying for him and told him that he was going to be okay. He had felt more than natural heat on his back where she had her hand as she prayed. Before they arrived at the hospital, he thought that his ankle was healed and that he was better, except the swelling still took another hour or so to go down. X-rays determined that he did not have a fracture.

A dentist I know went to provide free dental work to the poor of Mexico. He did that in the day and at night met them for Christian teaching and prayer. During one of these prayer times, a woman came to him carrying a child with impetigo. He prayed for her and simply prayed a blessing prayer for her child. He did not even pray a healing prayer. Within the next 15 minutes, he saw the woman with a group of other women pointing at him saying something in Spanish like: "He did it." My dentist friend did not know what she meant. She brought the child and showed him the change. The child no longer had runny eyes or a scabby chin. The impetigo had apparently been healed.

A patient recounted an experience with an abusive coach of a cheerleading team. She had been exercising as a part of her routines and had gotten shin splints. The coach pushed her to keep exercising as though she could work through it. It was so bad she ended up having to use a wheelchair. That night she had a prayer group pray for God to heal her. She was healed and able to walk away from that group without using the wheelchair and without pain.

Religious and Spiritual Miracle/Supernatural Events in the Bible

Food multiplication (Matthew 14:15–21 and Mark 8:1–9)
Being transported from one place to another (John 6:21, Acts 8:39)
Being healed of an illness (Matthew 9:32, Mark 1:34)
Being raised from the dead (John 11:44, John 20:1–17)
Being healed of a spiritual affliction (Mark 2:5–11, Matthew 8:28–33)

RELIGIOUS AND SPIRITUAL MIRACLE/ SUPERNATURAL EVENTS IN MY PERSONAL EXPERIENCE

Spiritual Feelings

When I was a young psychologist I had an experience in walking up the back hill above the garage on the farm where my mother grew up. I was walking to the little church on the hilltop, when in the middle of this cornfield I felt overcome with sadness without a known source. So I stopped and asked myself where it was coming from. Was it from me because of childhood nostalgia, having played and fished for crawdads in the creek below and having visited the farm during summers as a child? No. Was it about me from some other source? No. Was it feelings I was having for my mother? No. Was it feelings I was aware of which were my mother's feelings? Yes. That was it.

Years later, I relayed this story to my mother who began to cry and said that she knew what it was. Because of her mother's sudden death after her senior year in high school, and her mother's burial in the cemetery at the church on the hill top, my mother said that she never crossed the gate into the cemetery again during all the times she went to church. It became clear as Mother talked that her trauma became symbolized by the cemetery and the gate became a phobic object. Crossing it would be opening a door to her pain. This is what my story opened up in her. I realized it was not my feelings I was aware of, but my mother's, that overcame me. I was not feeling *for* my mother, nor having *empathic* feelings for my mother. I was suffering her pain. I believe this experience became the genesis for my developing the ability to feel another's emotional pain if they come into my presence feeling it, whether they are expressing it or trying to hide it. I believe that this is a spiritual gift that is beyond empathy.

Prophetic Vision

As a psychologist and a Christian, my religious and psychological traditions did not include an awareness of current experiences of prophetic visions. So, I was unprepared to believe what I experienced as really happening. I had had words with a woman who was trying to claim a parking space that we had been awaiting for several minutes. So as we went into the art and wine festival, I had a picture in my mind of our car being keyed or scratched, beginning at the front right fender and along the right side and doors to the rear fender. I was unprepared to believe what I was seeing and put it out of my mind. I thought I spontaneously psychologized it, just imaging it, because of the unpleasant encounter with the woman. When I returned to the car I was surprised to find that it had been keyed along the exact panels I had envisioned.

I have had several of these kinds of occurrences. Another occurred while I was praying with a group of people at the church we attend. We were in a room, removed from the worship center, and did not have any video or audio feeds on while we were praying. As we were praying, I saw a picture in my mind of a toolbox. I interpreted this as a symbol, so I prayed for the symbolic meaning of the tools God would use and the spiritual construction God would do in people's lives, and the skills of the pastor in this work. When we went to the worship service the next hour, I was amazed to see that the pastor had brought an actual toolbox onstage with him as a prop for his sermon.

Spiritual Dreams

I had a dream about opening an office for my psychology practice in a major city to the south, so that with the other clinician in my practice we would have two locations. My dream referred to my plans to open a second office as though I were driving a car. According to the dream, opening another office "would be the long way around" in getting to where I was going. I discounted this dream as having no predictive or revelatory meaning at the time. But within five years, I closed that other office, having concluded that I was unable to be a psychotherapist, a director of a clinic, a supervisor of other clinicians, and write. Writing, I believed, was my unfulfilled calling. Moreover, I reduced my work to a solo practice so I could have the time and energy to write.

Results from Prayer

One of the first results of prayer in my practice that seemed supernatural in origin regarded a schizophrenic woman I treated. She was particularly susceptible to her husband's power over her and so seemed to become psychotic as a way to deal with her anger and rage toward him or herself. During these episodes, she became Satan, in her view, or he became Satan. This woman moved away from the area, still lived with her husband, and came back to visit with me. Her face looked radiant and she was in the best emotional condition that I had ever seen her. So I asked what had happened. She said she had been meeting with her pastor who prayed for her. This was my first encounter with the potentially powerful effects of prayer on a patient.

One of my DID (Dissociative Identity Disorder) patients had integrated several of her alternative personalities through her therapy work. But she had many alternates who remained unintegrated. When visiting her brother, a pastor, they spent about 15 minutes praying for her. The result was that all of her remaining alters integrated into her core personality. Sometimes she misses them and her ability to dissociate to handle stress or emotional pain but her stability has persisted over the years of her continued therapy.

Another DID patient was hospitalized for cutting herself so badly that the hospital staff did not want her to traumatize or influence other patients in group therapy. She was also suicidal at the time. She appeared to be the acting out of one of her strongest alternate personalities, which was trying to be protective in a distorted way. Because of the threat, I resorted to a desperate measure: prayer. I asked her permission to involve this alternate personality in prayer. The patient was a Christian whose personal Christian faith, her spiritual and religious values, were consistent with my request. There was no overt active prayer done on behalf of this alternate. I simply invited this alternate personality to come into a room that in her imagination, inside herself, was filled with God's light. As the alternate personality did that, the nature and character of that alternate shifted from being harsh and antagonistic to being cooperative and helpful. Subsequently, the patient reacted to this event as though the alternate had died. The patient grieved the loss of strength that she had relied on from this alternate for years afterward. I had interpreted to this patient that her alter had not really disappeared, but had integrated its strength into her core personality with positive traits.

RELIGIOUS AND SPIRITUAL MIRACLE/ SUPERNATURAL EVENTS IN PSYCHOLOGICAL AND MEDICAL LITERATURE

After numerous searches in the medical and psychological literature, I am amazed to find so few topics related to spiritual life, recovery from death, NDEs (near-death experiences), and the like. In discussing these issues with physicians I know, I have concluded that a number of factors militate against reporting data in journals.

1. Supernaturalist language is excluded from scientific vocabulary as though such events do not exist or could not happen. Therefore science has not yet adopted words or terms to collect this kind of data.
2. An antisupernaturalist bias exists in healing communities of medical and related professionals. When we prayed for my daughter's healing from a brain tumor, my wife's physician was concerned that my wife was in denial about our daughter's condition because such things as supernatural healings "do not occur."
3. To deny the existence or occurrence of unexplained healings indicates a blind spot in one's research. We do not usually report data we have not figured out or researched well enough to explain.
4. Peer review of articles means that issues that do not have a replicable scientific explanation will not be accepted for publication in journals.

I suggest that a language be developed for miracle events. NDEs (near-death experiences) is an example of medical bias in the naming the category.

With NDE, it's not necessary to conclude that the person actually died, for presumably, that would be called ADE for after-death experience. NDE suggests that the person came close to dying, since they recovered and are currently alive to report their experience. I suggest a designation like FRAD for *full recovery after death* be made for people who are dead at least 15 minutes and are revived after death or are revived after a diagnosis of clinical death occurs and no functional impairment exists after coming back to life. The medical community understands that if coming back to life after death or a medical resuscitation does not occur within the first 10 minutes of loss of heartbeat or breathing, recovery without loss of functioning is not normally possible.

Perhaps a term like *LAD* for life after death could be adopted for any return to life after death. SNE might be a designation for a supernormal or supranormal experience that could refer to miracle, supernatural, or paranormal life experiences. SAB could refer to sighted after blindness. FAS could refer to functioning after a prolonged impairment from a stroke. I am sure the idea is clear. Healings and miracles occur and have not been recognized by the data categories of science. The scientific community needs diagnostic words as data catchers so that what happens can be categorized and commented on in medical and other scientific journals. I am not so concerned whether any of my ideas get picked up as categories, just that categories for healing, miracles, and the supernatural occurrences be adopted for the literature of medical and psychological research, reporting, and discussion.

RELIGIOUS AND SPIRITUAL MIRACLE/ SUPERNATURAL EVENTS REPORTED BY OTHER VERIFIABLE SOURCES

Dr. Chauncey Crandall

Dr. Chauncey Crandall is a physician in the Cardiovascular Clinic in Palm Beach Gardens and has served as a university instructor in schools of medicine at a number of universities. He describes a 53-year-old man who came to the hospital emergency room with a massive heart attack. His heart had stopped. The medical team worked with him for over 40 minutes and declared him dead. Dr. Crandall had been called in to evaluate at the end of this time while a nurse was preparing the body for the morgue. He states: "There was no life in the man. His face and feet and arms were completely black with death." He had felt compelled by the Holy Spirit to pray for this man so he went to the side of the stretcher where his body was being prepared and prayed. "Lord, Father, how am I going to pray for this man? He is dead. What can I do? All of a sudden these words came out of my mouth, 'Father, God, I cry out for the soul of this man. If he does not know you as his Lord and Savior, please raise him from the dead right now in Jesus' name.'"

"It was amazing as a couple of minutes later, we were looking at the monitor and all of a sudden a heartbeat showed up. It was a perfect beat; a normal beat; and then after a couple more minutes, he started moving and then his fingers were moving and then his toes began moving and then he started mumbling words. There was a nurse in the room. She was not a believer. She screamed out and said, 'Doctor Crandall, what have you done to this patient?' And I said, 'All I've done is cry out for his soul in Jesus' name.' We quickly rushed the gentleman down to the intensive care unit, and the hospital was by now buzzing about the fact that a dead man had been brought back to life. After a couple of days he woke up. He had an amazing story to tell after I had asked him, 'Where have you been and where were you on that day that you had that massive heart attack? You were gone and we prayed you back to life in Jesus' name.'" Dr. Crandall reports that he has seen three such people, who returned to life after death from cardiac arrest.[19]

Dr. Raquel Burgos

In an interview with Dr. Raquel Burgos, she remarked that the topic of healing and miracles "honestly, does not come up" among physicians. She expressed surprise if more than one or two out of a hundred physicians believed in supernatural healing or miracles. Her own experience was that she had a birth defect in her legs, part of which meant that one leg was two inches shorter than normal. Her mother took her to Kathryn Kuhlman healing services and as a result, the short leg grew out to match the longer one within a few days of healing prayer. She was in treatment to correct her leg by an orthopedist and so retains her medical records of what happened. She and a group of physicians started a group called H.E.A.L., standing for His Energy And Love. This group met to pray for the healing of their patients.

Dr. Jeannie Lindquist

Dr. Jeannie Lindquist cited a case she and her husband, both orthopedic physicians, had many years ago. This was during the early years of antibiotics. A man had come for treatment because of a knee injury and the infection that resulted in blood poisoning, sepsis. In order to treat the sepsis, they had to use massive doses of antibiotics, which resulted in kidney failure. They were going to send him for dialysis. Since they both shared the same Christian faith background, they asked him if he would mind if they prayed for him. He was glad to have them pray for his healing. Some time before the dialysis referral and after the prayer, they sent a sample to the lab. The lab thought they must have made a mistake because it was showing up with no kidney problem, unlike the previous sample. So they sent another sample that morning with the same results. A sudden healing had occurred in answer to prayer.

Keith G

A group of people from our church prayed for Keith G while he was a teenager, because he had such severe migraines continuously that he could not attend high school. While we prayed, I felt that I received assurance in my spirit that he would be healed. He moved with his family to the state of Washington. Years later, he went to the Healing Rooms in Spokane for prayer. During the first prayer time, the migraines disappeared, but they came back within a few days. Had the prayer not worked? Would he not be healed permanently? Prayer had brought the only relief he had experienced from the migraines so he decided to go back to the Healing Rooms for more prayer. This time, through prayer he was healed in a way that lasted. His ability to function in a way that permitted him to attend school was restored.

Mark Weber

Mark Weber is a Christian man who engages in healing prayer for people. While he believes he has seen thousands of people who have experienced healing as a result of prayer, he cited one as an example of a documented healing. This man had color blindness and was a third-generation male with that problem. For this problem to exist genetically there is almost certainly an absence of color receptor cones in his retina. He only saw in shades of grey. After prayer he could distinguish colors. Mark has also reported seeing scars up and down both arms of a woman who had been hospitalized with self-inflicted injuries disappear before their eyes as she received prayer.

Dick Patterson

Dick Patterson is a pastor whose integrity I know, a man who has accompanied Todd Bentley, a healing evangelist, on some of his trips to Africa to preach and pray for healing. He has been a part of many healings for which he has prayed. On one occasion there was a blind lady who recovered her sight in four stages in which she progressively regained more of her sight. After she could see, they took photos of her family dancing happily, because "grandma can see." Todd Bentley has documented many cases of people who regain their hearing after being deaf, and sight after being blind.[20]

Lorraine

Lorraine is a woman who experienced significant abuse from her mother and as a middle-aged adult is still recovering from it. She has an easier time attaching to animals than to people and is beginning to make the transition to being able to love and trust people. She had pet guinea pigs, one of whom was dying. She took him to the veterinarian and discovered that he had kidney failure. She was not ready to give up on her guinea pig, so she asked God to heal him. When she took him back to the veterinarian, the veterinarian was surprised and examined the pet twice to confirm that he no longer had kidney problems, was looking better, and had gained six ounces.

Gary Paltridge

Gary Paltridge is a layman who does pastoral and healing prayer work. A young man he worked with had an accident and was in chronic pain for which an implant was inserted to dispense morphine. After prayer, both Gary and the person he was praying for saw a mental picture of a demonic figure leaving the man's body. Simultaneously his pain was completely healed, necessitating the removal of the implant.

Ben

Ben has in his possession both an ultrasound and x-rays from his medical records. These show a mass in one picture, the ultrasound. He received healing prayer as the only intervention between the time of the ultrasound and the x-ray. When the x-ray was taken, no mass appeared on the x-ray. The growth had disappeared.

John G. Lake

John G. Lake was a man who lived in the early 1900s and had himself been healed. He became a man of great healing gifts. He lived in Spokane, Washington. He had a scientific bent and so participated in healing experiments so that the results could be observed by scientific instruments. He said that he kept track of and documented over 100,000 miraculous healings.[21] He founded the Healing Rooms Ministries, which has been revived today, so that now 623 healing rooms exist internationally, most of them in the United States of America, under the direction of Reverend Calvin Pierce.[22] There are currently 710 healing testimonies recorded on that Web site. Those testimonies are organized in medical diagnostic categories, but they are written by lay people without attention to the kind of verification that would be helpful to researchers.

Ricky Roberts

Ricky Roberts[23] was born severely retarded. At age 16, he weighed 300 pounds and was not able to do kindergarten work. The week of his healing from retardation, he went from kindergarten to tenth grade, and within that week was tutoring classmates in trigonometry. In a summary of her book,

A Walk Through Tears, his mother Dot Roberts writes: "In December 1977, a genuine modern-day miracle occurred.... God completely and instantaneously healed sixteen-year-old Ricky Roberts of severe mental retardation, a disability that has plagued him since birth." Today, Dr. Ricky Roberts has seven earned doctorate degrees, including two PhDs, and is the founder of True Light Ministries, a teaching and healing ministry based in Jacksonville, Florida. There appear to be hundreds of testimonies of healing on the True Light Web site.[24]

Harriet

In using prayer visualizations in psychotherapy with patients, I went from thinking that people were producing positive visions out of their imaginations, to believing that Jesus was actually communicating with them. Over many different people, patterns emerged in the manner in which Jesus communicated, sometimes saying things to the person about which the patient had an opposite position. I record the usage of prayer in psychotherapy in my paper presented at the convention of the Christian Association for Psychological Studies.[25] I not only have found it helpful with some people who are gifted and able to visualize, but believe that it is superior to my telling someone or having them come to a conclusion themselves when Jesus tells or shows someone something. Here's the background and the visioning experience of a woman I call Harriet in my book.

Her father was an angry man who picked fights with his family. She was the one who would stand up to him. She could not stand being around him. In fact, she hated him. As a teenager, she turned to athletics to douse the fire of her anger and bring calm. It brought order to her life, distanced her from disturbing and messy feelings, and kept her away from home. Liking herself seemed out of the question. Hating herself fit better.

She could tolerate all these angry feelings about herself and her father better if she just didn't think about herself. Even now, as a wife and mother, she still didn't like herself very well.

Instead of running away from her feelings, she was turning to face them. She didn't like what she saw. Some of what she saw she despised in herself. Would she ever be able to like herself, feel clean and whole, or forgive herself? It took all the power of will she had to face herself and these issues about how unworthy she felt. The truth was, she did not want to feel hopeful. She thought she didn't even deserve that much. She was, however, willing to open herself in prayer to what God might want to heal in her. While praying, she envisioned Jesus carrying his cross. She realized he was doing this for her. In her prayer picture, she walked alongside him, and as he looked at her his face became radiant and full of joy, because she was one of the people for whom he was doing this. She had trouble receiving the message of that radiance. She told Jesus, "I wish You would not do this for me. I am not worth it." She knew the anguished pain that lay ahead for him. She could see he was carrying a burden for her that she could not carry. She was glad He was doing something for her that she could not do. But she said, "Why are You doing that for me, when even my question is insignificant?" He looked lovingly at her and said, "It is the central point. It is the whole significance of what I am doing."[26]

John T. Dearborn, M.D.

John T. Dearborn, M.D., said:

A 63-year-old Asian woman who was otherwise healthy came to me for bilateral knee replacement surgery. I had no idea about her relationship with the Lord prior to operating on her. She had been exercising regularly to get ready for the surgery. Unfortunately, during the right knee surgery, her popliteal artery was injured. The injury was rapidly recognized and repaired by a vascular surgeon and within an hour her leg had normal blood flow restored. That should have been the end of the story. Unfortunately, the repair failed to maintain the blood flow through the vessel and she underwent a procedure in the angiography suite to reopen the vessel. That procedure also proved to be inadequate, and she subsequently went another full 12 hours with no documentable blood flow to her foot. Her foot and calf were ischemic and looked mummified when her leg was opened in the operating room by another vascular surgeon. Her blood pH was 7.1, not compatible with life for very long. The surgeon bypassed the clogged vessel and restored flow to what he, with 35 years of vascular surgery experience, felt was a lost cause.

He strongly felt over the subsequent hours that her leg should be amputated. Because I felt that amputation would be especially traumatic for this previously healthy patient and her family, I advocated that we wait. I agreed that if she began a downhill course or that if the limb became infected, amputation should be done immediately to save her life. In the meantime, I initiated a prayer chain with her family and our church family. It turned out that the patient and her family are also believers in Jesus. Her vascular repair held, blood flow returned, and despite the loss of much of the muscle in her calf, her skin remained viable and she kept her leg. The vascular surgeon called her course over the next several days "miraculous." She never recovered sensation or motor function below the knee, but she now can walk unassisted on her own foot instead of on a prosthesis.[27]

Leslie

A woman patient I will call Leslie attended a Christian women's conference: Fragrant Oil. While there was no specific prayer for her, she knew she had been healed of lactose intolerance. So she is now able to eat milk products without supplements.

Walter

A man I know whom I will call Walter had a snowboarding accident and as a result had severe testicular pain. This pain was too much to consider marrying his girlfriend. He went to a healing prayer session with someone with healing gifts and as a result had the pain reduced by about 95 percent, enough to get married and have a child.

Some Personal Experiences

I had a weakening of my acid enzymes when I was in my late forties that meant that I did not digest proteins properly. I took HCL (hydrochloric acid) supplements for years when I ate meat. During one time of extended prayer time and fasting, I knew that God had healed that problem, even though I never prayed for its healing during that time of prayer and fasting. It has been about 20 years since that time, and I have not had any more problem with insufficient stomach acidity to break down proteins.

I have a friend who told me of an experience that puzzled him. He was walking to a pool where his daughter was floating. He was walking and about 20 feet from the pool, and in the next step, he found himself instantly at the pool. When he leaned over, his three-year-old daughter who should have been floating on her back had flipped and was face down in the water. He was able to right her immediately. His wife at the time who observed his instant trip to the pool asked him, "How did you do that?" Of course he had no explanation.

I had an experience in a prayer group while speaking in tongues that was an obvious spiritual experience. Glossalalia or speaking in tongues is usually a very private prayer language experience. Different people sound different when speaking in tongues. You could not match someone else if you tried to. More than seven years earlier I had heard a certain kind of speaking in tongues that was unusual. It was distinctive. I had never heard it before, nor had I ever spoken in that kind of prayer language. In one prayer meeting of many county leaders and people of prayer, we were praying, when I heard myself and three other people instantly and simultaneously speaking in that particularly distinctive tongue.

I was in a meeting with Paul Cox that dealt with discernment of spiritual beings. He has a higher level of spiritual discernment than most Christians I know, and he was aware not only of angelic beings and demons present, but of powers also. He believes that powers carry an electromagnetic charge. He pointed to one place in the room where he believed a power to be present and then brought a compass out of his pocket. Outside the area where he believed the power to be present, the compass had one reading for north. But the needle changed about five degrees when he put it in the center of where he believed the power was.

Trent Cox

I have veterinarian friends, the Doctors Cox. While they lived in my family cottage, they were considering becoming missionaries, but Trent had such severe back problems that his wife had to help him to dress for months at a time during outbreaks of the problem. No mission board would have accepted them with his back condition as it was. He believes that prayer was the treatment that changed his condition. By the time they moved from our cottage, Trent's back was no longer incapacitating him.

Terry Burton

Pearl Burton's son Terry was born with hydrocephalus. This was confirmed with both x-rays and a CT scan. The doctor said, "Your son is severely brain damaged. The x-rays show that his brain is only the size of a walnut. I am afraid he will be a vegetable for the rest of his life." The doctor had said that the buildup of fluid in his head had severely damaged his brain cells. Pearl said, "I needed a miracle because medical science could give me no hope for my son." As she began to consider how to pray, she heard the voice of the Lord say in her spirit, "Pray that Terry will have the mind of Christ." Her prayer procedure was to pray in faith, laying her hands on him and confessing that he would have the mind of Christ and that he would receive the miracle of healing. She also got a developmental book that outlined normal growth in a baby. She began commanding in prayer that Terry's body would start doing the things that are normal for his age. In Terry's next visit to the neurologist, he couldn't understand how Terry could be walking since he did not have a brain to tell his body what to do. Pearl decided to see another neurologist who took a new x-ray of his brain, which showed a completely normal brain. She says she left the doctor's office rejoicing that "Jesus is the healer and is still in the healing business." Terry was tested in third grade as above average on an intelligence test. Terry is now an adult attending college on an academic scholarship.[28]

NOTES

1. Kim Vo (August 21, 2007), Faith Healing: Believers vs. Skeptics, *San Jose Mercury News*. Available online: www.mercurynews.com. Accessed March 15, 2008.

2. David Masci (August 27, 2007), *How the Public Resolves Conflicts between Faith and Science*, Pew Forum on Religion and Public Life. Available online: http://pewforum.org/docs/?DocID=243. Accessed March 15, 2008.

3. Phillip Yancey (2006), *Prayer: Does It Make Any Difference?*, Grand Rapids: Zondervan, 265.

4. Paul Vitz (March 2007), "Body and Relationship: Theological and Psychological Foundations of the Person" lecture, Christian Association for Psychological Studies International Convention.

5. Julian of Norwich (1966), *Revelations of Divine Love*, New York: Penguin.

6. Todd Bentley (2004), *Christ's Healing Touch*, vol. 1, Abbotsford, Canada: Fresh Fire Ministries.

7. Choo Thomas (2003), *Heaven Is So Real*, Lake Mary, FL: Creation House Press.

8. Bill Newcott (2007), Life after Death, *AARP The Magazine*, September/October, 73.

9. This is from the 1996 edition of the New International Version of The Bible.

10. Russ Llewellyn (2007), *Ultimate Worth*, unpublished book, 83.

11. Ibid., 83–4.

12. Bilquis Sheikh, with Richard H. Schneider (2002), *I Dared to Call Him Father*, Grand Rapids: Chosen Books, 35.

13. Phillip H. Wiebe (1997), *Visions of Jesus*, New York: Oxford University Press.

14. Anna Roundtree (2001), *The Priestly Bride*, Lake Mary, FL: Charisma House, 1–104.

15. Todd Bentley (2005), *The Reality of the Supernatural World*, Ladysmith, British Columbia: Sound of Fire Productions, 102.

16. Shawn Bolz (2004), *The Throne Room Company*, North Sutton, New Haven: Streams Publishing House.

17. Kathie Walters (1993), *Living in the Supernatural*, Macon, GA: Good News Fellowship Ministries, 60, 61.

18. Choo Thomas (2003), *Heaven Is So Real*, Lake Mary, FL: Creation House Press.

19. Dan Wooding (2007), Famed Heart Doctor Tells the Dramatic Story of How a Patient of His Was "Raised from the Dead" after Prayer, Assist News Service, accessed on March 15, 2008, from http://www.assistnews.net/Stories/2007/s07070094.htm

20. Todd Bentley (2003), *Journey into the Miraculous*, Ladysmith, British Columbia: Sound of Fire Productions.

21. John G. Lake (1994), *John G. Lake: His Life, His Sermons, His Boldness of Faith*, Fort Worth, TX: Kenneth Copeland Ministries.

22. The Healing Rooms (www.healingrooms.com) is a Web site of the International Association of Healing Rooms. Testimonies may be selected. Authors are individually noted for each testimony. Accessed on March 15, 2008.

23. Sid Roth's Messianic Vision Web site has video, audio, and text dealing with supernatural themes. Video interview is Sid Roth interviewing Dr. Ricky Roberts and his mother Dot Roberts on the subject: Healing from Severe Mental Retardation. Broadcast December 19–25, 2005. Accessed on March 15, 2008. http://www.sidroth.org/site/News2?abbr=tv_&page=NewsArticle&id=5694.

24. http://www.truelightministries.org (2008) is the Web site for the ministries of Dr. Ricky Roberts and Dot Roberts whose minsitries are located in Jacksonville, Florida. Once on site select bottom right "TLM" to enter home page. Open window for "Testimonies." Select "Healings" "Miracles." Accessed on March 15, 2008.

25. Russ Llewellyn (1996), The Therapeutic Use of Prayer in Psychotherapy, unpublished paper presented at a Christian Association for Psychological Studies International Convention, St. Louis, Missouri.

26. Llewellyn (2007), *Ultimate Worth*, 124, 125.

27. John T. Dearborn, MD, Director, Center for Joint Replacement, Palo Alto and Freemont, California, author's personal contact in August 19, 2007.

28. Pearl Burton (Winter, 1985), Thanks to God My Son Is a Walking Miracle, in *Manna*, Houston: Lakewood Church, 12–13.

REFERENCES

Bentley, Todd (2004), *Christ's Healing Touch*, vol. 1, Abbotsford, Canada: Fresh Fire Ministries.

Bentley, Todd (2003), *Journey into the Miraculous*, Ladysmith, British Columbia: Sound of Fire Productions.

Bentley, Todd (2005), *The Reality of the Supernatural World*, Ladysmith, British Columbia: Sound of Fire Productions, 102.

Bilquis Sheikh, with Richard H. Schneider (2002), *I Dared to Call Him Father*, Grand Rapids: Chosen Books, 35.

Bolz, Shawn (2004), *The Throne Room Company*, North Sutton, New Haven: Streams Publishing House.

Burton, Pearl (Winter, 1985), Thanks to God My Son Is a Walking Miracle, in *Manna*.

Julian of Norwich (1966), *Revelations of Divine Love*, New York: Penguin.

Lake John G. (1994), *John G. Lake: His Life, His Sermons, His Boldness of Faith*, Fort Worth: TX: Kenneth Copeland Ministries.

Llewellyn Russ (1996), The Therapeutic Use of Prayer in Psychotherapy, unpublished paper presented at a Christian Association for Psychological Studies International Convention, St. Louis, Missouri.

Llewellyn, Russ (2007), *Ultimate Worth*, unpublished book, 83.

Masci, David (August 27, 2007), *How the Public Resolves Conflicts between Faith and Science*, Pew Forum on Religion and Public Life. Available online: http://pewforum.org/docs?DocID=243. Accessed on March 15, 2008.

Newcott, Bill (2007), Life after Death, *AARP The Magazine*, September/October, 73.

Roundtree, Anna (2001), *The Priestly Bride*, Lake Mary, FL: Charisma House, 1–104.

Thomas, Choo (2003), *Heaven Is So Real*, Lake Mary, FL: Creation House Press.

Vitz, Paul (March 2007), Body and Relationship: Theological and Psychological Foundations of the Person, lecture, Christian Association for Psychological Studies International Convention.

Vo, Kim (August 21, 2007), Faith Healing: Believers vs. Skeptics, *San Jose Mercury News*. Available online: www.mercurynews.com, Accessed March 15, 2008.

Walters, Kathie (1993), *Living in the Supernatural*, Macon, GA: Good News Fellowship Ministries, 60, 61.

Wiebe, Phillip H. (1997), *Visions of Jesus*, New York: Oxford University Press, www.sidroth.org/site/News2?abbr=tv_&page=NewsArticle&id=5694.

Yancey, Phillip (2006), *Prayer: Does It Make Any Difference?* Grand Rapids: Zondervan.

CHAPTER 15

How Religious or Spiritual Miracle Events Happen Today

William P. Wilson

A miracle is an extraordinary event manifesting divine intervention in human affairs. This definition is often contested by those who do not believe that there is a supernatural God or, if he exists, that he intervenes in human affairs. Most of the leaders of Israel did not accept the miracles of Jesus even though they were empirical evidence of his divinity. Because he was God, Jesus could perform miracles. When asked if he was the Messiah by the disciples of John the Baptist, Jesus told them that the miracles he performed accredited his messiahship (Matthew 11:4–6). Interestingly he cited mostly healings. He said, "Go back and report to John what you hear and see: The blind receive sight, the lame walk, those who have leprosy are cleansed, the deaf hear, the dead are raised, and the good news is proclaimed to the poor." Miracles continued to occur after his death. Even as late as the fifth century after Jesus' death, St. Augustine in his *City of God*[1] cited 71 miracles occurring over a two-year period as testimony to the existence of God. Five of these were of raising of the dead. Because he called attention to them, one has to assume that most people in his day still did not believe miracles occurred.

EXPOSITION

Just as in Jesus' lifetime and in the apostolic period, there have been those who have denied the work of the Holy Spirit and his dispensation of gifts (John 14:12). More recently those called cessationists have averred that miracles ceased at the end of the apostolic period because they were only for the apostolic age. It is said that Calvin[2] and Warfield[3] were the major proponents of the cessationist's point of view. Miracles did not cease as they claimed. Throughout the centuries miracles have continued to be reported. Edward Gibbon, the historian, says that, "The Christian church, from the time of the Apostles and their disciples, has claimed an uninterrupted succession of miraculous powers, the gift of tongues, of visions and of prophecy, the power of expelling demons, of healing the sick and of raising the dead."[4] There is no question, though, that there are many in theology, science, and philosophy who still dogmatically state that miracles cannot and do not occur. Two most vocal philosophical critics in the recent past were Spinoza[5] and Hume.[6] At the present time Richard Dawkins[7] and Christopher Hitchens[8] have emphatically denied the existence of a creator God and the occurrence of miracles. Still there are continuing reports of documented miracles.

Before we attack the question posed by the title it is necessary to clarify the terms *religious* and *spiritual*. Many people use the terms synonymously, but they in reality have slightly different meanings. To be religious is to be devoted to religious beliefs and practices. The meaning of *spiritual* used here is the same, but we believe that miracles are empowered and thus effectuated by the Holy Spirit or by evil spirits. We will use the term *spiritual* as an etiologic descriptor of miracles since Paul in 1 Corinthians 12:10 states that one of the gifts of the Spirit is miraculous powers. Miracles happen by the power of the Spirit.

Others report miracles in our day. There are many books and articles relating to miracles in the medical literature. Many of them call some of the advances made in medical care miracles. A few report the occurrence of miracles in which God is purported to transcend nature and heal patients with diseases that are not treatable surgically or medically. The theological literature has many more references, but only a few report miracles in the world today. There is, however, one book entitled *Megashifts* by James Rutz[9] that reports many miracles including the raising of the dead in 52 countries of the world. He states that these are documented miracles and provides the evidence to support his contention. Even so, we still have to ask if miracles occur in our society, and if have we seen them and thus are able to witness to their reality.

Miracles have never ceased because Jesus deputized and empowered his disciples to perform miracles (Luke 9:1, 2 and Luke 10:1–9). Later he told them that they would do greater things than he had done (John 14:12). His prophecy came true since his disciples were the instruments of many miracles during their ministry, but their greatest miracle was the Christianizing of the Roman Empire.

If we define a miracle as an event that is above nature and has no natural explanation, we must have testimony to its occurrence and a description of its relationship to God's intervention if there is any. Thus the claim of a miracle has to have acceptable verification. It is for this reason that the Shrine at

Lourdes has a panel of 20 persons including physicians to evaluate and certify the occurrence of a miracle occurring there. The Catholic Church has officially recognized 68 miracles that have occurred. This is in light of the claim that over 4,000 cures have occurred. The miracles at Lourdes are said to have been examined and certified as authentic by the committee. For a cure to be recognized as a miracle, it must fulfill seven criteria. It is necessary to verify the illness, which must be serious, with an irrevocable prognosis. The illness must be organic or caused by injuries. There must be no treatment at the root of the cure. The latter must be sudden and instantaneous. Finally, the renewal of functions must be total and lasting, without convalescence. The certified miracles have occurred in the last 50 years. Their criteria are addressed to healing miracles.

Medicine has set criteria for healing with its treatments. It has used these to document its cures. Most cures are surgical. Medical treatments usually only control and ameliorate disease even though in the last 50 years we have cured infections. Modern medicine has developed what are called research protocols to document the effectiveness of a treatment or medicine. Most often they require two groups of patients. One of these is given the presumed active treatment, the other, a control group, is given a placebo. The data related to the effect of the treatment is collected and subjected to statistical analysis. To document the continuation of God's intervention in illnesses many demand that we conduct experiments using standard research protocols. This would mean that investigators would use what is called the scientific method for investigation. This method is defined as follows: (1) observation and description of a phenomenon or group of phenomena; (2) formulation of a hypothesis to explain the phenomena. In physics, the hypothesis often takes the form of a causal mechanism or a mathematical relation; (3) use of the hypothesis to predict the existence of other phenomena, or to predict quantitatively the results of new observations; (4) performance of experimental tests of the predictions by several independent experimenters and properly performed experiments.

It is obvious that miracles cannot be investigated by usual scientific methods since we cannot control the variables and perform experiments. Other religious phenomena can be investigated when the person becomes his/her own control. Thus we see papers on behavioral change after salvation or after other religious experiences that do not need statistical analysis although when the data is subjected to statistical analysis the results are significant. Any research on miracles could only have an n of one since they all differ. Even so, if the change is profound and instantaneous as a result of a spiritual intervention it is significant. In our reporting of miracles in the following paragraphs each person must have had a condition that had not responded to acceptable treatments or needed radical intervention, and there was a spiritual intervention that resulted in an immediate and dramatic healing or beginning of healing of the condition. No medical or surgical treatment was administered, and the change had to persist for an observational period that was more than 24 hours. In the case of medical diseases, there had to be structural or functional change demonstrated either by technical methods or by examination.

EXAMINATION OF MIRACLES

As Gibbon said, there is more to miracles than physical healing. The miraculous changes that take place in persons with salvation experiences are rarely if ever seen in ordinary life. There are, of course, self-actualization experiences that result in changes in personality and behavioral changes, but they are only in direction and not in fundamental personality characteristics.[10] Alcoholics become abstinent 35 percent of the time when they take part in the Alcoholics Anonymous (AA) program, but most of them continue to have serious neurotic problems. The AA program is religious (deistic) in content. In contrast, alcoholics who have an authentic conversion experience not only quit drinking and have no subsequent craving for alcohol, but their personality is also radically changed. They go from being selfish to being selfless. They become altruistic and are able to relate intimately in their relationships. The same is true for drug addicts.

William James[11] in his epochal book entitled *The Varieties of Religious Experience* said that the following changes take place with conversion: (1) there is a happy mood; (2) there is a perception of truths not perceived before; (3) there is a feeling of cleanliness within and without; (4) there is a new sense of purpose; (5) the person is now able to love more intimately than before. *All* of these changes do not occur with secular interventions, and even if *some* of them do occur they never take place instantaneously. These extraordinary changes take place only by divine intervention and results for the most part are permanent. Indeed it is a rare event that persons turn their backs on God or revert to their previous behavior if their conversion has the results described by James.

I have noted that Gibbon classified speaking in tongues, visions, and prophecy as miraculous powers. Tongues are indeed of divine origin, but they are so common in the Christian world today that we can remove them from the classification of miracles. They can also be demonic in origin. There is no question that visions and prophecy are also miraculous but their frequent occurrence removes them from the extraordinary classification. They are part of our supernatural communication with God who chooses to use these means.

Prophecy is a gift of the Spirit, but much of what is considered prophecy is treacle and of no significance. There were false prophets in the days when Isaiah, Jeremiah, and Ezekiel were prophesying. This is not to deny that there are legitimate prophets in the Christian world today, but they are few in number. David Atkinson, in an excellent monograph written for the Anglican church,[12] has defined prophecy as revealed in the Bible, and according to his criteria many of the "prophets" of today do not meet biblical criteria. Therefore, I will make no effort to cite prophetic utterances as evidence of miracles. I must add that one kind of prophecy described by Atkinson, the application of scripture to the condition of society today, is still being actively given.

The casting out of demons is a miraculous event. Satan has convinced most people in our society that he does not exist, so he is free to work his destructive influence on all who are susceptible to his influence.[13] All unregenerated persons are susceptible as well as those regenerated who have weaknesses. Many Christians have areas of habitual thinking that are contrary to God's laws, and are called strongholds. Using these, Satan infects them in three ways. They can become possessed, oppressed, and obsessed. The deliverance of persons from a possession state has been considered a miracle. Jesus gave his disciples the power to deliver infected people from possession.

Even though many claim that demon possession is explainable psychiatrically, the criteria for demon possession given by Nevius[14] clearly set apart the demonically possessed persons from people with psychiatric disease. These criteria are: (1) there is the automatic presentation in the victim of a new personality both cognitively and behaviorally. They have names and attributes that harmonize with their names. Also facial expressions, bodily movements and postures harmonize with their names; (2) the personality possesses supernatural strength, knowledge, and/or intellectual power; (3) there is a complete change of moral character; (4) there is hatred to God and especially to Christ. In the light of these criteria it is obvious that many psychologically determined problems attributed to demons today are not really due to demonization. Even so there are many people in our world and especially in the Third World who are truly possessed and manifest the characteristics listed by Nevius. Oppression and obsession are more common in our society.

God is still in the business of healing miraculously. Jesus made it clear that not only were his disciples to proclaim the Gospel, but they were also to heal the sick. He healed individuals, as well as groups as large as three thousand. The blind saw, the deaf heard, the mute spoke, the lame walked, lepers were cleansed, infections of all kinds were healed, and the mentally ill were normalized. His disciples did the same although not in the same numbers. As I have noted above, God has continued this activity up to the present.

Then there are dead people restored to life. Jesus raised several to life. The most notable was Lazarus. He also raised to life the son of the widow of Nain, and the synagogue leader's daughter. In Acts Paul raised up a boy who fell from a third-floor window. In this case it is not clear that he really was dead. Peter was responsible for the raising of Dorcas who was dead.

As I have previously noted, St. Augustine claimed to have seen five people raised from the dead. As reported by Rutz, Reinhard Bonnke, a German evangelist, was responsible for the resurrection of a man in Nigeria while he was preaching. Amazingly he did not know the corpse was in the building. This event along with interviews with the doctor and the mortician who attested to his resurrection was recorded on videotape.[15]

God heals in five ways. He heals: (1) by divine intervention; (2) using modern medical interventions; (3) with time; (4) by giving a person the ability to bear his "thorn in the flesh"; and (5) he heals when a person dies and receives his or her resurrection body. Although many medical miracles occur as a result of human intervention, we will cite only cases where God intervened when prayer entreated him to heal.

Physical Healing

Case 1

A Methodist pastor in his forties had been very successful but felt led by God to leave a small Wesleyan denomination and join the United Methodist Church. He did, and in a few years he was again successful. He then began having heart attacks. These were not treatable by catheterization, but he continued his work and received medication. In time he had a total of five hospitalizations for severe angina. He was finally told that he could not continue, and since nothing could be done for him because of the involvement of all the major arteries of his heart in extensive lesions, he would in time die.

His bishop finally told him that he was going to transfer him to a small dying inner-city congregation, and when he died the church would be closed. The minister did not take the church to have it close, so he worked at helping it come alive and it thrived. Finally after several years, he had another heart attack and was hospitalized. His physician catheterized him and found that he had 75% occlusion of his major arteries. The degree of occlusion was so extensive that he could not have stents put in to open them up. He was told he was going to die in the near future.

After the initial examination, he was lying in bed in the hospital when three couples from his church came into his room. After exchanging pleasantries they announced that they were going to pray for him to be healed. He told them that he would be pleased if they did, so they came around the bed, laid hands on him and began to pray. They prayed for nearly 3 hours when all of a sudden his pain abated, his heart rate normalized, and his breathing became less labored. At that moment he knew he was healed.

The next morning his doctor came in and was amazed to find him with almost all signs of cardiac decompensation gone. The next day he took him to the catheterization lab, recatheterized him, and found that all three vessels were now completely patent. The physician, who was not a Christian, had to admit that what had happened was a miracle. He had x-ray evidence that proved it.

In recounting the story, my friend, whom I met after the miracle occurred, told me that he had an extraordinarily high cholesterol (500+ mgm/dl) so that 10 years later he had to have three bypasses, but treatment of his hypercholesterolemia has prevented any further occlusion of his arteries and he is well 20 years later. He is now in his eighties. Thus he experienced both a divine miracle and a medical miracle.

Case 2

I was attending a weekend renewal conference where we usually had a healing service on Saturday night. There were several thousand people there so we had a large number of teams praying for healing. The organization believes in the priesthood of all believers, so most of the teams were made up of lay persons (as am I and my wife). I do not know how many people we had prayed for but there was a fairly large number when a young woman who was obviously pregnant came up and told us she was depressed and wanted prayer for her depression. She did not mention any other problems. Because she was a nurse, I was particularly moved to pray for her a little more fervently than usual. We did pray for her and nothing happened. Others were waiting so she left. I did not hear from her after the meeting even though she could have contacted me through the organization.

The next year we met in another town and again my wife and I were praying in the healing service. As we prayed I noticed an older woman with a cute little red-headed baby lying on a blanket in front of me. She had moved there from another part of the auditorium while we were praying. Finally, when we had finished praying for the many who wanted prayer, the woman beckoned to me. I went over to where she was sitting and she told me that the baby's mother wanted me to pray for her child. The mother was a nurse who was on duty and could not come. The child had asthmatic bronchitis from time to time and she hoped he could be healed.

I was tired so I told her that Dr. Francis MacNutt was still praying for people and maybe she should take the baby down to where he was ministering. She very quickly said, "No, his mother wants you to pray for him!" "Why?" I asked. She responded by telling me that his mother had been at our meeting the year before and I had prayed for her depression. She was instantly healed of the depression and at the same time her asthma that she had for almost 30 years was healed too. Whereas she had regular attacks of asthma before the conference, she did not have any after and discontinued all her medications.

I did not wish to disappoint his mother. I picked up the baby and prayed for him as fervently as I could. I do not know what happened since I saw neither the mother, grandmother, nor baby again. There was no doubt in the mind of the nurse or her mother that an unexpected miracle had occurred that night when I had prayed for her depression.

The next two cases were provided by Larry Eddings, MDiv, who has had a healing ministry for over 30 years.

Case 3

Bill, a 55-year-old heavy equipment operator, came forward during a Sunday service of worship and asked for prayer as he was scheduled for heart bypass surgery the following Tuesday. I, along with the congregation, asked God how we should pray for Bill. We sensed that God said to ask him to give Bill a new heart. That was our prayer, "God, we ask you to give Bill a new heart. Amen."

On Tuesday Bill phoned and asked to talk with me. I said, "Bill, aren't you supposed to be in surgery today for the bypass surgery?" He replied, "Yes, I was scheduled for it, but when I came in they ran the whole battery of tests again to make sure that I was ready for surgery. In the process the physician said to me, 'Bill, I don't know what has happened, but you have a new heart. You don't need surgery.'" Bill never did have to undergo bypass surgery and is still, several years later, strong and healthy.

An added note about Bill: He had received Jesus as his Savior two weeks prior to this event. He asked permission to stand in the pulpit the Sunday following his healing and share with the congregation what he "saw" when we were praying for him. He shared, "I saw Jesus standing before me. He reached into my chest, unhooked and removed my old heart. Then he reached toward heaven, took a new heart and placed it in my chest and hooked it up." He witnessed God doing a divine heart transplant. That was his testimony to the congregation regarding his healing.

Case 4

Gretta was a 70-year-old woman who came from Tucson, Arizona, and attended a week-long Christian family camp in Hawaii. She came off the plane in a wheelchair. She wore a neck brace, shoulder braces, and a body brace, and walked with two canes. She had been in a car accident in which someone ran a stop sign and demolished her car and her spine. She was an Orthodox Jewish woman who had recently accepted Jesus as her Messiah and had become a Christian. In the process her husband divorced her, her children disowned her, and they all considered her dead. She harbored much bitterness and unforgiveness in her heart because of the treatment she had received from her family and also against the person who caused the accident.

As she worked through the process of forgiveness of those who had offended her and sought God's forgiveness for her bitterness toward them, she began to experience healing and release within her body. After one day she was out of the wheelchair. On the second day she removed her neck and shoulder braces. On the third day she took off her body braces and put away her walking canes. On the fourth day she danced to the tune of a lively Israeli melody, giving praise to God for her physical and also emotional healing.

Added note on Gretta: When the camp was finished, she teamed up with a 25-year-old Jewish woman who had recently become Christian and the two of them went into Waikiki and witnessed to the Jewish business community there about Yeshua, the Messiah, and his healing power as evidenced in her life. We were back in Hawaii two years later and she was still on the streets of Waikiki doing ministry.

Healing and a Miraculous Escape from Prison

Case 5

Charles Stanley in his *In Touch* magazine[16] relates the story of Brother Yun, a Chinese house church leader who was imprisoned by the Chinese government for a third time. On this occasion his legs were beaten so badly that he could not walk. The bones were probably shattered. He was so crippled his friends had to carry him to the bathroom. One day he heard a voice telling him he must escape. He was, however, in the maximum security prison at Zhengzhou and any effort to escape would mean death. Still a voice in his mind said to him, "Go now, the God of Peter is with you." When he was taken to the bathroom he decided to go, got up on his feet and started walking. "Receive my spirit when the guards shoot me," he prayed as he walked out down the stairs and out a gate that was opened only long enough for him to get through. He walked by several guards who did not see him although they were looking at him. He continued to pray. He went through a large iron gate that was strangely unlocked, across an open courtyard to the main gate of the prison. It was open and unattended. He then disappeared in a yellow taxi that just happened to be standing there. The next day he was pedaling a bicycle to a shelter that a family had prepared for him after they were told in a dream he was coming.

Not only had Yun's legs been healed in his escape but God had made it possible for him to escape. It was the same as he had done for Peter as described in Acts 12. This story has three miracles in it. They are that his legs were miraculously healed, he was able on his healed legs to walk out of a maximum security prison, and the family was informed of his coming and their task to care for him.

We do not have x-ray evidence that the bones in his legs were shattered, but the fact that he had not been able to walk on them is documentation of a healing miracle. There were many witnesses to Yun's escape.

Case 6

I was speaking in a small church outside of Antananarivo, Madagascar. After the service I was asked to go to a nearby house to pray for a hopelessly crippled man. He could not leave the house even in a wheelchair, which he and his daughter could not afford. We drove the short distance to the red brick house where they lived and went inside. In a dark room on the north side of the house sat a man in a padded chair. Outside the open window was a pig pen with a pig inside. All through our stay, our conversation was punctuated by pig grunts. The man in the chair obviously had severe arthritis. It appeared to be ankylosing spondylitis. To confirm this diagnosis, I did a brief examination. I found that he had fixation of his joints in his back, his elbows, wrists, knees, and ankles. His knees and elbows were fixed at 90 degrees. His head was bowed forward onto his chest and he could not lift it up. In all his joints he had limited mobility. He had severe, advanced ankylosing spondylitis!

My interpreter explained to him why we were there. After the initial interchange, I asked him if he was a Christian. He said he was not. I then told him that my prayers would be more effective if he was a Christian and asked him if he would like to become one. He said he would. After he made the transaction, I told him we were now going to pray for his healing. I did not expect anything to happen since he was so crippled, but in obedience to the Lord's commandment to heal the sick, I prayed. As I did I visualized his joints being freed up. I could do this since I had worked with patients with his disease in the pain clinic at my hospital. It is difficult to chat through an interpreter, but we did the best we could to comfort him and departed. I thought no more about what we had done and in a few days came back to the United States.

Two years later I got an e-mail from the missionary I had worked with telling me that he had gone back to the church to preach. He noticed that there was a padded chair on the front row. Just before the service started the man we had prayed for walked in with his legs straightened and his arms swinging by his sides. He took his seat and participated enthusiastically in the worship service. It is a tradition in Madagascar to have prayers after the service with all the people in a circle holding hands. My missionary friend said that as they prayed the people began dancing. This is customary in their worship. He looked over to where our arthritic man was and noticed that he was dancing as enthusiastically as the other worshipers. He did not describe the position of his head. Curious, I wrote him back and asked him if he could lift up his head. He answered, "He lifted up his head!"

Conversion

Let us now turn to the miracles that occur with conversion. I am reluctant to cite these since they are so common. Yet I will describe the dramatic changes that occurred in two persons with whom I had professional contact and who were miraculously changed.

Case 7

A 29-year-old woman was a patient in the federal narcotics hospital in Lexington, Kentucky. I was conducting a research project on the family life of heroin addicts. I was interested in knowing what kind of homes they came from since I wanted to know if their parenting or lack of it in childhood was etiologic to their problem. At the end of my examination, I also had questions concerning any religious experiences or instruction they had and their hope for the future after their incarceration.

In my inquiry she told me that for five years she had been a prostitute supporting her pimp, her boyfriend, and herself. She also had come from a profoundly dysfunctional home. She had been sexually abused as a child and had been promiscuous before becoming hooked on heroin and becoming a prostitute to support her addiction. When I came to the questions concerning religious instruction she said she had none. When I asked her about any religious experiences, she said she had. I asked when it occurred. She said, "Yesterday." "In this place?" I asked surprised. "No not here," was her retort. Curious, I asked her to tell me about it.

"Well, we have this secretary on our unit who is a pastor's wife. She often would offer to take us to religious meetings. We would go just to get out of the place. Three days ago she asked us if we would like to go down to the Coliseum to hear a speaker. She could only take 11 of us so we had an election to see who could go and I got elected. It came time to go, and we got in the van and left. When we got there, the sign over the entrance said, 'David Wilkerson Crusade Here This Week.' I did not know who he was so I went in wondering what he was going to say." He was the founder of Teen Challenge, a ministry to addicted teens.

"After we got seated we sang a couple of songs and this man came out with a big black Bible and prayed. Then he began to speak. He first of all began to ask questions. They were the same questions I had been asking myself. The only difference was that he had answers that came from the Bible. I began to get scared, so as he talked I felt I had to get out of there. Finally he came to the end of his talk, and as he did he asked all those who wanted to give their lives to Christ come to the front. I thought, now is my chance. I will leave and wait in the foyer for the rest of the group. I got up and walked to the end of the row expecting to turn right and go out. But you know what, Doc? I couldn't turn right. I had to turn left and I didn't walk. I ran to the front! Tears were streaming down my face and I could hardly see, but when I looked around the other 10 girls were there too." She described her experience with tears again streaming down her face.

My next question was, "Do you have any hope for the future?" "You bet I do," she said, "I have Jesus."

"Where are you going when you get out?" "I don't know, but I am not going back to the street! God has a safe place for me." And she didn't go back. She went first to a Teen Challenge center and then to a rehabilitation farm they operated in Pennsylvania and in time went to college. I lost track of her then.

I need to point out that the average amount of time a patient stayed off drugs after discharge from Lexington was less than 6 months. She was off 3 years. Earlier I met others who had gone through the Teen Challenge program and had been off for 7 to 10 years. In my professional experience, the recidivism rate for heroin addiction was nearly 100 percent, but for Teen Challenge it is only 25 percent.

Case 8

One of my students at the seminary was a young black man who was outstanding as a student. At the beginning of the semester I asked the students to give their personal witness to the class. He told us that he grew up in a dysfunctional home and that in his late teen years he got addicted to marijuana and then to crack cocaine. He then became a street person, sleeping under bridges and eating out of dumpsters and garbage cans. He did this for three years when God sovereignly reached down and drew him to himself. He found shelter and in time got a job and a place to live. He joined a church where he was received with love. He then decided to go to college and enrolled in the top state university where he majored in sociology. After he got his degree he went to graduate school and got a master's degree in the same subject. Not satisfied with what he had learned, he came to the seminary and took all the counseling courses we offered. His thesis for his MTh degree was focused on counseling in the black church. He was incensed when he found that none of 40 pastors he interviewed did any counseling.

Demonization and Deliverance

Case 9

A 19-year-old ethnic Malagasy woman was brought to me because she would be violently thrown to the floor, whereupon two male voices would come out of her claiming to be former kings of Madagascar. They spoke Malagasy. This was unusual since she had been raised in France and only spoke French. Her parents, who taught in a French university, were a witch and a warlock. She had been sent back to Madagascar because of her spells, with the idea that her grandmother could find some help for her. None was available in France. She had come to a healing community where it was recognized that she was demon possessed, but the local people including the chaplain and physician could not bring about deliverance. After her history was presented, I had the names of the two kings written on the blackboard that was in the room. I then had her brought in and after I was introduced, I asked the interpreter to have her say, "Jesus is Lord."

She had barely begun to utter the sound of J when she was violently thrown to the floor, where she lay thrashing about. The locals got very excited and began yelling at the demons. I told them to stop since I knew demons were not deaf. I then called the demons by name and told them to come out and be taken away for disposition. I hardly got the words out of my mouth when she blinked her eyes and sat up. We helped her to her feet and had her sit in a chair next to me. I then, through my interpreter, told her that to maintain her freedom she needed to accept Christ as her Savior. She eagerly agreed and made the transaction. I brought her back the next day during my instruction period and had her say, "Jesus is Lord." She said, "Jesus really is my Lord!" She had no further spells during a follow-up period of one year.

Case 10

I gave a lecture in a local church on demonization and deliverance. At the end I asked any persons who wanted deliverance to come forward and

I would pray for them. A young couple did come up and as I started to pray for the woman, she rested in the Spirit before I could do any deliverance. I had not discerned that she was demon possessed. I then prayed for her husband and he too rested. As I was preparing to pray for the next person, she suddenly burst out alternately speaking in demonic tongues and screaming. I had to attend to her and prayed that what I thought was one demon to come out of her. She got quiet for a few seconds and then began to scream again. I commanded a second demon to come out and again she quieted for a few seconds before she screamed a third time. I then commanded a third demon to come out and she quieted, sat up, and was freed. I did not have time to find out what the demons' names were since she was screaming so loudly. I later found out that her father had sexually abused her when she was 15, and when she got pregnant, he forced her to have an abortion. She had lived a rebellious life since then. She was promiscuous, having had three illegitimate children and suffering from *pseudologia fantastica* (fantastic lying).

Since her deliverance she has been a different person, telling the truth and making an effort to learn how to be a good wife to her husband. She also had to give her life to Christ, and have her postabortion syndrome healed.

Multiplication of Food

Case 11

Father Richard Thomas, Society of Jesus, was appointed to Our Lady's Youth Center in El Paso, Texas. He had a professional staff of psychologists and social workers. His center was supported to a great extent by the United Fund. Shortly after he took over as director he returned to New Orleans, where he had graduated from seminary, to attend an alumni reunion. While there he attended a prayer meeting at the invitation of his classmate, Al Cohen. There they asked Father Thomas if they could pray for Mr. Cohen. He told them they could and they laid on hands and prayed. After they finished Father Thomas noted that he had a headache, so he went back to his room and went to bed. He awakened about 2:00 A.M. and the room was filled with a brilliant blue light. He also felt the presence of God so powerfully that he could hardly move. This finally left him and he went back to sleep. After the reunion he left for El Paso, but on the plane he had the impression that he was to terminate the employment of the psychologists and social workers and return any money from the United Fund that had not been spent. Back home he did this obediently.

Wondering what to do next, he felt compelled to go preach on the streets, although Catholic priests did not usually preach on the street. When he did, people got converted. His converts formed themselves into a group who met with him at the center as a small community. The community grew. When Christmas came his people wanted to do a project for the poor, so at the suggestion of a U.S. mail carrier who was a member, they decided to go across the border and feed the scavengers in the Juarez, Mexico, garbage dump.

From their preliminary observations they estimated that there would be 150 people. They prepared enough food for the 150. They went to the dump and set up their tables and called the people to come get the meal. Three hundred fifty people showed up. Dismayed, Father Thomas' people wondered what they were going to do. "Rick" (Father Richard) told them to feed the people until the food ran out. They began and they kept feeding until they had fed them all. When they looked at their remaining food supplies, they realized that they had as much food as they began with. The food had been multiplied. They then took the residuals and fed children in orphanages until the food really did run out.

This story is documented in a book called *Miracles in El Paso.*[17] However, the version I have rendered was related to me by Rick and verified by some of his people. There were many other miracles that occurred in Our Lady's Youth Center ministry, but this was the most dramatic.

THE BLIND SAW AND THE LAME WALKED

I belong to a group that sponsored major Holy Spirit conferences. We held one in New Orleans where about 25,000 people were in attendance. One of our plenary speakers was Reinhard Bonnke. On Saturday night things did not go well since one of the minor speakers spoke way beyond his allotted time and no one cut him off. Even so, Bonnke plunged in, giving a very evangelical teaching. At the end he asked for those who wanted healing to come forward. As we watched, four blind people were led forward and five wheelchairs were rolled up to the area in front of the stage. Bonnke went down to them and prayed for them and others. The blind saw and the lame got up out of their wheelchairs and walked. They all testified that they had indeed been blind and lame for years and that they now could see and walk. I was not able to examine these people before and after their healing, but their personal testimony and our witness of their healing verified God's intervention.

The most miraculous of the responses to Bonnke's presentation occurred earlier when he gave the attendees an invitation to accept Christ as their savior. It resulted in the positive response of over 2,000 Catholic nuns and priests. Bonnke thought that there had been a mistake. Surely they had misunderstood him. But no, it was no mistake, they really were seriously responding. The counselors were overwhelmed after the service by such a large group.

I can describe many other miracles such as visions and speaking in tongues, both real and unknown, but they are recorded elsewhere. The reader is referred to those resources that are readily available.

SUMMARY

The described miracles do not completely meet the criteria we set at the beginning. Some of these discrepancies have to do with our lack of knowledge concerning the course of the healing. For instance, we do not know how immediately the healing of the person with ankylosing spondylitis took place. We do know that no medical interventions were applied, so his healing had to be by God's intervention. I also do not know the circumstances of my student's healing from crack cocaine addiction since I was not a participant in his healing. I do know that there was no medical treatment. Also we have no knowledge of the amount of anatomical damage that the Jewish woman in Hawaii had. We do know that she had braces prescribed by her physicians, so they must have had evidence that she had anatomical damage.

The question, "Do religious or spiritual miracles occur today?" has been answered. Edward Gibbon has said that there is an unbroken succession of miraculous powers in the church throughout its history. In spite of the cessationist's view that miracles ceased at the end of the apostolic era, St. Augustine's report of miracles that he had witnessed gave the lie to that claim. Throughout time others have reported miracles in spite of constant denial of the verity of their claims. The author has reported a series of cases that he has personally been able to observe or verify by reliable witnesses. The answer to our question, then, is yes. Miracles do still happen today. Claims to the contrary are then based on passion or prejudice and are, therefore, not rational.

CONCLUSIONS

Miracles do occur in the world today. In spite of protestations by some scientists, documented events occur regularly both in this country and in the rest of the world. Most of the miracles are similar to if not replicas of the miracles Jesus did and those that have been reported through the entire history of the church. There is no reason why we should not expect them to continue.

NOTES

1. Aurelius Augustine (1950), *City of God*, Marcus Dods, trans., New York: Random House.

2. John Calvin (1960), *Institutes of the Christian Religion*, John T. McNeill, ed., Philadelphia: Westminster, 2, 1454.

3. Benjamin Breckinridge Warfield (1918), *Counterfeit Miracles*, New York: Charles Scribner's Sons.

4. Edward Gibbon (1993), *Decline and Fall of the Roman Empire*, with an introduction by Hugh Trevor-Roper, New York: Knopf, 1, 264, 288.

5. Benedictus de Spinoza (1951), *Theologico-Political Treatise*, R.H.M. Elwes, trans., New York: Dover.

6. David Hume (1963), *An Enquiry Concerning Human Understanding*, LaSalle, IL: Open Court.

7. Richard Dawkins (2006), *The God Delusion*, Boston: Houghton Mifflin.

8. Christopher Hitchens (2007), *God Is Not Great: How Religion Poisons Everything*, New York: Twelve/Hachette Book Group USA/Warner.

9. James Rutz (2005), *Megashifts*, Colorado Springs: Empowerment Press.

10. Abraham Maslow (1964), *Religions, Values, and Peak-Experiences*, Columbus: Ohio State University Press.

11. William James (1902), *The Varieties of Religious Experience: A Study in Human Nature*, New York: Longmans Green.

12. David Atkinson (1977), *Prophecy*, Bramcotes Not: Grove Books.

13. D. G. Barnhouse (1965), *The Invisible War*, Grand Rapids: Zondervan.

14. John Nevius (1968), *Demon Possession*, Grand Rapids: Kregel.

15. Rutz (2005), *Megashifts*, 9–13.

16. Erin Gieschen (April, 2007), The Heavenly Man, *In Touch*, 12–16.

17. Rene Laurentin (1982), *Miracles in El Paso*, Grand Rapids: Servant Books.

REFERENCES

Atkinson, David L. (1977), *Prophecy*, Bramcotes Not: Grove Books.

Augustine, Aurelius (1950), *City of God*, Marcus Dods, trans., New York: Random House.

Barnhouse, Donald G. (1965), *The Invisible War*, Grand Rapids: Zondervan.

Calvin, John (1960), *Institutes of the Christian Religion*, John T. McNeill, ed., Vol. 2., Philadelphia: Westminster.

Dawkins, Richard (2006), *The God Delusion*, Boston: Houghton Mifflin.

Gibbon, Edward (1993), *Decline and Fall of the Roman Empire*, with an introduction by Hugh Trevor-Roper, Vol. 1, New York: Knopf.

Gieschen, Erin (April, 2007), The Heavenly Man, *In Touch*, 12–16.

Hitchens, Christopher (2007), *God Is Not Great: How Religion Poisons Everything*, New York: Twelve/Hachette Book Group USA/Warner.

Hume, David (1963), *An Enquiry Concerning Human Understanding*, LaSalle, IL: Open Court.

James, William (1902), *The Varieties of Religious Experience: A Study in Human Nature*, New York: Longmans Green.

Laurentin, Rene (1982), *Miracles in El Paso*, Grand Rapids: Servant Books.

Maslow, Abraham (1964), *Religions, Values, and Peak-Experiences*, Columbus: Ohio State University Press.

Nevius, John L. (1968), *Demon Possession*, Grand Rapids: Kregel.

Rutz, James (2005), *Megashifts*, Colorado Springs: Empowerment Press.

Spinoza, Benedictus de (1951), *Theologico-Political Treatise*, R.H.M. Elwes, trans., New York: Dover.

Warfield, Benjamin Breckenridge (1918), *Counterfeit Miracles*, New York: Charles Scribner's Sons.

CHAPTER 16

ON THE LIMITS OF SCIENTIFIC INVESTIGATION: MIRACLES AND INTERCESSORY PRAYER

Richard L. Gorsuch

A common definition of miracles would be an event or condition produced by direct intervention of God. An example of a miracle in the New Testament is in the feeding of the 5,000. It occurred when Jesus was teaching a multitude of people. The disciples noted that it was late and suggested the people be dismissed so that they could find food. Jesus countered by asking them to share the food they had with the people. The amount they had to share was small. Yet after Jesus prayed over the food, not only was everyone fed but there were more baskets of food left over than they had when they started. This was impressive to the New Testament writers as it is reported multiple times in the New Testament (Mt 14:15–21, Mk 6:34–44, Lk 9:10–17, Jn 6:1–14).

The feeding of the 5,000 can be seen as a *miracle of the heart*. People saw Jesus and the disciples sharing, and so also shared their food. What food they did not absolutely need, they placed in the baskets for others to have. But how do we evaluate this event if we assume that (1) people did not have any significant amount of food to share, and (2) in his giving thanks for the food Jesus prayed that the food would multiply to feed all of the people? Could it have happened as a true miracle, that is, caused directly by God? To answer this question, we need to define further what is meant by natural laws that govern a causal chain of events and the limitations of that paradigm.

Supernatural intervention seems at variance with science, a prime source of truth in the contemporary world. When even the Templetons, who financially support research on religion, see the classical scientific experiment as the best method to establish truth, it would seem that the truth of miracles must be based in scientific experiments. Some experiments have been done on the efficacy of intercessory prayer. Do such studies prove or disprove miracles? Is there evidence that a supernatural force suspends natural laws to cause a miraculous outcome in answer to prayer? Is this the best way to phrase the question?

The purpose of this chapter is to evaluate whether science, and the natural laws that result, and miracles, to which history and experience seem to testify readily, are compatible paradigms. Are science and miracles both possible? If miracles are possible, then evaluating whether or when miracles have happened or are occurring is the task of scholars in the appropriate disciplines within the humanities.

THE NATURE OF SCIENCE

To understand how science may or may not be able to establish miracles, the nature of science needs to be understood. Is the nature of science such that it can examine miracles, or does its examining miracles remove the miraculous?

The nature of truth, even scientific truth, has been questioned in the current philosophical position of postmodernism (Murphy 1997). Postmodernism arises from the failure of modern philosophy to have found a basis on which truth can be logically built, that is, a secure base that no one can doubt. This skeptical analysis was found already in ancient Greek philosophy. It was dormant throughout the Middle Ages, which ignored the issue or assumed the foundation of all truth to be in divine revelation. Descartes (1701/1990) is the prototype for premodern philosophy in that he assumed God as the foundation of all truth, but he also raised the questions that led to postmodernism.

Descartes sought for a firm foundation for truth by seeking that which he could not doubt. He found that he could doubt virtually everything. Of course, it can be hard to doubt the existence of the chair on which one sits, but some doubt can always be suggested. For example, perhaps the chair is the result of a posthypnotic suggestion and an audience would see that he was just sitting on air. Obviously, this is unlikely but the quest for a firm foundation for knowledge is that it be completely unchallengeable at all levels.

Descartes found there was only one unchallengeable fact, and summarized it in his famous "Cogito, ergo sum." This is generally translated as "I think, therefore I am." The one undeniable fact was that he was thinking, for otherwise how could he challenge truths? I believe his equation as stated is too optimistic a position. It would be better translated as "thinking, therefore being," for "I" has no unchallengeable referent. Descartes quickly dismissed his own skepticism with reference to God and built his philosophy despite his skepticism, as had other medieval philosophers. Unlike Descartes, the post-modernists take this skepticism seriously. For the postmodernist all human intellectual enterprises are suspect because all conclusions can be doubted.

As postmodernism developed, Kuhn (1970) published his work on scientific revolutions. This is a historical treatise which suggests that paradigms—models of thought that attempt to describe reality—are important in science, and determine much of the field's activity. Our paradigms arise from our culture and from the history of the science and its past paradigms. These interact with the facts identified or data collected, and shape the expression of the facts in theories, thus specifying the range of research seen as legitimate. And the paradigms of science itself change over time, with scientific revolutions arising from the replacement of one paradigm with another.

Combining the skepticism inherent in intellectual enterprises with Kuhn's notion that science is determined in part by the intellectual enterprises of scientific paradigms raises a serious question about how we define science. Can it be defined sufficiently to encompass the most basic element of all scientific disciplines? What is it that distinctly separates it from nonscientific endeavors? Obviously, the distinction cannot lie in such characteristics as integrity, theory building, or paradigms, nor can it be in publishing scholarly articles. All academic disciplines share these.

I have suggested (Gorsuch 2002a, 2002/2007) that the identifying characteristic of science is seen in the research article. All disciplines that claim to be scientific have a distinctive element not found in papers in other disciplines: a methods section. The criterion for an adequate methods section is that it tells readers how they can replicate the study. Indeed, no finding is taken seriously until it is replicated. (In speaking tours at academic institutions, my audiences have always agreed that this is an essential characteristic of science.) Any conclusion is tentative until it has been replicated. For example, the Festinger, Riecken, and Schachter (1956) book, *When Prophecy Fails*, examined a group that had prophesied the end of the world. When that did not happen, the leaders decided it was because God had spared the world so that they could preach about a new era. However, others (Dein 2001) could not replicate this result with other such groups and so it has been dropped from many social psychology texts.

When sufficient replications occur, the consistency of the replicable data is referred to as a fact. It is then incorporated into theory, which is then tested in other experiments to see if results are consistent with the theory. Science finds that which can be replicated, and these are considered the norm for that phenomenon, natural laws. Gorsuch (2002a, 2002/2007) has labeled such truth as nomothetic. Only that which is nomothetic, that is, which is replicable and so law-like, is found by science. All nonreplicable events are considered unscientific, and unworthy of further scientific exploration. By the definition of miracles noted above, nomothetic science cannot address miracles, for the latter are violations of the nomothetic. The feeding of the 5,000, as miracle, is a nonreplicable event and so science lacks the tools to investigate whether it was a miracle.

REDUCTIONISTIC SCIENCE

Many psychologists have argued that religion and miracles are a function of nomothetic natural forces. They have sought to explain religion as a function of other variables. Of course religion is impacted by many forces, from the simplest, "how can they be saved if they have not heard," to the impact of one's family and community of origin. That is not the issue here. The issue is that of explaining away religion by attributing it to other variables having nothing to do with the truth of religion itself.

Freud is the most famous reductionist. It is questionable in what sense he should be called a scientist, in that he left us no explicit methods by which his work can be replicated. Such methods would need to control for alternative explanations, including, for example, post hoc interpretations. In the record of his work we do not have operational definitions to reduce the interpretation of just any data to support a complex theory. Nor does he give us the necessary checks against the problems of subjective evaluations. We need from him a methods section so there can be formal replication. However, he is accorded the status of a famous scientist by laypersons and professionals, alike.

Freud's argument in *The Future of an Illusion* (1927/1964) is that religion is a result of infantile projection of the father figure. Therefore, religion is, as the title suggests, an illusion. Faber (2002) has taken up Freud's psychoanalytic approach and his purpose is to demonstrate that "the supernatural is a human fabrication with no basis in reality" (p. 7). He argues that it is rooted entirely in human subjectivity. Others have taken reductionistic positions, but with a scientific base. In multiple studies of motivation, Cattell and Child (1975) considered religion as an attitude based in motivational needs.

There are two major problems with positions such as Freud and Cattell. It is well stated in the introduction to Freud's book. He *assumes* that religion is false (Freud 1927/1964), as does Cattell (Gorsuch 2002/2007). If it is false then it must be the function of wish fulfillment, anthropomorphizing, subjective motivation, or other such forces. That does not test the validity of religion. It merely rules it out of the arena of scientific investigations by assuming it to be unreality.

The second major problem with reductionism follows from the first: it fails to consider any evidence that religion is true. Nonetheless, for many of us, the truth of a religious proposition is of prime importance. Faber (2002) states that "The person who attempts to prove or disprove the naturalistic nature of religious experience in a manner similar to that which he would use to prove or disprove the heliocentric theory of the solar system or the molecular theory of chemical bonding will fall flat on his face" (p. 3). Of course this follows when one assumes religion is false. Such lack of concern for the evidence of religions permits Faber to talk about religion as a single class, with only minor reference to variations in religions. The reductionism of Freud and Cattell makes their work irrelevant to the task of understanding how miracles and science relate. Thus Freud, Cattell, Farber, and others in a reductionistic mode are irrelevant to the present task.

THE LIMITS OF SCIENCE

As science is nomothetic and so addresses that which replicates, all non-replicable events are not scientific. It is not that science rejects them but rather that they are outside the scope and paradigm of science so that science cannot even discuss them scientifically. To discuss them is to leave the area of replicable events. However, our question is, are there nonreplicate events? If there are, can they be studied? What would be the rules of evidence? Do they apply to miracles?

Gorsuch (2002a, 2002/2007) suggests that there are nonreplicable events. Consider any major event in a person's life, such as graduation from high school. Can a person replicate that event? No, as the prior experience of graduating would make it a different event for that person. In like manner, one can not replicate reading this book because the first reading changes the nature of the experience. Nor can anyone replicate any major historical event. The experiences of George Washington and his contributions to the founding of the United States cannot be replicated. They are unique to him and his times. Therefore they are outside of science. Indeed it seems that, by the definition of science, many of the most important events in a person's life are nonreplicable and so outside of the scope of scientific inquiry.

The humanities are disciplines that consider nonreplicable events (Gorsuch 2002). The most unique events are communicated by art and literature. The former communicates unique experiences in a nonverbal language form whereas the latter uses verbal language to communicate. History is the examination of nonreplicable events in other time periods.

Whereas science is referred to as nomothetic, nonreplicable events are referred to as ideothetic events (Gorsuch 2002a, 2002/2007). These include all the areas of the humanities, every discipline which does not use replication as its *modus operandum*.

Being ideothetic rather than nomothetic means that other evidence is used instead of replicable experiments. The courts are good examples of the search for truth in ideothetic situations. There is no way the crime can be replicated but truth is sought as to who committed the crime. Instead of replication, courts examine multiple sources of evidence, including credible witnesses, physical evidence, and circumstantial evidence. The circumstantial evidence used in ideothetic analysis generally includes the results of nomothetic science. If the evidence supports the defendant having violated the law, then he or she is convicted. As this court example implies, the important decisions that are made about a person's life may be primarily ideothetic. These include basic questions such as, "Does she or he love me?" "Shall I apply for this graduate school?" and "Am I ready to retire?"

ISSUES OF EVIDENCE

Circumstantial evidence is important in establishing ideothetic truth. Consider the case of the Old (OT) and New Testaments (NT). The life and times reported there are supported by considerable widely accepted circumstantial evidence. While the exact events are not recorded elsewhere, it is known that Jericho existed and had its walls destroyed on multiple occasions. The history of Jerusalem in other reports is consistent with the biblical record, as is the knowledge of Roman practices in the NT era. Jesus' trial and crucifixion ring true to the historians' expectation. The Dead Sea Scrolls are consistent with OT and NT. While circumstantial evidence is circumstantial, it is important evidence in building a case for the general accuracy of the Bible. This is in addition to the credible witnesses, those who told others of the events and of the many people involved.

Credible witnesses may include the many authors to whom books of the Bible are attributed. It may also include the canonization process, which involved many more people. While these were not witnesses to the original events, they could witness to the usage of these books as true in their own traditions. Since nothing can be completely proved beyond a doubt, some people accept and some reject the conclusions drawn by Christians from this evidence.

Contrasting with the circumstantial evidence for the Bible is the circumstantial evidence for the religion-like fervor of the German Nazis' notion of the divine ordination of the Aryan race to establish the thousand-year Reich and bring order and its "true destiny" to the world. There was no phenomenological, heuristic, or circumstantial evidence to vindicate any element of that worldview: no evidence for the existence of Uhr Menschen, no evidence of a divine mandate for Nazi or Prussian conquest, and no evidence for Jews being the counterforce to this divine order or the source of social evil. Circumstantial evidence is important in the search for ideothetic truth.

Miracles fall within the ideothetic realm as they are by definition nonreplicable events, but that does not mean they cannot be studied. As with any ideothetic event, they can be studied through credible witnesses and circumstantial evidence. What makes a witness credible is the experience of the person and how we perceive that experience. Who are credible witnesses for discussing miracles? That will vary depending on one's paradigm. If one is a Christian, then the NT writings are credible witnesses. The feeding of the 5,000 is accepted as a miracle because credible witnesses have reported it. Note that the scriptures do not discriminate between the two types of miracles that may underlie the feeding of the 5,000. Whether it is a miracle of the heart or an actual physical miracle will depend upon the judgment of the reader and the reader's religious paradigm.

Might there be conditions under which a nomothetic event has ideographic underpinnings? Actually this is a major position of some who pray for miracles. Murphy (1997) formalizes this by means of a model in which God works at the quantum physics level. The quantum physics level is characterized by its lacking the property of any predictability. In her view, God's intervention is at this level and it works its way up the causal chain to help the person. The observed cause is just the last step of the original divine action at the quantum level of the ideothetic event.

The view that God may work through nomothetic chains appears common. Casteel's (1955) classical approach assumes God works through the chain of events: "Even the simplest of our requests may entail the changing of a great many very powerful factors before an answer can come" (p. 117). Perhaps the feeding of the 5,000 was a miracle both in that people had food to bring and that they shared it, and that God multiplied the total quantity to insure that it was more than adequate. In illness, people do pray for the physician and other factors in the perceived causal chain of events that may cure an illness. Ideothetic and nomothetic are not mutually exclusive.

RESEARCH ON INTERCESSORY PRAYER

Nomothetic research on miracles can study many facets of it. Who reports miracles? What kind of miracles do they report? What are the conditions under which miracles are reported? What are the antecedents of reported miracles? What is the impact of the reported miracle on that person and on others? Such questions have been raised in regards to prayer. Research on multiple aspects of prayer can be found in Brown (1994) and Frances and Astley (2001).

There are several systems to classify prayer that have been used in research. Some systems are concerned with types of prayer, as historically classified. Casteel discusses prayer as adoration, confession, thanksgiving, and prayer as asking and receiving. The last divides into petitions for oneself and intercession for others. This is similar to Poloma and Gallup's (1991) division into ritual, petitionary, conversational, and meditative; or to Hood, Morris, and Harvey's (1993) contemplative and liturgical. Their model includes two forms of petitionary prayer, in which the goal of one is blessings and the goal of the other, material things. Others categorize prayer as to what it is based

on and whether it is inward (self), outward (others), or upward (divine) oriented (Ladd and Spilka 2002, 2006).

While each of these systems is appropriate in its context, this current
project needs a somewhat different perspective. It needs to categorize prayer
in terms of the source of the effect, and whether that effect can be nomothetic
or ideothetic. Only the latter would include miracles.

Prayer may have effects through two sources that would be replicable.
Together these two have been referred to as subjective effects, although
whether that refers to subject effects or effects only seen subjectively is
open to interpretation. This category consists of two subcategories. First
are the effects on the person who is being prayed for, the *personal effect* of
prayer. Do they feel the prayer has been effective? This is the only criterion
when the intercessory prayer is for inner healing of emotional and spiritual
health.

If the conditions under which the person feels the prayer is helpful are
replicated, then a personal effect has been found. This may be the placebo effect. The placebo effect is found in research on drugs, which finds that many
people feel they are helped even when they are in a control group given a
placebo, a physiologically inert substance resembling the pill being tested.
These are rather large effects and are nontrivial, but they occur from the
psychological impact of believing that one may be receiving a helping drug.
In many research designs, these are not distinguished from spontaneous recovery; to separate them would require two control groups for which no one
prayed, one believing someone is praying for them and another group who
were not told the researchers would pray for them. These effects may occur
with all types of prayer, including intercessory prayer.

In addition to personal effects, there may also be *social effects*. This effect
would arise from the impact of the prayers on the person's social network.
Thus a congregation may be more supportive when they are all praying for
a person, and that may lead to helpful communication or other support provided by the social network. The support could be psychological or physical.
These effects would occur to the extent that the community knows about the
praying.

There is one effect that is both social and personal: when a person knows
that others are praying for him or her. The effect is social in that communication of the praying is necessary for the effect and personal in that it affects
the person psychologically and is open to a placebo interpretation.

Personal and some social effects have been investigated by psychologists
for a long time. Brown (1994) and Frances and Astley (2001) are appropriate introductions to that literature. Ladd (2007) has laid out a system for
examining prayer psychologically. It encompasses the motivation to prayer,
the qualities of prayer including physical postures, the experiential content
of prayer, and the ramifications of prayer. While he recognizes a possible

supernatural efficacy of prayer, that is external to the psychological model. The psychological model is restricted to nomothetic processes.

With intercessory prayer, there need not be a personal or social effect. The effect may happen without the person knowing it and without involving the person's social network. Such an effect would be objective. Some have tried to research intercessory prayer for such effects.

CURRENT INTERCESSORY PRAYER RESEARCH

The purpose of intercessory prayer research is to determine if prayer has an objective effect. It is researchable and several studies have been conducted. However these studies are not without their problems.

Research Design

The purpose of a research design to test for the effect of intercessory prayer is to eliminate alternative explanations for the effect if found. First, control must be made for other conditions that might affect the outcome. For example, Galton (1872/2001) concluded that prayer showed no effects because the sovereigns, who were prayed for by everyone in the nation, lived only 64 years, which is the shortest of 11 groups reported, who were not prayed for by everyone. Of course, there were other differences between the lives of sovereigns and other occupations of that time. It may be that the sovereigns, having often intermarried with each other, had a different genetic base. Or perhaps they ate only the best meats, which in that time would be the fatty meats. Of course, there are a host of other differences that could affect the health of one group compared to another. There are so many alternative explanations for Galton's results that they cannot be informative. The study is only useful in showing the need for controlled studies.

The problems of Galton's study are now answered by using randomly assigned intervention and control groups. The control group does not receive the intervention, in this case, intercessory prayer, but, because of the random assignment, will not on the average differ from the intervention group. The random assignment controls for all possible influences that need to be controlled regardless of our knowledge of them.

Other alternative explanations that must be addressed in prayer research concern the fact that research design must control for the alternative explanation of the placebo effect, in this case, an effect on the person from knowing that prayers are being offered for him or her. This can be controlled either by having a group that thinks they may be prayed for when no such prayers are being made or by not telling people in the intervention group that they are being prayed for. They are blind as to whether they are in the intervention group.

Research on intercessory prayer needs to control for someone, including physicians and nurses when health is the issue, treating the patient differently because prayers are being given for them. Hence people involved with the person must be blind as to whether they are in the experimental or control group. Evaluating the outcome also must be controlled. A person reading a file for outcome data may make different assumptions and mistakes if he or she knows which person is in which group. Hence the evaluations must also be blind.

Therefore a study needs to randomly assign participants to the intervention group and to at least one control group who believe they may be prayed for just as much as the intervention group. A second random control group would be useful to establish recovery rates for people who have not been told they may have someone praying for them. The study needs to be blind to the condition of the participants in three senses: the participants are blind, others who interact with the participants are blind, and those who enter and process the data are blind to the conditions of each participant.

The Criterion Problem

Prayer research has only investigated areas in which the outcomes would be generally viewed the same by all observers, such as survival of illness and quick recovery. If the research moves to other areas, then who is praying for what may matter. I succumbed to the temptation to pray that the Cowboys, in an important football game, would intercept the opponent's pass on the next play. To my delight it happened! However, there may have been some mighty prayers on the other side for, a couple of plays later, the Cowboys fumbled the ball and the opponent recovered. Such trivial cases aside, the answer to one person's prayer may be offset by another's. An example would be of a prayer for speedy recovery of the patient that is offset by others praying for a nurse, a prayer that God could answer by having the patient stay in the hospital a few more days to help the nurse. These effects are countered by random assignment but may result in lower effect outcomes.

The answer to prayer is assumed in these studies to be a reduced death rate. It is used as the primary criterion in the studies of prayer noted below. However, is this criterion always the best? Consider the case of a child with major trauma to the brain followed by irreversible coma. It was obvious that doctors accepted that the boy would never recover most brain functions. What is the prayer in this case? My prayer was for either a healing miracle or that the boy would "go to be with God." He died, and I believe that was an appropriate answer to prayer in this case. But prayer research finds that to be evidence against prayer.

The criterion of survival is problematic because Christians may not pray for life in times when others would expect them to do so. Consider Htu Htu

Lay, a Christian Karen leader against the oppression of his people by the Burmese military government (FreeBurmaRangers.org). Given that his life may often be in danger, we on the outside would expect him to pray for safety. That is not what he prays for. Instead he prays "not that I may live a long time, for we all must die. I pray that when I die I shall be doing God's work." Long life is not the criterion that is the most relevant to many Christians.

Gorsuch (2002/2007) notes that one Christian perspective is that God is less concerned with long life and more concerned with how that life is lived and with suffering. Jesus in the Garden (Luke 22) prayed for release from the task that led to the crucifixion, but added, "Your will be done." Suffering on the cross was the result of that prayer. How would this be judged in research on intercessory prayer?

The NT has virtually no passages that tell us how to live longer. Nor does it address this topic at a length suggesting it is a major issue. Yet there are passages about comforting the afflicted and visiting the sick. Healing is a topic and a focus of Jesus' miracles, but these were mostly with long-term infirmities and only occasionally about critical illness. Even Jesus lived a short life (33 years), and died with minimal suffering for a crucifixion. God seems more concerned with suffering than with long life. Perhaps some deaths should be put in the "God answered prayer" category.

Whether a prayer is answered is always open to the post hoc problem. One may consider a yes or a no to be the answer to a prayer. Such situations are common in ideothetic life. Numerous questions can be considered answered with either response. These include an application to graduate school, taking a driving license test, and proposing marriage. However, these are simple questions with relatively objective answers. For prayers with numerous possible answers, such as "God, what major should I study?" measuring the outcome of the prayer is probably too subjective and ideothetic to be able to use it as a criterion for research at this time.

Present Intercessory Prayer Research

Hodge (2007) has reported a meta-analysis of the literature testing intercessory prayer using 17 studies found through multiple searches of the literature. Meta-analysis is an excellent method of summarizing studies. Instead of subjectively comparing studies, meta-analysis summarizes studies statistically. Effect sizes are entered for each study, along with other information such as the number of participants. The studies are weighted by that number and an overall effect size is computed and tested.

Hodge (2007) reports a significant effect of $p < .02$. The effect size was .17. However this is based on the published studies. It is possible that studies of prayer are more likely to be published if there are significant results. Journal editors are more receptive to significant studies. Authors are more likely to work to get significant studies published. Fortunately, meta-analysis includes a procedure by which one can determine the number of unpublished studies needed to reduce the observed effect size to nonsignificance, assuming only nonsignificant studies go unreported. Hodges reports that it would require 32 unreported nonsignificant studies to reduce the effect size to nonsignificance.

Note the small effect size requires a large number of participants distributed equally between a prayed-for group and control group(s), in order to be significant. If the number were just enough for a .17 to be significant, half the studies would fall below this mean of .17. Therefore an even larger number is needed. Details of the study would need to be examined in a power analysis to estimate the number needed as well as the investigator's tolerance for Type II errors, but it would seem that at least 300 are needed to have a chance of finding a significant effect with both Type I and Type II errors held to the .05 level.

The small effect size may be a function of uncontrolled variables, such as low reliability of measures or the impart of other events not reported in the study. With some outcome criteria, the results may be heavily skewed in that almost all may be healed and so the number not healed is small. This also makes effect sizes smaller although meta-analysis can correct for such restrictions of range. Other elements often found in a meta-analysis are not reported by Hodge. Meta-analysis can also correct effect sizes for unreliability, which means that Hodge's effect sizes are smaller and less significant than if they had been so weighted.

Another set of unreported analyses of considerable importance is that of comparing different types of studies for whether they produced the same results. Probably due to the limited number of empirical studies of intercessory prayer, Hodge did not evaluate whether triple blind studies, in which neither the patient, those evaluating the outcome, nor the medical staff knew who was in the prayer or control groups, found different results than single blind or nonblind studies.

We can examine the results for studies that used at least double blind procedures and had a reasonable number of participants. Here they are:

- Benson, Duseck, Sherwood, Lam, Betha, Caperter, and others (2006), not significant ($N = 1,201$).
- Alves, Whelan, Hernke, Williams, Kenny, and O'Fallon (2001), not significant trend ($N = 799$).
- Harris, Thoresen, McCullough, and Larson (1999), significant. ($N = 990$).
- Byrd (1988), significant ($N = 393$).
- Leibovici (2001), significant ($N = 3,393$).

Hodge did not publish the effect sizes for these but each is large enough to find significant a much smaller correlation than .17. It appears that when the studies are limited to only the better ones, there is limited support for a positive, though small, prayer effect.

So far the effects, if any, are small. In fact they are so small, that giving the patients a drug placebo may be more effective. There could be some increase in effect size upon investigating parameters in which the studies differ. These include the number, type, and nature of the prayers as well as the characteristics of those who are praying.

A problem that future research in this area may wish to address is what other prayers are being offered. In a study with 1,000 patients, random assignment assures that there are few differences between the control and experimental groups. The other prayers by the patient and by those who know the patient will average out to be the same. But yet other prayers, which could be measured by asking the patents about their own prayers and those in their religious support system, could be measured and parceled out statistically. The result would be a more accurate effect size, possibly raising it above a trivial effect.

Another question not examined in Hodge's meta-analysis was whether there were dosage effects. In medicine, strong doses of a medicine are generally found to have more powerful effects than weaker doses, additional evidence that the intervention is successful. In the studies, what was meant by a prayer varied widely, as did the characteristics of those praying. They were all religiously committed, but the number in Hodge's (2007) summary of the studies varies from one person praying for the list of patients to 15 Christians praying for individuals, to rotation among a group of 40 that included multiple faiths such as Buddhists, Christians, shamans, and secular people praying. Such a diversity of interventions makes the overall test from the total set of studies difficult to interpret.

The research on prayer needs to consider each person's religious motivation. That may be Intrinsic Religiosity (Allport and Ross 1967), in which the person prays as a part of his or her religious life, or Extrinsic and Personal (Gorsuch and McPherson 1989; Kirkpatrick 1989). The latter do not pray as a part of their religious life but pray because they have a problem. The problem leads to the prayer. Extrinsic religion generally relates to negatives about one's life. On the other hand, Intrinsic motivation is associated with positives in one's life. Just correlating prayer with other personal or social outcome measures is not meaningful, for the correlation will suggest negatives if the sample contains primarily Extrinsics or positives if the sample contains primary Intrinsics. With sizable proportions of each in the sample, they would offset so that the correlation would be zero. Measuring the type of religious motivation clarifies the situation, and one may well find both a positive and a negative correlation with a dependent variable from the two types of motivation.

The nomothetic research on prayer is not yet sufficient to decide whether there is an objective effect. The effect, if any, may be stronger if some of the considerations mentioned above are controlled in the study.

Nomothetic Considerations in Intercessory Prayer

The purpose of this chapter is broader than just whether research has or has not found intercessory prayer to be effective. Instead the purpose is to examine the possible meanings of such studies given the nomothetic and ideothetic distinction explained above. The following discussion uses the intercessory prayer research as a starting point for that discussion.

Casteel (1955) includes the following as problems with intercessory prayer: (1) It may be that God only acts through natural law. Then there is no ideothetic action and theology has become deistic with a creator who is no longer in charge of his creation. In this case, miracles as generally defined do not happen and so will not be found in nomothetic research. (2) It can be argued that God, loving his people, already knows and so provides for them, but this becomes a theological determinism taking people out of the decision making. No parent would always do the best for their child by making all the decisions without the child's input, so why should God? (3) Then there is the criterion problem we noted above: what is an answer to a prayer? If the answer is yes, it is clearly identified. But the answer may be given in multiple ways. The answer could be "no," "wait," or "here is a better answer for your need than what you prayed for." In the eyes of faith, all prayers have an answer even if the answer is, "no comment." These are all problems for nomothetic intercessory research.

Another question can be raised about intercessory prayer. Does God wish to pay attention to the researcher's prayers? Somehow adding one person or even a set of people to pray for a stranger seems less important than the many Christians already praying for that person who know them well. Moreover, there are the thousands of general prayers said each day, praying for all those who are sick. Only if one sees the research's people as special mediators between the divine and the human would the effect be large enough to not be drowned in the sea of other prayers. The only other option is to assume that God just adds up the number of prayers and then helps those with the most so that adding the research team prayers would add sufficiently to all those being said for a few people that it would put them over the top. This is in keeping with theologies that sponsor prayer wheels so that the prayers are made sufficiently often to manipulate a spiritual force into doing what we desire, but this is a poor fit with Christian theology.

Brown (1994) raises the question of who is to blame if an action fails. If an experiment fails to find an established effect, then Brown suggests the experimenter may be blamed, whether it be the fault of failed apparatus, the experimental design, too few subjects, or other such causes. The ineffectiveness of prayer research may be caused by experimenter-linked phenomena. There are answers that are too readily given for the perceived failure of prayer, "you did not have enough faith," but Brown's point is that this is a consideration from within a religious community and tradition.

There are those who hold that intercessory prayer is not testable but for other reasons than the nomothetic-ideothetic distinction of this chapter. Brown (1994) presents several of these from multiple sources. The most prominent argument is to suggest that the purpose of prayer is less petitions that treat prayer as magic, than prayer as a relationship with God. This, however, changes it from an intercessory prayer to another type of prayer.

Would establishing intercessory prayer on a nomothetic base place prayer in the realm of magic? "Any technology is magic to those whose culture does not understand the technology" is a phrase that could be used to illustrate the problem. How does magic differ from technology? General usage suggests several differences. First, magic is based in arbitrary words and movements, such as "abra cadabra" and waving a wand over a top hat. Another difference is the source of the power that underlies the action. Magic is considered to be a force that has powers over events that are not directly related to the words said or motions made. But these do not seem sufficient critiques, for there are devices such as computers that can be programmed to respond to verbal commands and motions. These devices can have considerable power, such as sending missiles with nuclear bombs.

For magic, other than the illusions of a magician, the difference appears to be having powers over a spiritual force, a spirit that understands and can hear language even though it shows no physical presence. So far, science has not needed spirits as an explanatory principle, and our paradigms are marked by action through a chain of physical events rather than the action of invisible spirits. This may change as more Third World people become involved in scholarship, for the nonbelief in spirits is not universal.

Inclusion of the Leibovici (2001) study along with other intercessory prayer research may be controversial because it was retrospective. A person gave a prayer for half the patients after treatment was completed but before the outcomes were examined. This is unusual because one of the conditions normally expected in assuming that an intervention caused the results is that the cause be prior to the outcome. Leibovici was following a different line of thought: God is outside of space and time, and so can act in prior times as well as current ones. The limitation is that God does not change an outcome after we have observed it.

Note that God could only perform a miracle post hoc before those praying know the results. Hence one can pray post hoc for events that are completed until one knows the outcome. This begins to feel like a good basis for a science fiction story. What, for example, might happen if we pray for a completed event for which we already knew the outcome? If God is independent of time, he could change it; this would be an answer to the prayer. While God may be able to track parallel time lines, we cannot. So if he answered such a prayer, we would remember it as it has been changed, and have no memory of our prayer that changed it. Then there would be no prayer to influence God to change it, and so no answer to any prayer. It is best to go with Leibovici and keep the discussion to those results that we do not yet know.

Is retrospective intercessory prayer legitimate science? By the definition in this chapter that science examines that which replicates, the answer lies in others applying this easy methodology to more cases. If it replicates, science should take it seriously. Before we reject post hoc prayer, we need to realize that physics is not quite as certain about cause and effect, at least at the quantum level, as often implied. In quantum physics, Schroeder's cat may not be said to be alive or dead until someone checks to see, which is after the quantum event. This is the same line of thinking as in Leibovici.

A nomothetic definition of science contains no assumption that a cause precedes an event. The only problem is the interpretation of cause when the cause comes after the event. But attempting to solve a problem before there is replication of the results, to assure that there is a problem, is not a good use of our time. Therefore judgment on the interpretation of post hoc prayer needs to await replication of Leibovici (2001).

Science normally accepts replicated data consistencies as facts when they fit within a paradigm providing a physical vector for action. Light produces action by the light streaming from the source, which can be followed and measured at any point. Of course, the major question about a replicable prayer effect is the interpretation of the causal agent. Religious people immediately say the cause is God, while nonreligious people posit a hidden unknown cause or something more general. James (1902/1985) posited an unknown force whereas Cattell (1938) laid out a theory of a theopsyche, a psychological force that operates as if there were a supernatural force. Not having a known vector for the action is not an unknown problem in science. Despite the discussions of graviton waves, there is no known physical vector by which gravity operates. In the last volume of his treatises, Newton makes exactly this point and suggests that it shows God acting (Simpson 1992). If there is a replicable nomothetic effect in prayer studies, then a search for a physical vector or action would be warranted. This would be part of the effect of the function of God as creator, and not a miracle as normally defined.

Nomothetic research can only establish replicable data consistencies and so prayer only as a natural phenomenon. This does not mean it is not, as in Christian theology, from God, but that it is a consistent effect. However, being natural, it would operate by some mechanism, which would be the object of further research, and would not be considered a miracle by our standard definition.

Ideothetic Considerations in Intercessory Prayer

The traditional definition for a miracle is always open to a god-of-the-gaps effect. When little was known of the nomothetic principles of medicine, any healing could have been attributed to a unique event outside of natural law, and so a miracle. Thus a person's not getting cholera in the medieval era may have been seen as an answer to prayer but might be explained today by that person following the custom of only drinking tea brewed the old-fashioned way, heat the water until it is at a rolling boil, which would have had the then-unknown effect of killing the cholera germs in the water.

On the other hand, few areas of medicine are so well developed that only the nomothetic seems to apply. People respond differently to illness and medications when physicians treat by general nomothetic principles. "The research shows successful results in 82 percent of the cases, so let's try it," which may leave God room to intervene in the other 18 percent. A conversation with any medical doctor will turn up many cases of unusual results. This may be interpreted as possible miracles by the religious or as variations on undocumented nomothetic principles in the case of the nonreligious, both of which are, of course, equally post hoc explanations. Whether there is an ideothetic event that can be labeled a miracle would need to be evaluated by ideothetic standards. These are set by the theologians of each faith that wishes to address the issue of miraculous answers to prayers.

Interaction between Nomothetic and Ideographic

There is no reason for an event being just nomothetic or just ideothetic. Joint events happen in everyday life. A unique event such as a successful birth has nomothetic aspects; the course of the pregnancy is well known for the average woman, as are the effects of medical interventions to control a wide range of possible problems. Yet, for that mother, the birth is a very ideographic event and may also be ideothetic for the physician if unusual situations arise. Events can be both nomothetic and ideothetic. Therefore it is possible to have miracles combining with nomothetic events. Every science-based clinical treatment, whether by physicians or psychologists, is based on bringing the nomothetic of science into the ideothetic of a person's life. God may also bring the ideothetic into a nomothetic event.

If there is an obvious cause for the answer to the prayer, that may or may not be considered an answer to prayer. Some Christians consider a prayer for healing to be answered if the doctor changes the patient's prescription and the new one is more effective. Indeed, it is common for people to pray for the doctor to make the best decisions for the patient. Few limit an answer to prayer to just those events that cannot be explained any other way.

Interpreting normally nomothetic events to be answers for a prayer distinguishes between *direct causation* and *sanctioning*. Smith and Gorsuch (1987) note that courts use this distinction. The physical cause is that which is the direct physical agent. The sanctioning agent is that which guarantees the outcome by this physical agent or, if that is not effective, by another physical agent. When one prays for improved health, the physical cause may be from the taking of a medicine, from a surgeon's skill, or from a set of radiation treatments. The sanctioning agent is the doctor who selects between these physical causal agents. If the first physical causal agent selected by the doctor is ineffective, the doctor selects another physical agent. The physician may try several approaches until one works. Surely God can do the same. The prayer is for God to sanction the healing by assuring that some physical agent produces the healing. Is it any less of a miracle if God works through a physician? Indeed, is that not the task of a Christian physician, to heal people in response to God's desires for all to be healed?

This approach means the ideothetic intervention can take place in any of the events leading up to the answer to a prayer. It may be, as Murphy suggests, in the randomness of quantum physics. Or it could be in helping a physician recall a critical article at the most appropriate time. Or it could be in having a cab handy to take a woman suddenly going into labor to the hospital. All of these look nomothetic, only when we look just to the immediate cause, and forget that God as a sanctioning agent may work through dozens of physical agents.

From an ideothetic perspective, God can work miracles at all levels of causal chains and outside of causal chains. This means that God can work along with natural law, and that it may be difficult to separate the nomothetic from ideothetic interventions.

CONCLUSION

Science only works with replicable events; and miracles, being nonreplicable, are outside the scope or domain of what have been called the exact sciences. However, the normal definition of *miracle* makes the mistake of creating a false dichotomy. It implies things must result from either an immediate natural cause or a completely ideothetic intervention. With our distinction between nomothetic and ideothetic, there is ample reason to suggest that both are widely involved in our lives. Both scientific interventions and God's actions flowing from sanctioning a given result may well be the correct understanding; and our definition of miracle may need to shift to take that into account.

What happened at the feeding of the 5,000? God may have been a direct cause by multiplying the loaves and fish; or he may also been a sanctioning cause by reminding a number of the people at the start of the day to bring plenty of food, and motivating them to share it. Indeed, God may have done all those things at once. The appropriate disciplines need to define miracles so that both are recognized as acts of God, one by direct cause and one through sanctioning. Who of us is ready to limit God as to the natural and transcendental channels through which he can and may operate? This is his world and all the channels, presumably, are open to his action.

REFERENCES

Allport, G. W., and J. M. Ross (1967), Personal Religious Orientation and Prejudice, *Journal of Personality and Social Psychology* 5, 432–43.

Aviles, J. M., E. Whelan, D. A. Hernke, B. A. Williams, K. E. Kenny, W. M. O'Fallon, et al. (2001), Intercessory Prayer and Cardiovascular Disease Progression in Coronary Care Unit Population: A Randomized Controlled Trial, *Mayo Clinic Proceedings* 76, 1192–98.

Benson, H., J. A. Duseck, J. B. Sherwood, P. Lam, C. F. Bethea, W. Capenter, et al. (2006), Study of the Therapeutic Effects of Intercessory Prayer (STEP) in Cardiac Bypass Patients: A Multi-center Randomized Trial of Uncertainty of Receiving Intercessory Prayer, *American Heart Journal* 151, 934–42.

Brown, R. (1994), *The Human Side of Prayer*, Birmingham: Religious Education Press.

Byrd, R. C. (1988), Positive Therapeutic Effects of Intercessory Prayer in a Coronary Care Unit Population, *Southern Medical Journal* 81, 826–29.

Casteel, J. C. (1955), *Rediscovering Prayer*, New York: Association Press.

Cattell, R. B. (1938), *Psychology and the Religious Quest*, London: Thomas Nelson & Sons.

Cattell, R. B., and D. Child (1975), *Motivation and Dynamic Structure*, New York: Halstead Press.

Dein, Simon (2001), What Really Happens when Prophecy Fails: The Case of Lubavitch, *Sociology of Religion* 62, 383–402.

Descartes, R. (1701, reissued in 1990), Discourse on the Method of Rightly Conducting the Reason, in *Great Books of the Western World*, P. W. Goetz, ed., Vol. 28, Chicago: Encyclopedia Britannica.

Faber, M. D. (2002), *The Magic of Prayer*, Westport, CT: Praeger.

Festinger, L., H. Riecken, and S. Schachter (1956), *When Prophecy Fails*, Minneapolis: University of Minnesota Press.

Frances, L. J., and J. Astley (2001), *Psychological Perspectives on Prayer*, Herdfordshire: Gracewing.

Freud, Sigmund (1927/1964), *The Future of an Illusion*, rev. ed., Garden City: Doubleday.

Galton, F. (1872/2001), Statistical Inquiries into the Efficacy of Prayer, in L. J. Frances and J. Astley, eds., *Psychological Perspectives on Prayer*, Herdfordshire: Gracewing.

Gorsuch, R. L. (2002a), The Pyramids of Sciences and of Humanities, *American Behavioral Scientist* 45, 1822–38. Reprinted in A. Dueck (2006), *Integrating Psychology and Theology*, Pasadena: Fuller Seminary Press.

Gorsuch, R. L. (2002/2007), *Integrating Psychology and Spirituality?* Westport, CT: Praeger, 2002; Pasadena: Fuller Seminary Press, 2007.

Gorsuch, R. L., and S. E. McPherson (1989), Intrinsic/Extrinsic Measurement: I/E Revised and Single-item Scales, *Journal for the Scientific Study of Religion (JSST)* 28, 348–54.

Harris, A., C. E. Thoresen, M. E. McCullough, and D. B. Larson (1999), Spiritually and Religiously Oriented Health Interventions, *Journal Health Psychology* 4, 413–33.

Hodge, D. R. (2007), A Systematic Review of the Empirical Literature on Intercessory Prayer, *Research on Social Work Practice* 17, 174–187.

Hood, R., R. Morris, and P. Harvey (1993/2001), Prayer Experience and Religious Orientation, in L. J. Frances and J. Astley, eds., *Psychological Perspectives on Prayer*, Herdfordshire: Gracewing.

James, W. (1902/1985), *The Works of William James: The Varieties of Religious Experience*, Vol. 15, Cambridge: Harvard University Press.

Kirkpatrick, L. A. (1989), A Psychometric Analysis of the Allport-Ross and Feagin Measures of Intrinsic-Extrinsic Religious Orientation, in D. O. Moberg and M. L. Lynn, eds., *Research in the Social Scientific Study of Religion (RSSSR)*, Vol. 1., Greenwich, CT: JAI Press.

Kuhn, T. S. (1970), *The Structure of Scientific Revolutions*, 2nd edition (1989), Chicago: University of Chicago Press.

Ladd, K. L. (2007), *Inward, Outward, Upward Prayer: Links to Attachment Theory*, American Psychological Association annual meeting, August 17, 2007.

Ladd, K. L., and B. Spilka (2002), Inward, Outward, Upward: Cognitive Aspects of Prayer, *Journal for the Scientific Study of Religion (JSSR)* 41, 3, 475–84.

Ladd, K. L., and B. Spilka (2006), Inward, Outward, Upward Prayer: Scale Reliability and Validation, *Journal for the Scientific Study of Religion (JSSR)* 45, 2, 233–51.

Leibovici, L. (2001), Effects of Remote, Retroactive Intercessory Prayer on Outcomes in Patients with Bloodstream Infection: Randomized Controlled Trial, *British Medical Journal* 323, 1450–51.

Murphy, N. (1997), *Anglo-American Postmodernity*. Boulder: Westview Press.

Poloma, M., and G. Gallup (1991), *The Varieties of Prayer*, Philadelphia: Trinity Press International.

Simpson, T. K. (1992), Science as Mystery: A Speculative Reading of Newton's *Principia*, in M. J. Adler, ed., *The Great Ideas Today*, Chicago: Encyclopaedia Britannica.

Smith, C. S., and R. L. Gorsuch (1987), Sanctioning and Causal Attributions to God: A Function of Theological Position and Actors' Characteristics, in M. L. Lynn and D. O. Moberg, eds., *Research in the Social Scientific Study of Religion (RSSSR)*, Vol. 1., 133–52, Greenwich, CT: JAI Press.

CONCLUSION

J. Harold Ellens

The sixteen chapters in this volume represent the careful work of 17 scholars, representing a number of different countries in North America and Europe. Moreover, they present the perspectives of serious-minded analysts of both science and the Bible. These perspectives vary as widely as the continuum of human imagination and analysis can stretch. This work has been made urgently necessary because of the fact that inadequate cooperation has been achieved, so far, between the contribution that the empirical sciences and the biblical and theological sciences can bring to bear upon the study of miracles in the ancient world and in our own day. The exact sciences and the psychosocial sciences have tended to follow a trajectory of investigation in one direction and the biblical and theological or spiritual investigations have tended along a different track. The former, understandably, follows the avenue of the hermeneutic of suspicion, while the latter, also understandably, holds itself open to a hermeneutic of analytical but less suspicious and more affirming inquiry.

The virtual absence of pages or sections in professional and scientific journals devoted to religious, spiritual, or theological perspectives, on issues dealing with paranormal human experiences, is most unfortunate. *The Journal for Psychology and Christianity* and *The Journal for Psychology and Theology* are virtually alone in the American world, as sophisticated professional journals that regularly seek and publish empirical and clinical research on phenomena in the fields of psychosocial science and spirituality or religion. In the European Community the *Journal of Empirical Theology* has undertaken similar concerns. Division 36 of the American Psychological Association also deals continually with interests in these matters.

Of course, the function of peer-reviewed journals is to publish replicable research results. However, perhaps a section in each professional journal should be devoted to reporting incidents of the paranormal so that a universe of discourse and a vehicle for discussion could be developed for taking such date into consideration. At present it is not discussed in the scientific realm because no instrument is available for collecting and processing the data. It is important to create a culture of openness to the paranormal experiences humans have regularly and really, so that the frequency of such events can be understood more clearly, recorded, described, named, categorized, and analyzed.

We may discover, if we create such instruments for raising our consciousness level and increasing our information base, that there are eight things that strike us with surprising urgency. First, we may discover that the incidents of paranormal events are more frequent, should I say more normal, than we think. Second, we may discover that they fit into specific patterns that can be categorized and even analyzed more readily than we have imagined. Third, that may bring to the surface of our thought processes insights about the nature and sources of paranormal events that are currently ignored because we have not reduced our mystification about them, simply because we have not done the first and second steps above.

Fourth, we may find that the paranormal events are apparently more normal, in terms of the frequency and universality with which humans experience them, than are the normal. Fifth, we may discover that we can establish criteria for sorting out the real from the unreal in what we are now referring to as the mystifying paranormal. Sixth, we may discover that a solicitation of anecdotal reports will produce such a wealth of information as to give rise to an entirely new arena for productive research. If the spirit of God is communicating with our spirits by way of paranormal experiences, presumably it is because God thinks we can hear and interpret the content, making unmystifying sense of it if we study it carefully, just like we have of the stuff of this world that we have mastered by our science. Seventh, not all truth is empirical data. A great deal of our understanding of the truth about this mundane world we know from phenomenological investigations and heuristic interpretations. These seem to be trustworthy instruments of research that are particularly suited to investigation of the reported experiences humans have of the paranormal. We should be able by means of them to create useful theories, data collection and management systems, hypotheses, and laws regarding the human experiences of the paranormal.

Eighth, if one assumes the existence of God and God's relationship with the material world, immediately a great deal of data is evident within the worldview of that hypothesis, suggesting a good deal of available knowledge about God. Much of this is derived from the nature of the universe itself. Much of the evidence for God's nature and behavior, within that model of investigation, is replicable, predictable, testable, and the like. Why would we not assume the same is true of the world of the paranormal, if we studied it thoroughly and systematically? We call it paranormal only because we have not yet discovered or created a framework of analysis by which its data can be collected and managed.

Some decades ago a great deal was made of chaos theory and entropy in interpreting the unknown aspects of the material world, particularly in the field of astrophysics and cosmology. It turned out that we always think that things just beyond our model and grasp are chaotic. That is only because we do not understand them, not because they are not coherent, lawful, and predictable. We think things just beyond our ken are chaotic because our paradigm is too limited to manage the data out there. Life is always a process of that kind of growth that requires constant expansion of our paradigms. When we cannot expand our paradigm to take in the next larger world that we are discovering, either because of our fear or blockheadedness, we shrink and wither, and our scientific systems go down.

At this very moment we stand upon a threshold demanding an expansion of our scientific paradigm to take in the data of the paranormal in a manner that it can be brought into new but coherent models of knowledge and understanding. William Wilson said in chapter 15 that part of the difficulty in studying the spiritual and related paranormal data lies in the fact that each event is intensely personal and unique. Each scientific exploration of that event must deal with an equation in which n is 1. That makes scientific extrapolations impossible. I suggest, however, that if we undertook the program I propose above, we might well discover that n is much more than 1, and in that case we would be off and running along a trajectory that would teach us how to expand our present limited scientific paradigms to take in the additional real data. We have attempted to begin that enterprise with this volume of scholarly investigation.

Index

ABOUT THE EDITOR
AND ADVISERS

EDITOR

J. Harold Ellens is a research scholar at the University of Michigan, Department of Near Eastern Studies. He is a retired Presbyterian theologian and ordained minister, a retired U.S. Army colonel, and a retired professor of philosophy, theology, and psychology. He has authored, coauthored, or edited 165 books and 167 professional journal articles. He served 15 years as executive director of the Christian Association for Psychological Studies and as founding editor and editor-in-chief of the *Journal of Psychology and Christianity*. He holds a PhD from Wayne State University in the Psychology of Human Communication, a PhD from the University of Michigan in Biblical and Near Eastern Studies, and master's degrees from Calvin Theological Seminary, Princeton Theological Seminary, and the University of Michigan. He was born in Michigan, grew up in a Dutch-German immigrant community, and determined at age seven to enter the Christian Ministry as a means to help his people with the great amount of suffering he perceived all around him. His life's work has focused on the interface of psychology and religion.

ADVISERS

LeRoy H. Aden is professor emeritus of Pastoral Theology at the Lutheran Theological Seminary in Philadelphia, Pennsylvania. He taught full-time at the seminary from 1967 to 1994 and part-time from 1994 to 2001. He served as visiting lecturer at Princeton Theological Seminary, Princeton, New Jersey, on a regular basis. In 2002, he coauthored *Preaching God's Compassion: Comforting Those Who Suffer* with Robert G. Hughes. Previously, he edited four books in a Psychology and Christianity series with J. Harold Ellens and David G. Benner. He served on the board of directors of the Christian Association for Psychological Studies for six years.

Alfred John Eppens was born and raised in Michigan. He attended Western Michigan University, studying history under Ernst A. Breisach, and received a BA (summa cum laude) and an MA. He continued his studies at the University of Michigan, were he was awarded a JD in 1981. He is an adjunct professor at Oakland University and at Oakland Community College, as well as an active church musician and director. He is a director and officer of the Michigan Center for Early Christian Studies, as well as a founding member of the New American Lyceum.

Edmund S. Meltzer was born in Brooklyn, New York. He attended the University of Chicago, where he received his BA in Near Eastern Languages and Civilizations. He pursued graduate studies at the University of Toronto, earning his MA and PhD in Near Eastern Studies. He worked in Egypt as a member of the Akhenaten Temple Project/East Karnak Excavation and as a Fellow of the American Research Center. Returning to the United States, he taught at the University of North Carolina—Chapel Hill and at The Claremont Graduate School (now University), where he served as associate chair of the Department of Religion. Meltzer taught at Northeast Normal University in Changchun from 1990 to 1996. He has been teaching German and Spanish in the Wisconsin public school system and English as a Second Language in summer programs of the University of Wisconsin. He has lectured extensively, published numerous articles and reviews in scholarly journals, and has contributed to and edited a number of books.

Jack Miles is the author of the 1996 Pulitzer Prize winner, *God: A Biography.* After publishing *Christ: A Crisis in the Life of God* in 2001, Miles was named a MacArthur Fellow in 2002. Now Senior Advisor to the President at J. Paul Getty Trust, he earned a PhD in Near Eastern languages from Harvard University in 1971 and has been a regents lecturer at the University of California, director of the Humanities Center at Claremont Graduate University, and visiting professor of humanities at the California Institute of Technology. He has authored articles that have appeared in numerous national publications, including the *Atlantic Monthly*, the *New York Times*, the *Boston Globe*, the *Washington Post*, and the *Los Angeles Times*, where he served for 10 years as literary editor and as a member of the newspaper's editorial board.

Wayne G. Rollins is professor emeritus of Biblical Studies at Assumption College, Worcester, Massachusetts, and adjunct professor of Scripture at Hartford Seminary, Hartford, Connecticut. His writings include *The Gospels: Portraits of Christ* (1964), *Jung and the Bible* (1983), and *Soul and Psyche: The Bible in Psychological Perspective* (1999). He received his PhD in New Testament Studies from Yale University and is the founder and chairman (1990–2000) of the Society of Biblical Literature Section on Psychology and Biblical Studies.

Grant R. Shafer was educated at Wayne State University, Harvard University, and the University of Michigan, where he received his doctorate in Early Christianity. A summary of his dissertation, "St. Stephen and the Samaritans," was published in the proceedings of the 1996 meeting of the Société d'Etudes Samaritaines. He has taught at Washtenaw Community College, Siena Heights University, and Eastern Michigan University. He is presently a visiting scholar at the University of Michigan.

ABOUT THE CONTRIBUTORS

Benjamin Beit-Hallahmi is the author, coauthor, editor, or coeditor of 17 books and monographs on the psychology of religion, social identity, and personality development. Among his best-known publications are *The Psychology of Religious Behaviour, Belief and Experience, The Psychoanalytic Study of Religion,* and *Psychoanalysis, Identity, and Ideology.* In 1993 he was the recipient of the William James Award (Division 36 of the American Psychological Association) for his contributions to the psychology of religion.

Kamila Blessing has been an Episcopal priest for 25 years and has served a number of Episcopal parishes and 13 other denominations. She has been applying Murray Bowen's Family Systems Theory to all kinds of organizations for over 20 years. Blessing holds a PhD in New Testament with a minor in Semitic studies from Duke University and further degrees in Systems Science from the University of Pittsburgh. She was licensed as a mediator by the Lombard Mennonite Peace Center and has become known as a "turnaround specialist." She is the founder and president of Blessing Transitions Consultants (www.Mediate.com/Blessing), working to heal crises, transition problems, and conflicts for parishes, families, communities, and organizations. She has been involved in healing by prayer for 40 years and has had a national healing ministry for much of that time. Her book, *It Was a Miracle: Stories of Ordinary People and Extraordinary Healing* (Augsburg Fortress, 1999) demonstrates the essence of that ministry as well as the extraordinary relevance of the Bible for modern people.

Richard L. Gorsuch is senior professor of psychology at the Fuller Graduate School of Psychology and a prolific researcher, best known for his studies in the psychology of religion, substance abuse, social psychology, and statistics. A member of the School of Psychology faculty since 1979, he is known across the social sciences for his publication of *Factor Analysis* (1983), and is the developer of the statistical software program Unimult. Gorsuch is a licensed social psychologist, an active member of the Religious Research Association, and a fellow of the Society for the Scientific Study of Religion and the American Psychological Association. He has served in editorial capacities for journals including *Journal for the Scientific Study of Religion and Educational and Psychological Measurement* and has authored and contributed chapters to over 20 books. Current projects include *Integrating Psychology and Spirituality: An Introduction* and his next book is *Building Peace, the 3 Pillars Approach*. He has also been listed among the 2,000 Outstanding Scholars of the 21st Century by England's International Biographical Centre.

Louis Hoffman is a core faculty member at the Colorado School of Professional Psychology, a college of the University of the Rockies, and an adjunct assistant professor of psychology at the Graduate School of Psychology at Fuller Theological Seminary. He serves on the editorial board of the *Journal of Humanistic Psychology* and *PsycCRITIQUES: APA Review of Books*, and is coauthor of *Spirituality and Psychological Health, The God Image Handbook for Spiritual Counseling and Psychotherapy: Theory, Research, and Practice*, and the forthcoming book *Brilliant Sanity: Buddhist Approaches to Psychotherapy*. Dr. Hoffman is active in writing and presenting on existential-integrative psychotherapy, religious and spiritual issues in therapy, theoretical and philosophical issues in psychology, and diversity issues.

Erkki Koskenniemi is adjunct professor at the Finnish universities of Helsinki, Joensuu, and Åbo Akademi. He has contributed to the research of Classical Antiquity and Theology (Early Judaism and New Testament). He is the author of many books.

Antti Laato is professor in Old Testament exegesis and Jewish Studies in Theological Faculty at Åbo Akademi University in Turku, Finland. He has written several books. His current research interests are Rewritten Bible, Jewish-Christian encounters, and the Children of Abraham.

Andre LaCocque is professor emeritus of Hebrew Scripture and former director of the Center for Jewish-Christian Studies at Chicago Theological Seminary. He is the coauthor (with Paul Ricoeur) of *Thinking Biblically: Exegetical and Hermeneutical Studies;* (with Pierre-Emmanuel LaCocque) of *Jonah:*

A Psycho-Religious Approach to the Prophet; contributor to *Psychology and the Bible* and *Psychological Insight into the Bible;* he is the author of *The Trial of Innocence: Adam, Eve, and the Yahwist;* as well as of *Onslaught against Innocence: Cain, Abel, and the Yahwist* (in press), among others.

Russ Llewellyn received his biblical and theological training at Bryan College, Dallas Theological Seminary, for his ThM, as well as studying at Fuller Theological Seminary. He received his scientific training at Fuller Graduate School of psychology where he received his PhD degree in clinical psychology. He has been in practice as a clinical psychologist for 31 years now, until recently, full-time. He started a church when he was fresh out of seminary. His long-time professional memberships have been in the Christian Association for Psychological Studies, where he has been a presenter, and the American Association of Christian Counselors. He is a writer and has produced two books: *Ultimate Worth,* and *Gaining Life's Prize.* Both deal with the issues of self-esteem from the standpoint of God's eternal perspective. The second deals with how our glory is shaped by adversity.

Katherine McGuire studied at the University of Innsbruck, Austria, and the University of San Francisco, earning a BA in English. She also holds a diploma from the St. Ignatius Institute, a Great Books, philosophy, and theology program. She received her MS in Elementary Education and has taught at the elementary and college level, which included two years of teaching in Ankara, Turkey. She is currently a doctoral student pursuing a degree in clinical psychology at the Colorado School of Professional Psychology, a college of the University of the Rockies.

Patrick McNamara is director of the Evolutionary Neurobehavior Laboratory in the Department of Neurology at the Boston University School of Medicine and the VA New England Healthcare System. Upon graduating from the Behavioral Neuroscience Program at Boston University in 1991, he trained at the Aphasia Research Center at the Boston VA Medical Center in neurolinguistics and brain-cognitive correlation techniques. He then began developing an evolutionary approach to problems of brain and behavior and currently is studying the evolution of the frontal lobes, the evolution of the two mammalian sleep states (REM and NREM), and the evolution of religion in human cultures.

Petri Merenlahti received his PhD from the University of Helsinki, Finland, and is currently working as postdoctoral researcher in its Department of Biblical Studies. His fields of specialization include New Testament studies, narrative criticism, and psychological biblical criticism. His publications include

Poetics for the Gospels? Rethinking Narrative Criticism (2002), "Reading as a Little Child: On the Model Reader of the Gospels" (*Literature and Theology,* 2004) and "So Who Really Needs Therapy? On Psychological Exegesis and Its Subject" (*Svensk Exegetisk Årsbok,* 2007).

John W. Miller is professor emeritus of Religious Studies at Conrad Grebel University College, University of Waterloo, Ontario, Canada. His ThD is from the University of Basel. His current fields of specialization are in the canon history of the Bible. He was cofounder and cochair of the Historical Jesus Section in the Society of Biblical Literature. He also served as director of Psychiatric Rehabilitation Services at Chicago State Hospital. His writings include *Meet the Prophets: A Beginner's Guide to the Books of the Biblical Prophets—Their Meaning Then and Now* (1987); *The Origins of the Bible: Rethinking Canon History* (1994); *Jesus at Thirty: A Psychological and Historical Portrait* (1997); *Calling God "Father": Essays on the Bible, Fatherhood & Culture* (1999); *How the Bible Came to Be: Exploring the Narrative and Message* (2004); and a commentary on *Proverbs* (2004). In publication is a Bible study program (*The Ecumenical Bible Study*) introducing the Bible in the light of the intentions of those who created it.

Stephen J. Pullum is professor of Communication Studies at the University of North Carolina, Wilmington, where he teaches courses in Communication Theory, Intercultural Communication, and the Rhetoric of Faith Healing, among others. He is the author of *"Foul Demons, Come Out!": The Rhetoric of Twentieth-Century, American Faith Healers.* Dr. Pullum has won UNCW's Distinguished Teaching Professorship and the Chancellor's Teaching Excellence Award.

Wayne G. Rollins is professor emeritus of Biblical Studies at Assumption College, Worcester, Massachusetts, and adjunct professor of Scripture at Hartford Seminary, Hartford, Connecticut. He has also taught at Princeton University and Wellesley College and served as visiting professor at Mount Holyoke College, Yale College, College of the Holy Cross, and Colgate Rochester Divinity School. His writings include *The Gospels: Portraits of Christ* (1964), *Jung and the Bible* (1983), and *Soul and Psyche: The Bible in Psychological Perspective* (1999). He coedited four volumes of essays with J. Harold Ellens, *Psychology and the Bible: A New Way to Read the Scriptures* (2004) and a volume on *Psychological Insight into the Bible: Texts and Readings* (2007) with D. Andrew Kille. He received his PhD in New Testament Studies from Yale University and is the founder and chairman (1990–2000) of the Society of Biblical Literature Section on Psychology and Biblical Studies.

Reka Szent-Imrey is a student in psychology at University of Massachusetts at Boston and a research associate at the Institute for the Biocultural Study of Religion in Boston, Massachusetts.

William P. Wilson is professor emeritus of Psychiatry at Duke University Medical Center and is currently distinguished professor of counseling at Carolina Evangelical Divinity School. He has been active in evangelical circles for the last 40 years. He has lectured in 31 countries in Africa, Asia, and Europe on Christian psychiatry. He has published numerous articles on the subject of neuroscience, psychopharmacology, psychopathology, and the psychology of the Christian religion. He is the author of *The Grace to Grow* and *The Nuts and Bolts of Discipleship*.